the
BAKER IDI
Wellness Plan

Baker IDI Heart and Diabetes Institute is an independent, internationally-renowned medical research facility, with a history spanning more than 90 years. The Institute's work extends from the laboratory to wide-scale community studies with a focus on diagnosis, prevention and treatment of diabetes and cardiovascular disease.

The comprehensive range of research undertaken to target these deadly diseases, combined with the flexibility and innovation to respond to changing health and community needs, is unique and sets Baker IDI apart from other health and medical research institutes.

The Institute's mission is to reduce death and disability from cardiovascular disease, diabetes and related disorders; two prevalent and complex diseases responsible for the most deaths and the highest health costs in the world.

With Australia facing an ageing population and rapidly growing rates of chronic disease, Baker IDI's work has never been more important to Australian communities, as well as the global communities in which it operates.

Baker IDI is well positioned to address these challenges, with multidisciplinary teams comprising medical specialists, scientists and public health experts all focused on translating laboratory findings into new approaches to prevention, treatment and care.

The Institute's main laboratory facilities are located on the Alfred Medical Research and Education Precinct in Melbourne, Australia. Baker IDI also runs a national Aboriginal Health program dedicated to addressing the profound health disadvantage experienced by Aboriginal Australians, with a dedicated campus in Alice Springs in Central Australia.

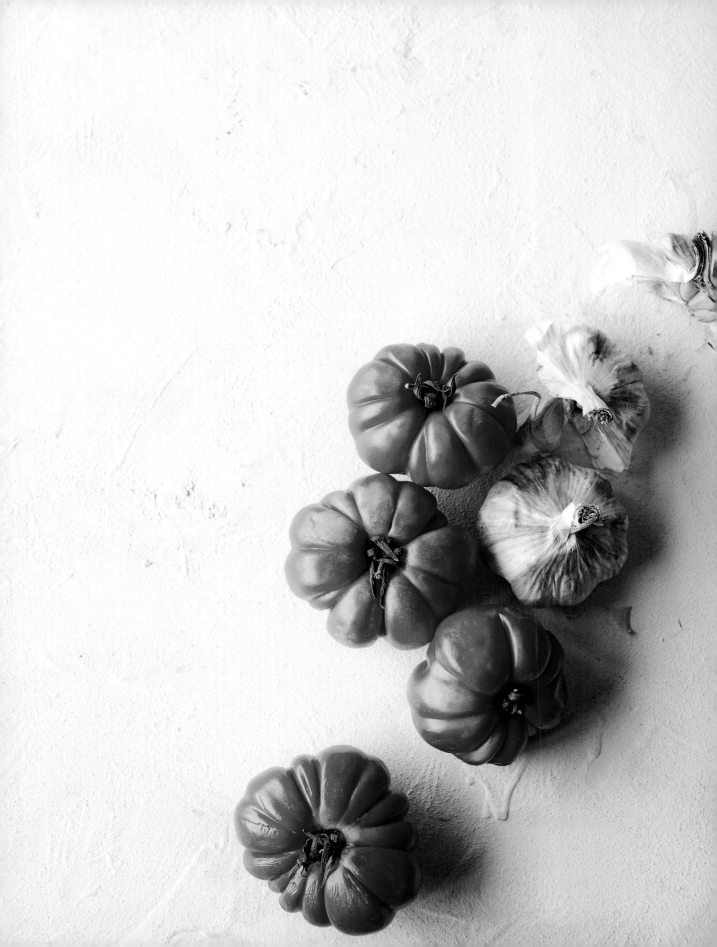

the
BAKER IDI
Wellness
Plan

Scientific secrets for a long
and healthy life

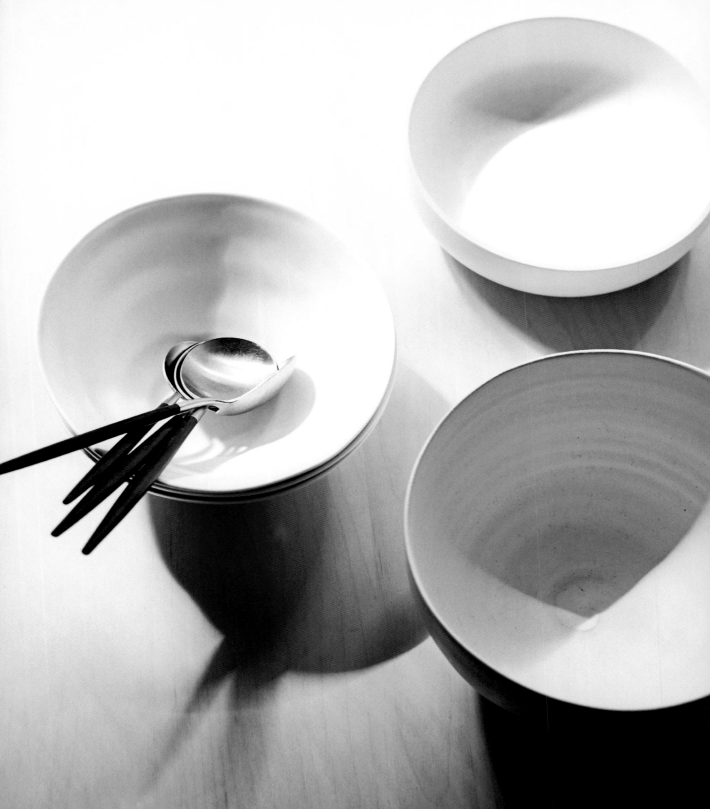

CONTENTS

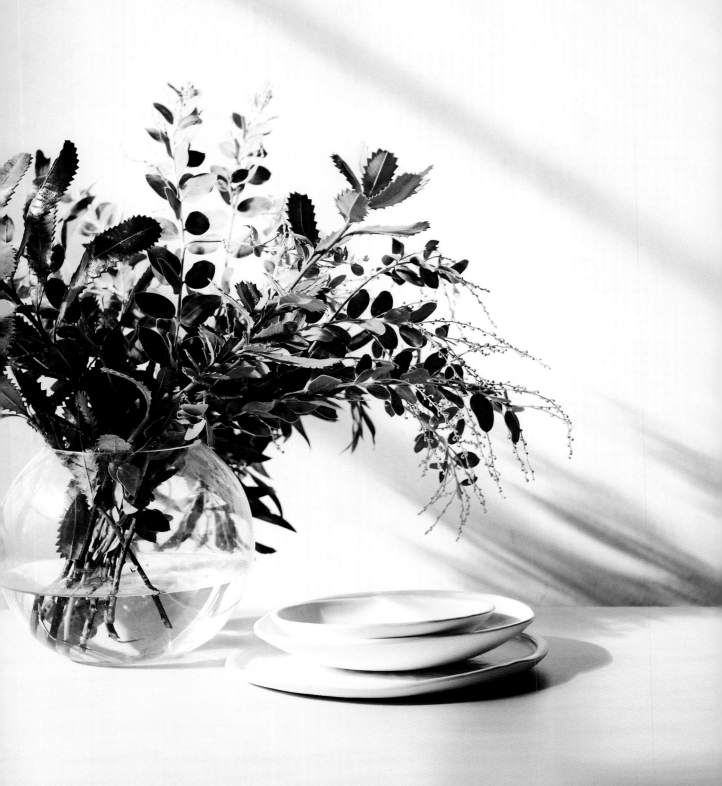

FOREWORD

In the last few decades, there has been more and more interest in the concept of wellbeing. It is now widely recognised that this state of comfort, health and happiness encompasses a broader definition of health and is one that we should all aim for. However, despite all the talk of wellbeing, in our increasingly affluent society many people feel dissatisfied, perhaps most in the sense of their general health. From my clinical experience, the major manifestations are fatigue, lack of energy, decreased ability or an inability to be physically active, and depression.

In general, these symptoms are a consequence of lifestyle factors in our modern, post-industrial society, including inactivity, sedentariness, excessive sugar and alcohol intake, poor sleep patterns, and being overweight. These features are the risk factors for cardio-metabolic disease, a group of conditions that are having an increasing impact, not only in the developed but increasingly in the developing world. Simply put, inactivity and excessive calories – especially sugar and animal fat – lead to weight gain, type 2 diabetes, high blood pressure, blood vessel damage and eventually, a group of predominantly vascular diseases that remain the commonest causes of death and disability in our society – heart attacks, stroke, heart failure and peripheral vascular disease.

The researchers at Baker IDI Heart and Diabetes Institute are focused on ways of preventing these conditions and improving health outcomes when these conditions strike. In this book, our experts explain how to take healthy steps towards a state of wellbeing, and avoid or reverse the lifestyle factors that lead to disease.

Engaging with healthy lifestyle behaviours is of course more complicated than might be apparent at a superficial level. After all, we do unhealthy things instead of the healthy alternative because the unhealthy behaviour seems interesting or attractive. Dealing with the problems requires recognition and understanding by an individual, and lifestyle guidance about specific strategies to overcome them. Such strategies may include medical care, but more commonly requires the lifestyle changes recommended in this book, involving diet, activity, sleep habits and mental health.

Understanding and dealing with cardio-metabolic risk, the risk of having a stroke or developing conditions such as heart disease or type 2 diabetes, represents one of the major health challenges of our generation. We hope that you and your family will benefit from a better understanding of how to keep yourself well, avoid disease and live a long and healthy life.

Professor Thomas Marwick
Director and Chief Executive of Baker IDI
Heart and Diabetes Institute

PART 1

WELLBEING

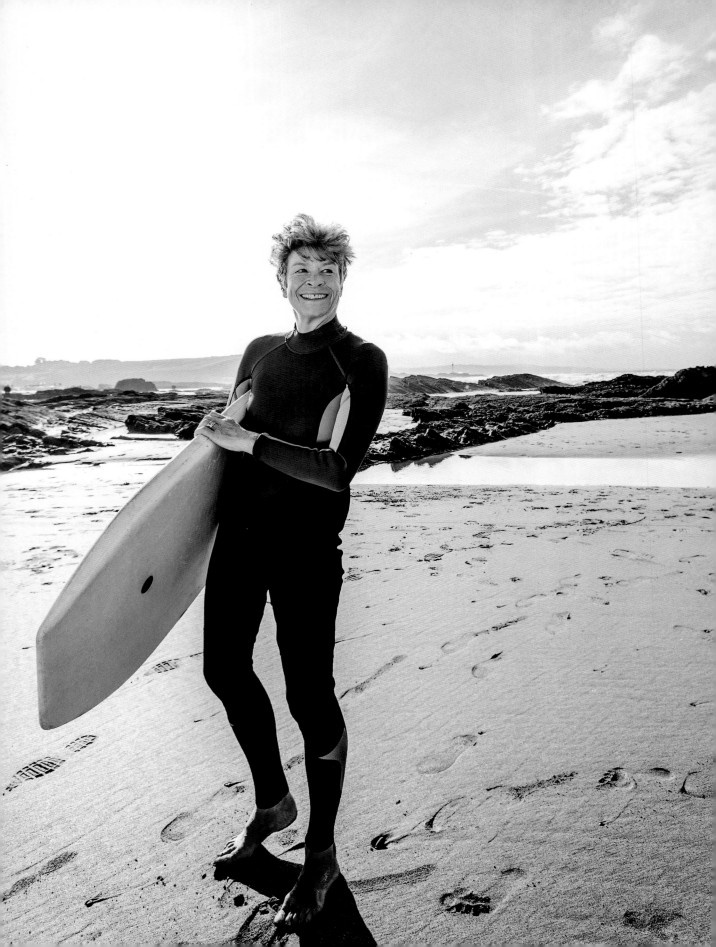

1

WHAT IS WELLBEING?

If you asked one hundred people what they think 'wellbeing' is, you would get a hundred different answers. We all have an idea of what it means – that we feel okay – but what does it really mean? What aspects of our life does it encompass? How much control do we have over it? How important is it in our lives? And – how do we obtain our own version of 'wellbeing'?

A general definition of wellbeing is that it is an overall picture of a person's mood. It includes components such as a person's feelings of satisfaction, how fulfilled they feel, their levels of happiness, their ability to carry out daily tasks, their equilibrium and their resilience.

The pathway to wellbeing in our society often encounters some road bumps. In this era of reality TV, six-minute doctor consultations and sound bites from our politicians on the nightly news – we want it all, we want it now and we want every solution to be simple. Unfortunately, there is no quick fix for 'wellbeing'. There is no pill we can pop, no superfood we can sprinkle on our cereal, or no spa retreat that can instantly inject it into you.

To achieve an overall wellbeing, we collectively need to invest in all aspects of life; the physical, the psychological and the emotional. And while the steps to healthy wellbeing can be simple, they need to become lifetime habits for us to truly see results. With lifestyle-related disease now the leading cause of death across much of the world, there is much we can do to protect our health for now and into the future.

Defining wellbeing

Recently, a new definition of wellbeing suggested that we can think of it as the balance point for a person between their resources (such as time, money and coping skills) and the challenges they face (such as job loss, relationship breakdown or ill health). See the figure on following page. This definition is useful, because it allows us to understand a person is in a state of stable wellbeing when they have the psychological, social and physical resources they need to meet a particular psychological, social or physical challenge.

With this definition, people roll out of a state of wellbeing if they are experiencing more challenges than they have resources to deal with. For example, a person who has good health, a supportive network of friends and colleagues and is in a strong financial position is likely to have a smaller loss of wellbeing when faced with a job loss than the person who does not have these resources.

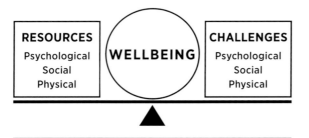

A stable state of wellbeing (Source: Dodge, Daly, Huyton and Sanders, The challenge of defining wellbeing, 2012)

In this context, it is obvious that good wellbeing comes both from increasing your resources and limiting the challenges you face. Wellbeing, seen in this way, is a continual and dynamic interaction between you and your environment.

So what do we know about what gives people greater individual resources, be they psychological, social or physical?

Many factors contribute to the resources a person has to use throughout their life, and many of those resources are built in early life. Those who start with greater resources are more likely to experience greater wellbeing and physical health later in life.

THE IMPORTANCE OF A GOOD START

We know that health and wellbeing in later life can be predicted by a child's start in life, including their genetics, the health and wellbeing of their parents, the nutrition they receive in their early life, their environment, the type of community they live in and the stability of their home life.

The Australian Institute of Health and Welfare's (AIHW) *A Picture of Australia's Children* sets out the 19 key indicators of child health, development and wellbeing. These include in utero conditions, such as maternal smoking or alcohol consumption and birth weight; health indicators, such as presence of a chronic condition like asthma or type 2 diabetes; family indicators like whether a child is breastfed or read to or exposed to cigarette smoke in the home; markers of learning and development at school; and the safety and security of the child both at home and within the community. In 2012, the indicator report card showed that most of these indicators have been improving over time. So, are we seeing improvements in wellbeing too?

We know that life expectancy has increased enormously over the past 100 years or so, from about 55 years in the early 1900s to around 82 years in 2016. In Australia, we also know that our perception of how good our health is has also increased in recent years, with the vast majority of Australians rating their own health as excellent, very good or good (AIHW, *Australia's Health*, 2014). However, there is no regular measure of wellbeing, or happiness over time and we know that some aspects of today's world are rapidly changing and can negatively affect our wellbeing.

Of course death is not the only health-related outcome we are interested in preventing. Another measure reflects the number of years of life impaired by disability. In Australia the leading causes of disability-adjusted life years (DALYs) are cancer (19%) and cardiovascular disease (15%), followed by mental and substance abuse disorders (12%), musculoskeletal conditions (12%), and injuries (9%).

Factors that affect our wellbeing

We know that at the broader societal and environmental level, many factors increase the risk of poor wellbeing. A number of factors have been rapidly changing over past decades, including our connection with the natural world, our social structures and cohesion, and our work patterns. Studies have consistently shown that greater exposure to nature is associated with greater wellbeing. This includes seeing and/or being close to water (such as lakes or the ocean), as well as having access to greenery, walking spaces and open spaces with natural elements. One interesting recent study of residents living near the Great Barrier Reef found that they felt that the health of the reef was more important for their wellbeing than the jobs and income associated with development. In modern urban settings the ratio of concrete to nature has increased relentlessly. In Australia, since the early 1990s, the proportion of new buildings that are multi-unit dwellings, such as apartment blocks, has almost doubled. At the same time block sizes have shrunk and house sizes have increased.

We have also seen large changes in our social structures, with high sustained divorce rates, low birth rates, universal car use, increasing frequency of house moves, and the increasing prominence of information technology in our social lives. As Hugh Mackay indicated in *The Art of Belonging* (2014), we absolutely depend on communities to nurture us and sustain us and the point that we sometimes overlook in the march of individualism is that communities also need us to nurture and sustain them.

CHOICE AT WORK

Work patterns have also changed markedly. In Australia we have seen large increases in part-time work, and increases in variable and flexible working arrangements. This has been accompanied by some reports of increases in hours worked and perceived increases in work stress. We know that employment is generally associated with good self-reported health compared to unemployment. A person's employment conditions also play a part, and wellbeing seems to have a link to the level of choice that a person feels they have with their work pattern. It is not only the number of hours that a person works that is important, but also the amount of flexibility and control that is available to the individual worker.

REGULAR EXERCISE

At the personal level, there are a number of health or risk factors that have been changing unfavourably over recent decades that are likely to challenge our wellbeing. We know that most elements of having a healthy lifestyle (such as having regular physical activity, a healthy diet, being a non-smoker and a moderate alcohol consumption) all act to improve our physical health, our

mental wellbeing and our social connectivity. In recent decades, physical activity, and healthy diets have come into sharp focus as levels of obesity and type 2 diabetes have increased alarmingly.

There are reams of evidence that every form of physical activity improves our outlook on life. It is a natural form of endorphins, improves our strength and fitness, and often involves social interaction. So, we know it is good for us, but how do we fit it in to our busy, car-bound and office-bound lives? A good motto with physical activity is 'every little bit counts'. Whatever works for you, try to make it routine and share it with your friends and family.

EATING WELL

Similar to physical activity, it is clear that the changes in our food environment over past decades have made consumption of an unhealthy diet more and more likely. We are surrounded by limitless options of cheap, tasty food wherever we go. Our on-the-go food options are almost all high in kilojoules but low in nutritional quality or a capacity to satisfy us. Yet it is not just the traditional junk foods that are the problem. Many of the foods we think of as healthy are really unhealthy foods in disguise. Breakfast cereals are a typical example. Many breakfast cereals are high in sugar or salt and not very high in fibre. Children's breakfast cereals are among the least nutritious choices to buy.

What do we know about how a diet high in sugar, fat or salt affects our wellbeing? It leads to obesity, type 2 diabetes and diseases such as hypertension, heart disease and dental decay. But the quality of our diet has also been shown to have a link to our mental health, cognitive health and wellbeing.

We also know that food has long fulfilled a social function. Preparing, eating and sharing food provides pleasure and has been one of the key social pillars in all societies around the world. Traditionally food has been shared, representing traditions, generosity and respect, and it's often the time when families or whole villages come together. We all recognise how much our eating habits and meal times have changed over the

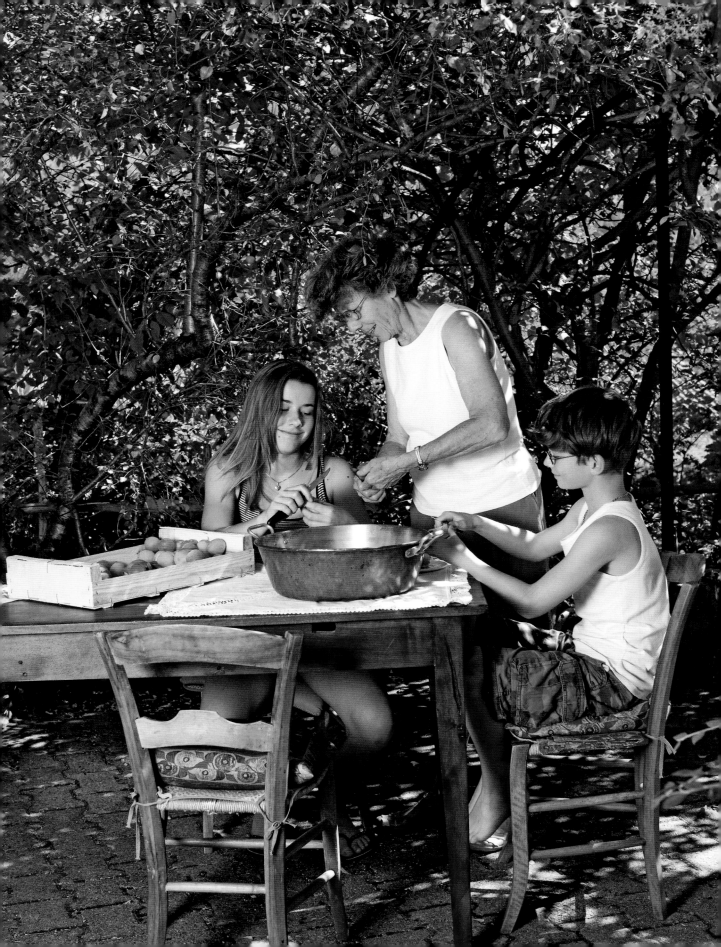

last few generations. We have seen large decreases in the time spent together in food preparation, the time spent eating together and our collective understanding of food, cooking and meal preparation. With an increase in snack, or on-the-go meals and food consumption outside the home, the role of food as a source of social wellbeing is weakened. Recent initiatives that support a central, social role of food (including growing, preparing or eating it) have shown clear positive benefits for wellbeing.

How the Baker IDI Wellness Plan can work for you

In today's busy world, we all need to make a conscious effort if we are to increase our levels of wellbeing. We need to think cleverly about how to make nature, friends and family, and a healthy lifestyle routine elements of our daily lives. And we need to share our ideas with our friends, families, colleagues and broader communities so that good wellbeing moves from being a rueful wish to an accepted norm.

In *The Baker IDI Wellness Plan*, we have gathered our experts to help unravel the myths around healthy living for you. We will explain fad diets and healthy meal plans, how much and what kind of physical activity you need, and advice on achieving good mental health. You will also learn how experiencing just one or a combination of risk factors – whether you are overweight or have high cholesterol – can put you on the path to serious health consequences if left unchecked.

We want this book to help empower you on your quest for wellness, so importantly we will explain how you can monitor your risk of disease, how to reduce this risk and why early action is best.

What can we do to increase our wellbeing?

- Interact with nature in some way every day: appreciate the clouds or the sunset, go for a walk through gardens, along a creek or the beach, enjoy your local park, play sport with the kids on the local oval.
- Spend time with people who are important to you.
- Get to know the people in your community.
- Look after your mental health.
- To the best of your ability, figure out the work pattern that suits your life best.
- Be physically active: there are lots of great resources to help you find an activity you enjoy that you can add into your routine every week. This could be a walk with a friend, a ride to work or school, a swim somewhere you love, or simply taking the stairs at work.
- Break up long periods of sitting: get out of your chair and move around, or perhaps do some of your work standing up.
- Eat a healthy diet: there are lots of great resources to help work out healthy meals and snacks for you and your family that fit with your tastes, lifestyle and culture. Find the ones that work for you and use them to get tips and ideas for easy, healthy meals and snacks. See chapter 10 for information on healthy eating.
- Make some of your meals a time to sit down with friends or family.

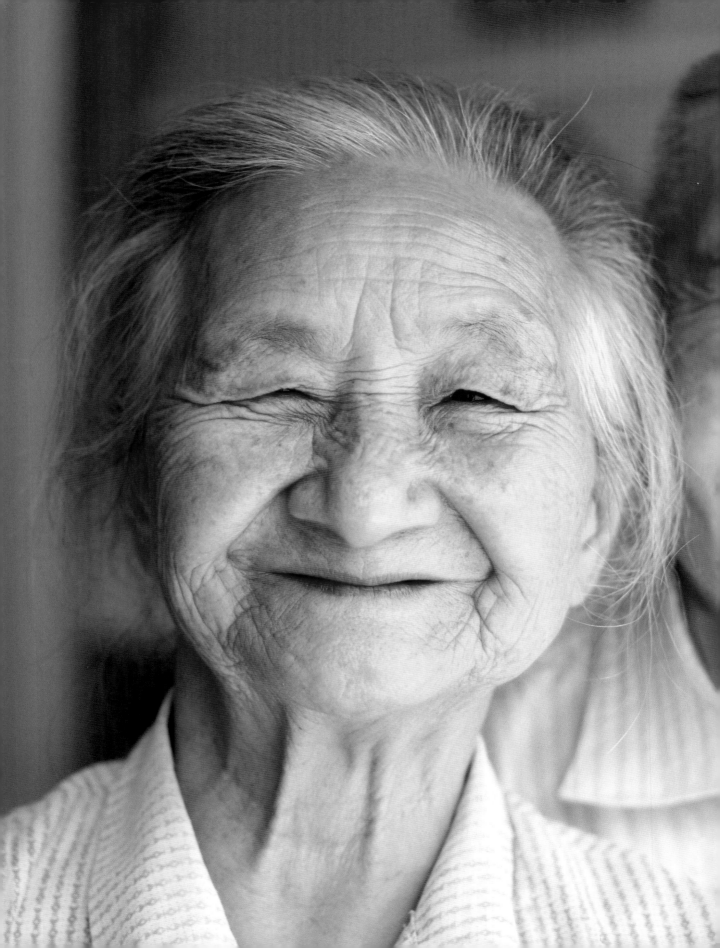

2

WELLBEING AT EVERY LIFE STAGE

Australians are living longer than ever so it's important to learn how to be well throughout your potentially long lifespan. By 2060, the number of Australians aged over 75 will increase by four million people, jumping from about 6.4 to 14.4% of the population. One in 100 babies born this year will live to reach 100. A female born today will (on average) live for 94 years, while a male born today is likely to reach his 91st birthday. Because people will be living longer, they are also likely to be living with chronic diseases for long stretches of their life. In all probability, they will be living with multiple conditions.

The odds are that we are in this for the long haul – if we look after ourselves, that is. To do this we need to understand and monitor the risks to our health at different life stages. We need to eat and drink in moderation, and focus on choosing healthy foods. We need to move more and stress less.

The cycle of wellbeing

Wellness is a cycle. Often, that cycle is in the shape of a downwards spiral. If we are unhappy, it is a challenge to eat well. It's difficult to find energy

for exercise, so we might turn to alcohol as a comfort and then our sleep suffers. We gain weight. Whatever the start of the cycle, it's a hard trajectory to break away from.

The benefits of wellness don't just bring renewed energy, thirst for life and contentment in the here and now. They also have positive long-term consequences later in life. They also affect the health of your offspring and their offspring.

'SEVEN STAGES OF MAN' . . . AND WOMAN

Our wellbeing is affected by different lifestyle factors at different stages of our life.

William Shakespeare wrote about the 'seven stages of man', where each life stage has its own exit and entrance in a person's life. Different health risks and preventative messages are more relevant at different ages, but making positive changes at the earliest opportunity gives us the best chance of staying healthy throughout life.

FROM THE WOMB TO CHILDHOOD

A fascinating emerging field of science called epigenetics shows how genes are switched on and off in response to our environment. The old maxim 'we are what we eat' has been well established by an ever-increasing number of studies in this field. Astonishingly, epigenetics now demonstrates that we are also what our parents and our grandparents ate.

The first evidence of the long-term effect of what we eat came from the 1944 Dutch famine, where people who were exposed to poor nutrition while in the womb were at greater risk of obesity, heart disease, type 2 diabetes and preferred eating a high-fat diet in middle age. These effects were also passed on to the next generation.

Further research is showing that our weight, the likelihood of developing allergies and metabolic conditions later in life can all be influenced by our parents' lifestyle. Their life choices – such as whether they smoked, how active they were and their weight – affected their genes, which subsequently affect our genes. Maternal obesity prior to conception not only reduces fertility, it affects the health of the human baby in the womb and puts the mother at greater risk of gestational diabetes. This, in turn, increases the risk of type 2 diabetes and obesity in the child. These epigenetic factors and childhood influences may set us on our path in life, but this trajectory doesn't have to be our destiny.

Mental health, body image, substance abuse, accidents and risk-taking behaviours are typically the biggest challenges to wellbeing at this life stage. About three-quarters of cases of mental illness starts before the age of 24, while suicide accounts for almost one in five adolescent deaths.

It is important that during this time young adults are educated and supported in establishing healthy habits. This includes developing good sleep hygiene, such as removing technology from the bedroom and setting regular sleep patterns. They also need to understand the physical and psychological risks of drugs and binge drinking.

Good nutrition is vital for the developing brain. Participation in regular physical activity will help maintain a healthy weight and develop strong bones, heart, lungs and muscles.

ADULTHOOD

Physically and mentally, we should be in our prime upon reaching adulthood. Wellbeing at this stage means forging a strong sense of identity and coping skills, having the physical capabilities to live the life you want, and remaining disease-free.

However, at this life stage we are also shouldered with added responsibilities including careers, study and caring roles. These eat into time

Genes and environment

In the past, we tended to think of genes and environment as having separate effects on our body and health. These two factors are no longer considered to be unrelated, thanks to epigenetics. Certainly, some rare diseases are almost entirely genetic. However, those that are clearly genetically based will often appear differently in members of the family who share the same gene disorder.

Families also share habits, not just genes. They share meals, portion sizes, leisure time and attitudes. We know that overweight children are more likely to become overweight adults. Type 2 diabetes was once referred to as 'adult-onset diabetes'. Not anymore. The number of obese children being diagnosed with this lifestyle-related condition has changed the definition. It's very hard for one member of a family to eat well and be active on their own.

In Part 2 we will explore healthy habits, eating and exercise tips that will benefit the whole family.

we once had for planned physical activity, sleep, relaxation and preparing healthy meals. The stress that comes from juggling these extra responsibilities can push people towards unhealthy habits such as smoking, binge drinking and drugs. Our incidental activity throughout the day suffers. Sleep is compromised. Our weight can balloon.

Then as we enter middle age, new risks emerge. Our bodies change. Muscles shrink and become less flexible if we don't challenge them. Our metabolism slows. The heart starts to pump less. Blood vessels and arteries become stiffer, causing the heart to work harder with each beat.

Health checks for adults

Many risk factors for serious disease such as high cholesterol, high blood pressure and high levels of fat in the blood, are invisible. All adults should know their cholesterol levels, blood pressure, blood glucose and waist girth. These simple checks can be done by your doctor.

Heart disease and cancers – such as prostate, bowel and breast – start to become more common, making regular checks important. Ensure the check-ups and tests you and your doctor discuss are based on evidence not fads. We will explore the pros and cons of particular tests in chapter 6.

Carrying excess weight, unhealthy diets, smoking and alcohol consumption, can multiply the risks that are associated with high blood pressure, both types of diabetes and cholesterol, which if left unchecked can have serious consequences such as heart disease and stroke.

And the effects can have a domino effect. People with high blood pressure are 60% more likely to develop type 2 diabetes. About 70 to 80% of those with type 1 or 2 diabetes will eventually die of cardiovascular disease.

Health care plans

You are not a passive participant in your health care. It is important you develop a health care plan with your doctor to ensure you understand the purpose of medication and get advice on taking it as prescribed. This also applies to the use of supplements or alternative therapies, many of which impact the effectiveness of medications. It is best

to keep your doctor and pharmacist informed of any additional therapies that you are taking. Unfortunately, you can't believe everything health-related on the internet, so stick to authoritative sources. Some of these reliable sources are listed in the Resources list on page 298.

For some people, medications may be part of the health plan you create with your doctor to reduce the risk of further damage. There are many factors that can influence whether someone stays the course of a prescribed medication, such as cost or not appreciating the benefit of the treatment. It is important to discuss these factors with your doctor.

OLDER ADULTS

Wellbeing at this stage of life means maintaining independence, retaining good mental function and memory, and moving without pain and restriction. As we age, our bones, muscles, ligaments and tendons aren't as strong. Wear and tear on the joints, such as knees, becomes common. Our metabolism slows.

Throughout life, men develop lifestyle-related risk factors such as high blood pressure and cholesterol at higher rates than women, until menopause hits. Then women catch up.

And because women tend to live longer, more will be diagnosed with these lifestyle-related conditions later in life.

Psychological wellbeing becomes an issue in older age as families disperse, social connections can be lost, and retirement brings up questions of identity and purpose.

Degenerative brain disease like Alzheimer's disease and dementia are often the biggest fear for people as they age. There is an inextricable link between dementia and high blood pressure, high cholesterol, type 2 diabetes and smoking. Research is showing that regular physical activity throughout life can help reduce the onset of these neurological conditions.

As well as doing the crossword to ward off dementia, your best bet is to invest in a good diet, take regular exercise and avoid smoking throughout your life to help ward off the lifestyle-related conditions that will bump up your risk.

What affects wellbeing?

Regardless of our life stage, wellbeing is affected by the following elements.

WEIGHT

Why does it seem that one person walks past a cake shop and puts on five kilograms, while another can eat like a horse and never gain weight? Australian researchers are among those looking at why two people can be on the same exercise and diet plan and yet yield very different results. By uncovering the way our individual set of genes influences our response to physical activity and diet, they are aiming to prescribe the right combination of physical activity and food for individual results.

But in the meantime, it's a simple message we need to abide by: move more, and (if we are overweight) eat less.

We sit in the car to work, we sit all day at desks, we drive home to sit in front of the TV. Our lives have become sedentary in the extreme. And it is our weight that suffers.

We maintain our weight by equalling the energy we consume through food with the energy we burn through exercise and bodily functions. To lose weight, we need to burn more than we consume.

The effect of being overweight

If we are overweight or obese, we are more likely to develop a whole range of conditions such as type 2 diabetes, high blood pressure, blood fat abnormalities that lead to metabolic conditions, cancer and skeletal problems. Overweight people are weight lifters. For every three kilograms of weight you put on, you put on one kilogram of muscle to carry it around. This is hard on our joints. It increases the risk of developing osteoarthritis by 15 times.

Fat is also toxic to our organs and blood. The classic 'apple' body shape, where fat is mainly stored around the abdomen, is the most dangerous in terms of increasing your risk of metabolic conditions.

Fat is not inert. Research is showing that it can switch on inflammatory processes that damage organs, upset metabolism and blood clotting systems, and cause the heart to work overtime by narrowing the arteries. Some of this is genetic but there is a major contribution from lifestyle. Chapter 7 has some tips on making lifestyle changes.

Healthy eating

A common myth is that we can lose large amounts of weight through exercise alone. A healthy diet is critical to achieving an optimal weight. We need to eat a nutritionally balanced diet and not turn to a fad diet for long-term weight management.

Why belly fat is dangerous

People who put on fat around organs like the gut, liver and heart and get a pot belly are at greater risk than those who put weight on at the hips. This is because abdominal fat is more metabolically active.

It attracts infiltration of a particular form of white blood cell called macrophages. These are responsible for the release of molecules associated with inflammation.

They circulate through the body causing tissues to become resistant to the normal role of insulin, which helps glucose move into cells and act as fuel. This puts strain on the pancreas to make more insulin and increases the risk of type 2 diabetes.

Other effects of these inflammatory molecules include increasing the level of triglycerides in the blood and lower levels of the beneficial form of cholesterol, high density lipoprotein (HDL). The consequence is a greater risk of cancer, cardiovascular disease and other conditions that we know are associated with obesity.

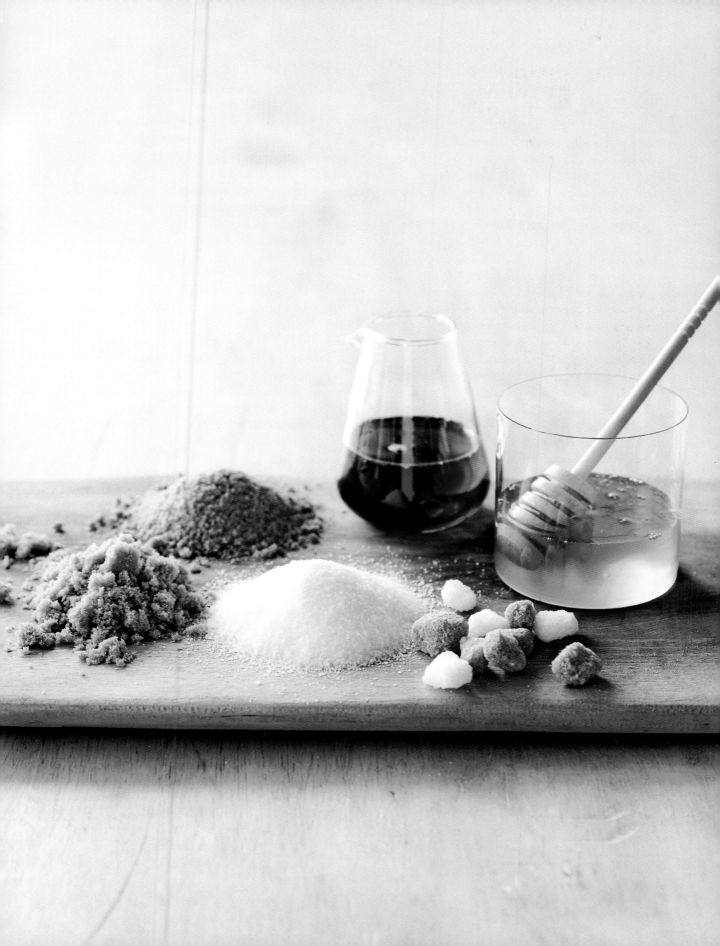

How can you achieve a healthy weight? The best way to do this is through eating moderately and keeping fit throughout your life. Be careful of big portions, especially when you are eating out, and fill up with healthy fruit, vegetables, low-fat dairy foods and cereals rather than sugars and fats in prepared food and drink. It is much easier to prevent weight gain this way than to get excess weight off once you've put it on. However, it is never too late to make healthy changes to your diet.

SMOKING

There is no safe level of smoking cigarettes. Tobacco contains thousands of chemicals, with about 70 of these having known links to cancer. The effects of smoking on the body are wide-ranging. These include stained teeth and tarred fingers, decreased bone density and increased risk of macular degeneration (which is the leading cause of blindness in Australian adults).

The chemicals in smoking make it harder for muscles to work because carbon monoxide replaces some of the oxygen in the blood. It also interferes with blood flow, causing an increased risk of stroke. Of the three million smokers in Australia, two-in-three will die from causes directly related to smoking. One-fifth of cancers in Australia are attributed to smoking.

Smoking also has effects on some of the damaging mechanisms caused by being overweight. So if smokers are carrying extra weight, or already have high cholesterol, they are not just adding to their risk of poor health, they are multiplying it.

The Quitline gives good advice on how to stop smoking. You can access the Quitline by dialling 13 7848 (13 QUIT) from anywhere inside Australia. It might take a few goes at quitting before you achieve long-term success – so do not ever be discouraged and never give up trying. Your doctor or pharmacist can give you advice on products that can help some people.

ALCOHOL

Unlike smoking, there is probably a minimum level of alcohol consumption that's healthy.

At light levels of consumption (around one standard drink each day), alcohol may reduce your risk of developing or dying from heart disease or type 2 diabetes. Aside from exercise, alcohol is one of the few things that will raise your level of high density lipoprotein (HDL, or 'good' cholesterol), which is associated with greater protection against heart disease. Whether you drink spirits, red or white wine or beer, the benefit is likely to lie in the alcohol component, regardless of the type of drink. Balance and moderation is the key to preserving any health benefits.

But the risks associated with over-consumption are undisputed. High levels of alcohol consumption, no more than two standard drinks each day, can damage the liver and brain, muscles can waste away, hearts can fail, gastritis becomes common and the risk of cancers and stroke increases.

Even at moderate levels, alcohol is highly dense in kilojoules. This means it carries significant energy. The health conscious worry about the carbohydrates and sugar in beer, and beverage companies are spending millions of dollars to promote the tipple as essentially 'sugar-free'.

It is the alcohol that carries the kilojoules, and 'liquid kilojoules' like this – also found in smoothies, fruit juices and soft drinks – are potentially more dangerous to dieters. They don't trigger the same mechanisms as solid food to leave you with the same feeling of fullness. Hence we eat more and gain weight.

Have a look through chapter 7 for healthy habits regarding alcohol consumption.

SUGAR

Sugar-free diets have taken their place alongside fasting, lemon detoxes and restricting kilojoules in the list of fad nutrition regimes.

But is sugar as toxic as alcohol and tobacco, as some health experts claim?

Sugar has clear links with obesity, given its kilojoules are unaccompanied by nutrients. High consumption, particularly of sugar-sweetened beverages, can cause erosion of tooth enamel and lead to decay. But beyond this, the harmful effects of sugar are not fully understood.

Studies have linked high sugar diets and refined

(rather than unprocessed) starch to a higher chance of dying from heart disease, and developing type 2 diabetes or metabolic syndrome.

Other studies in animal models suggest Western diets – which are high in saturated fats and sugar – cause damage to the brain's appetite control, overriding its ability to prevent overeating.

The Australian Dietary Guidelines have been updated to include recommendations to limit intake of sugary drinks. The concern is understandable, given that home cooking has largely made way for processed and pre-prepared foods, most of which have added sugars as flavour or preservative. This includes sauces, cereals, bread, juices and even tinned vegetables.

But the jury is still out on whether table sugar – known scientifically as sucrose (which is made up of glucose and fructose) causes damage beyond its impact on the waist line and in the mouth.

Artificial sweeteners may not be the saviour. Studies in animals and a small number of humans suggest that common sugar substitutes can alter bacteria in the gut and impair metabolism, increasing the risk of the very metabolic diseases dieters are trying to avoid.

Not all sugars are bad. They occur naturally in foods such as fruit and dairy foods and we know these can be part of a healthy diet. Really high intake of added sugars in processed foods has become a problem and is what we need to be mindful of. Common sugar substitutes like honey, coconut sugar, brown rice sugar and maple syrup have no health advantages over ordinary sugar.

Chapter 10 has lots of good advice on getting the best balance of nutrients in your diet.

SLEEP

It is not completely understood why we need sleep. Studies in animal models have recently uncovered a process called glymphatic system that suggests sleep helps restore the brain by flushing out toxins that accumulate when we are awake.

What is clear is that we cannot live without it. The amount we need varies for each person, with just over eight hours the average for adults. School-age children generally need more, about nine to eleven hours a night, with older adults supplementing disrupted night-time sleep with naps during the day.

Any compromise on our individual requirement, however, leaves us exhausted and unable to perform as well during the day. Studies in Australian shift workers, such as truck drivers and nurses, show they can close their eyes for up to 15 seconds during driving simulation exercises following typical patterns of deprived sleep. We can feel these effects by getting less than six hours sleep.

In chapter 7 we explore ways to promote healthy sleep habits such as setting regular bed times and creating a conducive environment for sleep.

INACTIVITY

Research continues to emerge on the dangers of sitting for long periods of time.

It was once thought that just TV watching was the enemy, that this passive pastime was driving shorter life expectancies. But we now understand it is the passive act of sitting across the full day that is the issue. Research by our Institute and others, has shown that watching TV for three hours or more each day is associated with increased risk of death.

And while you try to counteract this with an hour running the dogs or on the gym exercise bike at night, this will help make you fitter and stronger, but it won't negate all of the damage from being sedentary during the day.

There are strong links emerging between a sedentary lifestyle and heart disease, weight gain and type 2 diabetes. Sitting for long periods of time causes your metabolism to slow, and because energy expenditure is low then the breakdown of fat also reduces. We stop relying on our postural muscles and there is evidence that this leads to reduced glucose uptake and a shut-down of the processes that control cholesterol production.

Reducing the amount of time that you sit during the day is ideal, but breaking up the time when you do sit is a good start. See page 64 for some ideas on how to reduce your sitting time.

The encouraging news is that our research is showing that you can reduce your risk and improve blood glucose levels after a short period of time with regular breaks from sitting during the day.

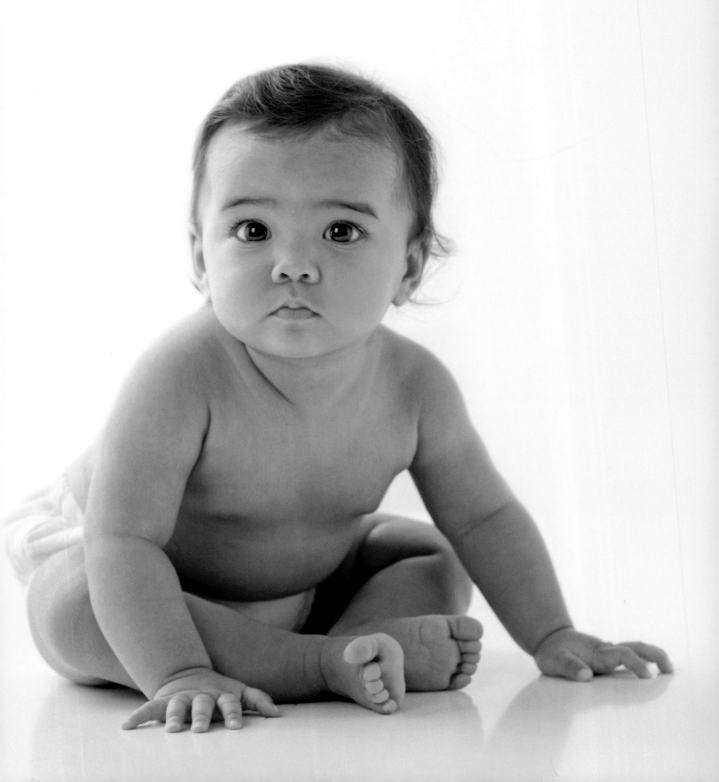

3

THE WELLBEING SPIRAL

Chronic diseases such as depression, arthritis, type 2 diabetes, heart failure and even acute catastrophic events like heart attack and stroke do not come out of nowhere.

There are pointers throughout life that will determine the likelihood of these problems affecting your wellbeing. Sometimes these indicators are your genes and having a strong family history of a particular problem. More often they are related to your individual habits, choices and practices. Understanding the small daily steps that can lead you toward disease, means that you can take action now to ensure you have the best possible chance of health and wellbeing in the years to come.

The health spiral

Over a lifetime, a person's wellbeing often takes the shape of a spiral. For many people, this is a downward movement, with factors that are small to begin with growing into larger problems. However, by adopting some healthy choices and practices, this spiral can be transformed into an upwards-moving one. It's never too late to take action, and the Wellness Action Plan on page 56 suggests specific steps that you can take to maintain health and wellbeing.

To understand how the health spiral works, let's look at various milestones in a typical person's lifespan. Factors that can have an cumulative effect on your health can begin as far back as your time in the womb. In this section, we will outline some of the risk factors, and provide information about how you can make healthier choices for you and your family.

PREGNANCY AND INFANCY

As described in chapter 1, there is an association between small birth weight and chronic disease later in life. Sometimes babies are small because their genes made them and others in their family that way. Babies that are small due to poor nutrition, smoking or other lifestyle choices of their mother are the ones who face difficulties later on. Under-nutrition (not getting enough healthy food during pregnancy) or over-nutrition (consuming too much sugar, salt and fat which can be associated with too much weight gain and high blood pressure during pregnancy) can all be associated with a low birth weight.

Keeping mother and baby healthy

- Pregnancy is not the time to start vigorous exercise for the first time, diet or try to lose weight. But all women who are pregnant without complications should participate in aerobic and strength training of moderate to vigorous intensity, for 30 minutes, five days a week.
- Steady weight gain is important over the pregnancy, but gaining too much weight can be harmful to mum and baby. See chapter 6 for advice on weight gain during pregnancy.
- Pregnant women don't need to 'eat for two', but they do particularly need to increase their intake of grains and cereal foods in the second and third trimester, as well as eat foods that are high in iron and iodine. The focus should be increasing nutrient dense foods, rather than increasing kilojoule intake. A pregnancy multivitamin for at least one month prior to conception and for the duration of the pregnancy will ensure enough essential nutrients for the baby.
- There is no safe level of alcohol consumption during pregnancy.
- Smoking during pregnancy increases the risk of ectopic pregnancy, miscarriage, premature labour and low birth weight babies, who are at greater risk of infection, respiratory problems and death.
- Having a baby is an exciting time but it can also be challenging. Remember to ask for help and give yourself time to learn parenting skills.
- Spend time working out what recharges you and make some time to do this.

THE TEENAGE YEARS

Small birth weight babies rapidly catch up in body size in the first few years of their life. Indeed, they can become overweight children and adolescents. It is as if the body somehow senses the mismatch between what it needed for energy and growth in the womb and what is being provided. Often this pattern is associated with disadvantage of one kind or another. It could be social, economic or societal in nature. Disadvantage increases the risk of risk-taking behaviours in adolescence, such as smoking tobacco, binge-drinking alcohol, taking other harmful drugs or risky driving. The early signs of depression or other mental illness might also be present.

Keeping teenagers healthy

- Ensure your teenager makes time to be active each day, whether that be riding to school, walking the dog, playing sport, or spending time outside with friends.
- Encourage your teenager to practise good sleep habits: aim for 8–10 hours of sleep each night, ensure the bedroom is dark at night with blockout blinds or eye masks and let natural light in each morning to help them wake up. Remove phones, computers and TVs from bedrooms, and help them set daily wind-down rituals before bed such as showering, reading or writing to encourage sleep.
- Provide access to healthy meals including two serves of fruit and five serves of vegetables, encourage breakfast daily, and limit takeaway foods and soft drink.
- Reduce your teenager's risk of depression and anxiety by:

- making time to talk with them each day
- expressing affection for them
- encouraging them to develop a wide range of interests to help develop self-confidence
- being involved in their life but avoiding them being too dependent on you
- minimising conflict and criticism between family members
- matching your expectations of them to their capabilities, interests and personality.
- Researchers at Monash and Melbourne Universities have developed strategies to help parents safeguard their child's mental health. See www.parentingstrategies.net/depression.

ADULTHOOD

In one's late twenties and thirties, weight becomes a dominant issue. Two-thirds of Australians in this age bracket are now overweight or obese. This is a very new phenomenon. When heart disease was at its peak some decades ago, the typical sufferer was a thin smoker. Now it is the overweight adult with glucose intolerance leading to type 2 diabetes, high blood pressure and abnormal blood fats. If a person continues to smoke, the risk of these is multiplied several-fold.

None of these conditions are very obvious at first. You don't know your blood pressure unless you have it measured, nor your blood glucose or blood cholesterol. In most people, these conditions do not cause symptoms, so the incentive to make major changes to lifestyle or to take medications long term – and probably forever – is not very strong. It would be though if people understood the risks they are facing; not just for heart disease, but for various forms of cancer, muscle and skeletal problems, stroke and dementia. Knowing your absolute risk (see page 47) at the

Keeping adults healthy

- Use key transition points in life (such as leaving school, becoming a parent, relationship breakdown or retirement) as health 'stocktakes'. Use these milestones as a reminder to check in with a doctor or counsellor to assess your health status, risk factors and ways to improve your health.
- Keep up-to-date with screening tests that are appropriate for your age. (See page 296 for our Health tests checklist, which will help you decide what tests are right for you at each stage of your life.)
- Take a check of your own mental health and that of your partner and family. Men particularly are more likely to focus on physical symptoms of depression such as tiredness and weight loss, and ignore they are feeling 'down', angry or irritable.
- Learn ways to manage stress as your responsibilities increase throughout adulthood. Identify what triggers stress for you to assess if there are ways around these scenarios. Organise your time better by making lists, learn when to say no and get to know what part of the day you are most productive.
- Spend time working out what gives you energy. Where possible, make lifestyle changes such as sticking to physical activity or social appointments, regularly do things that relax you, and give yourself regular breaks.
- To the best of your ability, figure out the work pattern that suits your character, strengths and commitments best.

age of 45 and understanding what it means is a very important and useful thing to do. (More information about absolute risk can be found in chapter 6.)

As described in chapter 2, obesity sets off a whole range of responses in the immune system which damage other organs of the body. High blood glucose and obesity also act on similar damaging pathways. The immune and hormonal consequences of obesity cause an increased risk of cancer, but more commonly damages large and small arteries. In the eyes, this can lead to blindness. In the kidneys, this can lead to chronic kidney disease. In the heart, this can lead to coronary heart disease. In the leg arteries, this can lead to walking difficulties and even gangrene.

High blood pressure is the primary risk factor for stroke, and a 10 millimetre of mercury (mmHg) increase in blood pressure can be associated with a 20-fold increase in risk. It is also one of the three main risk factors for coronary heart disease, particularly for heart failure. It also makes the consequences of either form of diabetes and kidney disease even worse.

Abnormal blood fats, especially high LDL cholesterol, is the other major risk factor for atherosclerosis (the underlying cause of most heart attacks and stroke). Most importantly, atherosclerosis of the coronary arteries (which supply blood and oxygen to the heart) leads to heart attack, while atherosclerosis of the carotid arteries (which supply the brain) leads to stroke. It is not clear why atherosclerosis (which is a problem that can affect all of the arteries in the body) picks out the coronary artery in one person, the leg arteries in another, and an artery to the brain in someone else. Certainly, high blood pressure has a predilection for stroke. People with leg artery disease are more often smokers and or have either type of diabetes.

OLDER AGE

Having survived all of this, the next problems many people face are the chronic diseases of ageing. These include heart failure, one of the consequences of previous damage to the heart. Heart failure is as malignant as many common cancers, but importantly, it also leads to widespread disability among the three-quarters of a million Australians who live with it.

Heart failure is a major cause of hospitalisation in the elderly and it is hugely expensive for the health system. Modern medications, other treatments

Keeping older adults healthy

- Assess your fall risk. Get care givers to help clear trip hazards and uneven or slippery surfaces from your home, ensure there is adequate lighting and railings on the entrance and exit to your home, and take part in exercise that improves your muscle strength and balance.
- Stay independent and mobile for longer through regular exercise. Start slowly and aim for gradual improvement in your strength, stamina, balance and flexibility.
- Maximise your brain health by keeping active, enjoying a healthy diet, challenging your brain through new activities, keeping social, and looking after your physical health by reducing high blood pressure, high cholesterol, type 2 diabetes and your weight.
- A reduced appetite or ability to buy and make healthy meals can put older adults at risk of missing out on vital protein, vitamins, minerals and fibre. Calcium is particularly crucial for keeping bones strong in older age, as is fibre for encouraging regular bowel habits.
- Spend time with people who are important to you and get to know the people in your community.
- Consider volunteering in your community.
- Where possible, spend some time each day doing something for yourself.

and disease management programs are proving very effective. However, it's much better to take active steps early to remain healthy and prevent heart disease, such as quitting smoking or losing weight.

The rates of most cancers are directly related to age, particularly lung, breast, prostate and bowel cancers. Early awareness of symptoms and signs, and in some cases effective screening programs, are the key here.

Osteoarthritis can be very limiting for older people. The causes of osteoarthritis are sown early in life, through inadequate nutrition, not getting enough calcium into the bones or inadequate physical activity to strengthen them. Maintaining physical activity throughout life not only has positive effects on many risk factors, but also strengthens muscles in the back. This can help prevent or reduce pain in the back, legs and arms, and it provides for more active participation in the activities of daily life.

Another common and increasing problem associated with ageing is atrial fibrillation, which doubles in frequency every decade after the age of 70. This is an irregularity of the heart rhythm which may occur in conjunction with some other heart condition or high blood pressure. In many people though, it appears as an isolated problem in someone who otherwise has a healthy heart. Sometimes the pulse rate is very rapid, irregular and uncomfortable, and it can be associated with reduced physical capacity. However, the real problem is the risk of stroke associated with atrial fibrillation. It is a factor in about one-quarter to one-third of strokes in our community. If the risk of stroke is moderate or high, people are given blood-thinning medications, which can dramatically reduce the risk of a future stroke (though at the cost of a slight increase in bleeding tendency).

Dementia is already a major human burden for individuals, their families and the general community, because of the cost of providing care to our ageing population. About one-third of dementia is caused by problems that affect the blood vessels (such as type 2 diabetes, high blood pressure and stroke). It has all the same causes that lead to vascular problems (such as coronary heart disease) elsewhere in the body.

The most common type of dementia is Alzheimer's disease. This is associated with major parts of the brain accumulating tangles of a protein called amyloid. For reasons that are not well understood, the very same risk factors that are associated with cardiovascular disease, including high blood pressure, type 2 diabetes and smoking, increase the chance of Alzheimer's disease.

The other main type of dementia is called vascular dementia. This arises from past damage to the brain from vascular causes, especially large and small strokes or high blood pressure. Not surprisingly, it has the same risk factors that precede Alzheimer's. As with heart failure, coronary disease, stroke and many cancers, we know that action earlier in life, well before the disease becomes obvious, can stop the trajectory and lead to a healthier ageing.

Turning the spiral upwards

There is nothing inevitable about a person experiencing a downward health spiral. Balanced nutrition, avoiding tobacco and other harmful substances, regular physical activity, immunisation and health checks as recommended, and attending to the early signs of an emerging problem are so important to have the best chance of living a long and healthy life, and contributing to the health of our community.

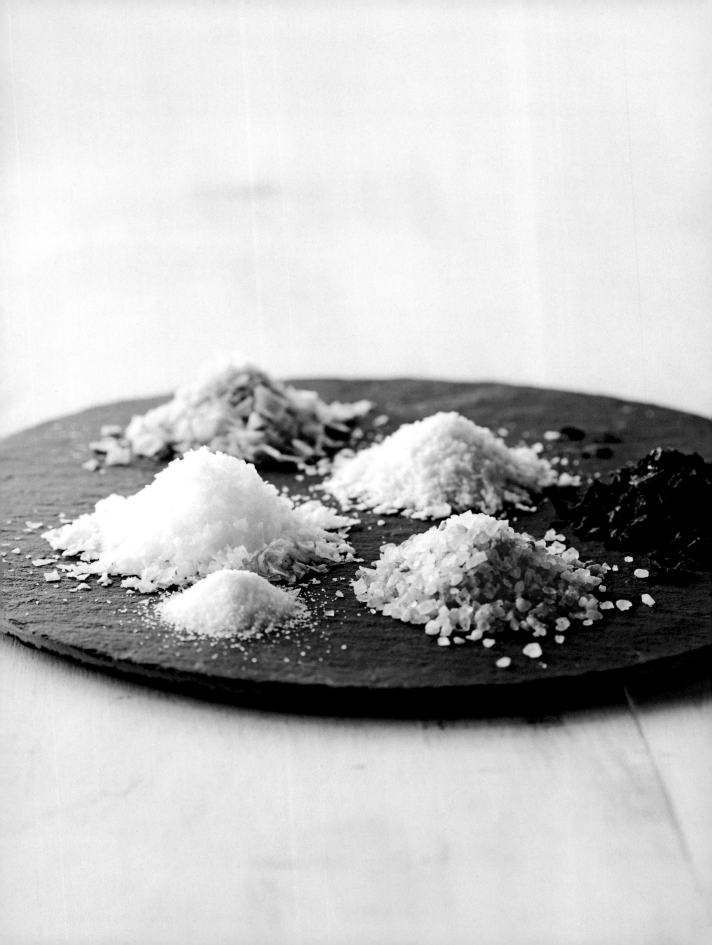

4

DEMYSTIFYING RISK FACTORS AND DISEASE

To stay well, we need to understand and monitor the factors that put our wellbeing at risk. These are often silent – even perhaps hidden– but if we know they are there we can act on them at the stage where our wellbeing is not being diminished. This is much better than waiting for health to be affected, even with all the wonderful treatments that are available. When we talk about risk factors, we are talking about the statistical probability that a person will be affected by a condition. This is a calculation – it is not inevitable that a particular person will definitely be affected. A person can be at risk of developing a disease, but may never go on to develop that disease. On the other hand, people with no apparent risks will be affected. Other times, people with a full hand of risk factors will emerge unscathed.

Most Australians have at least one risk factor putting them at risk of some type of chronic disease. The world's leading risk factors for death are high blood pressure (responsible for 13% of deaths), tobacco use (9%), high blood glucose (6%), physical inactivity (6%), and overweight and obesity (5%).

The major risk factors

Eight risk factors (alcohol use, tobacco use, high blood pressure, high body mass index, high cholesterol, high blood glucose, low fruit and vegetable intake, and physical inactivity) account for over 60% of heart, stroke and vascular disease deaths. Mental stress has also been associated with heart attack risk.

The more risk factors a person carries, the higher their likelihood of developing coronary heart disease and certain other diseases. Men who have at least five risk factors have a three-fold increase in developing chronic lung disease such as emphysema or bronchitis. Women with multiple risk factors are three times more likely to have a stroke, and more than twice as likely to develop depression than a woman with two or less risk factors.

Some risk factors tend to cluster together, adding to the chance of disease. A person who is obese is less likely to get enough physical activity. Someone who is a heavy drinker is also more likely to smoke. Engaging in poor health habits are also more common in areas of social disadvantage.

However, you can develop protective strategies to reduce the likelihood of disease.

High blood pressure usually does not have visible symptoms, despite it being the most common and largely preventable major risk factor for stroke and heart disease. About one-third of Australian adults have high blood pressure – also called hypertension – but half will not know they are at risk. Hypertension is much more common with age.

What is blood pressure?

Blood pressure is the force of blood against the inside wall of arteries as it is delivers oxygen-rich blood around the body. This pressure fluctuates throughout the day to cater for different bodily functions such as sleeping, exercise and emotional states. With each heartbeat, your blood pressure rises and falls in a wave pattern. Blood pressure rises when your main arteries expand as blood leaves the heart and it contracts. This is called the 'systole' reading. It is the first number in a blood-pressure reading, and what you feel when you take your pulse.

Blood pressure drops when your heart relaxes and fills with blood. This is called the 'diastole' reading. It is the second number in a blood-pressure reading, However, blood pressure varies minute to minute, day to day, depending on circumstances.

A blood pressure reading is taken by a blood pressure cuff being placed on the upper arm. Normal blood pressure is 120 mmHg (millimetres of mercury) over 80 mmHg. This is usually stated as 120/80.

Hypertension is defined by a systolic reading over 140 mmHg and a diastolic reading of more than 90 mmHg. This is usually stated as 140/90. If pressure remains high, blood vessels aren't able to regulate how they deliver blood around the body and this can damage the heart, kidneys and brain.

What raises blood pressure?

You may develop high blood pressure because it is a factor in your family's medical history. Smoking causes an acute rise in blood pressure and heart rate, and can also make blood vessels become stiff, which then puts stress on the heart.

Regular alcohol intake is associated with a small rise in blood pressure. Binge or heavy drinking can often lead to significant blood pressure rises that can be enough to cause stroke. Being overweight, obese or having a sedentary lifestyle is another risk.

Hormones like adrenaline and noradrenaline or cortisol cause elevated blood pressure levels during times of stress. There has been a long-standing debate on whether these short-term changes in blood pressure can become sustained with chronic stress. Baker IDI research has shown that in some people this is the cause of their high blood pressure, but there are many other causes.

In people with type 2 diabetes, blood pressure can also rise when high insulin levels cause the body to store more salt and water in the kidneys. Kidney disease is another major cause of hypertension. Most people with type 2 diabetes have hypertension.

The influence of salt

A high-salt diet can also raise blood pressure. Recent studies suggest that reducing the amount of salt consumed daily by 3000 mg would prevent 3000–6000 deaths in Australia each year. Adults should limit daily salt intake from all sources to less than 6000 mg (this is about 1 teaspoon). It's easy to be unaware of the amount of salt we are eating as 3/4 of our salt intake comes from processed foods. Foods that contribute the most are bread, meat, poultry and game products, including processed meat, snacks and cereal products and cereal-based dishes such as biscuits and pizza. You can tell how much by looking at the label. If it has less than 120 mg sodium per 100 g, it is low in salt. If it has more than 400 mg of sodium per 100 g, it is high in salt. Salt is a preservative – to avoid it, it's best to eat more fresh foods.

The effect of pressure

High blood pressure has obvious pressure-related consequences, such as putting so much stress on the artery walls that they break down and rupture. If this happens in the brain, it triggers a stroke due to bleeding in the brain called cerebral haemorrhage. Similarly, the heart may fail if it has to pump against a very high pressure for many years.

The other consequences of high blood pressure are more insidious, such as the propensity for coronary heart disease and heart attack. Coupling with other risk factors, it can cause fatty deposits to build up inside arteries. This is known as atherosclerosis.

Managing your risk

The good news is that making healthy lifestyle changes to your diet, weight and physical activity, as well as the strategic use of medications (such as ACE inhibitors, calcium-blockers and diuretics) are very effective at reducing risk.

We will discuss how to measure your risk in chapter 6.

METABOLIC SYNDROME

Metabolic syndrome is a collection of risk factors that usually occur together and increase the risk of heart disease, stroke and type 2 diabetes. It is estimated that more than one-third of Australian adults suffer from this.

You are diagnosed with metabolic syndrome if you have at least three of the following risk factors:

- abdominal obesity: excess fat stored around the stomach, like the classic 'apple' body shape
- hypertension
- high blood triglycerides
- low levels of high-density lipoproteins (HDL), the 'good' cholesterol, which protects against fatty deposits building up inside blood vessels
- higher than normal blood glucose levels and resistance of the body to some actions of insulin.

Triglycerides make up the bulk of dietary fats, and once digested they circulate in the blood to be used as fuel for energy. Leftovers are stored as body fat.

If we regularly consume more foods that are high in sugar and saturated fats than we burn off through exercise, this encourages weight gain around the stomach and may raise triglyceride levels in our blood. Foods high in saturated fats include processed meats, fat and skin on meats, full-fat dairy products, cakes and biscuits, and deep-fried foods.

The medical term for abnormal blood fats such as triglycerides or cholesterol levels is 'dyslipidaemia'. Many people with high triglycerides also have low levels of 'good' HDL cholesterol, which helps remove fat from the arteries.

Just like with high blood pressure, abnormal blood fats can also lead to fatty plaques building up on the walls of blood vessels, a process called atherosclerosis. This restricts blood flow, and a complete blockage can cause a heart attack or stroke.

Healthy nutrition and regular exercise are the keys to avoiding the development of metabolic syndrome. If adopting a healthy diet and exercise lifestyle are not as effective as they need to be to combat metabolic syndrome, medications are also available through your doctor.

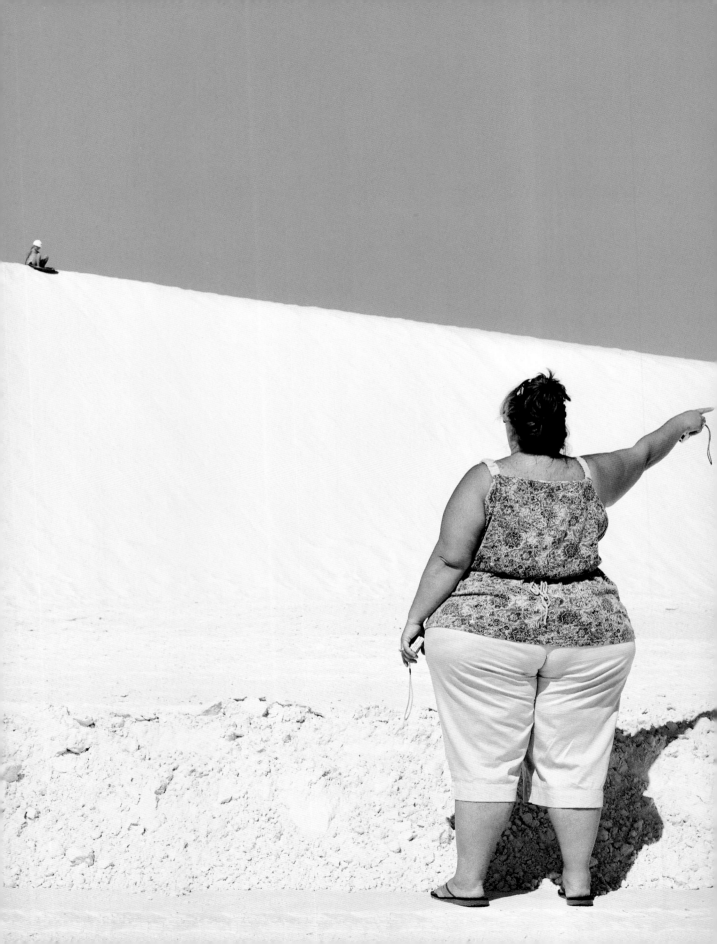

Metabolic diseases

Metabolic diseases are conditions where the body is unable to control critical biochemical reactions involving the processing or transport of proteins (amino acids), carbohydrates (sugars and starches), or fats (fatty acids). Some metabolic diseases are the result of rare genetic disorders but more common examples include diabetes, metabolic syndrome and obesity, where the body is unable to manage fat and carbohydrate metabolism in a healthy way. Apart from type 1 diabetes, there are many lifestyle changes you can make to reduce your risk of developing these diseases or lessen the severity of them.

TYPE 2 DIABETES

Insulin is a hormone made by the pancreas, a gland just below the stomach. Insulin allows the glucose we consume in food to move from the blood into cells. Glucose is the body's main source of energy. Diabetes sets off a range of damaging inflammation processes in the body, particularly affecting the arteries and nerves. Consequently, it's a common cause of blindness, gangrene in the legs and kidney damage. Baker IDI research is also showing an emerging relationship between both types of diabetes and increased cancer risk.

In type 1 diabetes, the body's own immune system destroys the pancreatic cells that make insulin. Without daily insulin injections, this leads to a toxic build-up of glucose in the blood.

Type 2 diabetes is often referred to as 'lifestyle-related diabetes', and accounts for about 85% of diabetes cases. Up to 60% of type 2 cases can be prevented with healthy lifestyle changes.

In this condition, the pancreas doesn't make enough insulin or the insulin produced doesn't do its job properly (a condition called insulin resistance).

'Pre-diabetes' is a term when blood glucose levels are higher than normal but not high enough to be diagnosed with full-blown type 2 diabetes. This is diagnosed through an Oral Glucose Tolerance Test. This test can diagnose both pre-diabetes and type 2 diabetes.

Risk factors

Those most at risk of type 2 diabetes include:
- people with pre-diabetes
- Aboriginal or Torres Strait Islanders, Pacific Islanders, Maori, Asian, Middle Eastern, North African and Southern European adults aged over 35
- people over 45 who are obese, overweight, have high blood pressure or have an immediate relative with the condition
- people aged 55 or over
- people with cardiovascular disease
- women with polycystic ovarian syndrome who are also overweight
- women who have had gestational diabetes
- people taking some antipsychotic or corticosteroid medications.

You can reduce your lifestyle risk factors through:
- maintaining a healthy weight
- exercising regularly
- eating a healthy diet
- maintaining a normal blood pressure and cholesterol level
- not smoking.

OBESITY

Whether obesity is a disease in its own right or is a risk factor remains controversial. The problem is that if obesity is not considered a disease, it becomes easier for the community, policy makers and family members to laden blame and responsibility onto the individual. There is a tendency to do nothing about obesity prevention at the community level because it's a 'person's own fault' and they should 'have more willpower'. This is a recipe for inaction. It's increasingly becoming understood that there are many drivers for obesity, including environmental, socio-economic and genetic factors.

But what is indisputable is obesity's link to disease and its effect on life expectancy. Studies show that people who are obese lose on average 2–4 years of life, and 8–10 years for the severely obese. As far as heart disease or stroke is concerned, obesity is not as strong a risk factor as is smoking or high blood pressure. But it is a very important factor for cancer, particularly colorectal, kidney, pancreas, esophageal, uterine and breast cancer. Obesity is also the major risk factor for type 2 diabetes. The more fatty tissue you carry, the more your cells become resistant to insulin.

The new normal?

Being overweight is not unusual now. Two-thirds of Australian adults are overweight or obese. High income earners are 40% less likely to be obese than those on low incomes.

There is no quick fix for obesity but a healthy balanced diet and lifelong physical activity will avoid its complications.

Cardiovascular disease

Cardiovascular disease is the umbrella term given to diseases of the heart and blood vessels. It includes heart failure, heart attack, valve disease, angina, cardiomyopathy, coronary heart disease, congenital heart disease, arrhythmias such as atrial fibrillation and stroke.

Many of these diseases can be life-threatening. They remain Australia's leading cause of death.

RISK FACTORS

The three main risk factors of cardiovascular disease are:

- Cholesterol: The build-up of these fatty deposits inside arteries over time cause a blockage, known as atherosclerosis, or a hardening of the arteries. This can trigger a blood clot to form. When arteries that supply the heart with blood are blocked this can cause heart attack. When arteries to the brain are affected, this can trigger a stroke.
- High blood pressure (hypertension): High blood pressure can weaken artery walls, causing them to rupture and haemorrhage. If this happens in the brain, this can lead to a stroke. When combined with high cholesterol, and its build-up of fatty plaques inside the artery walls, it can lead to an aneurysm. The risk of heart failure is 6–10%, double the general risk for people aged over

65, when blood pressure is over 160/90. Reducing systolic pressure by 10mmHg (the first number in a blood pressure reading) can halve the risk of heart failure.
- Smoking: This is an important risk factor for all forms of vascular disease including stroke. Over time, the toxins in cigarettes allow fatty plaque deposits to build up on the inside of vessels that supply oxygen-rich blood to the body. This narrowing makes the blood vessels stiffen, which puts more stress on the heart and can lead to a heart attack, stroke or coronary artery disease (CAD). Having CAD gives you a one-in-three chance of developing Peripheral Arterial Disease, a particular problem in smokers in which blood flow is blocked to the legs causing numbness, pain and even gangrene.

You are also at risk of cardiovascular disease if you are obese, are physically inactive, have type 2 diabetes or a family history of cardiovascular disease.

LINKS TO DIABETES

Increasingly, doctors are seeing obese people develop type 2 diabetes that leads to heart disease. About three-quarters of patients on acute cardiac wards in Australian hospitals either have either type 2 diabetes or pre-diabetes.

The good news is that heart disease is largely preventable through healthy lifestyle change.

Dementia

Dementia describes a number of symptoms caused by brain disorders. It is not a word that describes one specific disease. Dementia can affect behaviour, personality, decision-making, memory and the ability to carry out daily tasks.

The most common types of dementia include Alzheimer's disease, vascular dementia, Parkinson's disease, Lewy body disease, alcohol-related dementia (also known as Korsakoff's syndrome) and Creutzfeldt-Jacob disease. There is no effective prevention or cure for dementia. Current treatments only target the symptoms.

There is some good news. Australian patients with early stage Alzheimer's disease have been among the first in the world to trial a new class of drug. This drug has shown promise in not just improving memory but also – for the first time – slowing disease progression in animal models.

But until the time that such drugs become widely available, we must rely on making healthy lifestyle changes to reduce our risk.

WAYS TO TAKE ACTION NOW

The physical changes in the brain – the build-up of amyloid plaque and tau tangles that lead to cell death and brain shrinkage that cause dementia – can start 20 years before any symptoms appear.

Middle age is a vital time to start implementing healthy lifestyle changes. You can reduce your risk of dementia by up to 40% by:
- maintaining a healthy weight
- keeping your heart healthy by controlling your blood pressure and cholesterol
- avoiding developing type 2 diabetes
- not smoking
- getting the recommended amount of exercise
- managing depression
- avoiding serious head injury
- being socially and mentally active.

Age-related risk factors

YOUNG PEOPLE

Youth is a time that is associated with a higher incidence of harm resulting from risky behaviours, such as dangerous or risky driving, excessive drinking and using drugs in a social manner. Injury is the major cause of death for Victorians aged 15–24 years, mainly from suicide and road transport accidents. Young men are two to three times more likely to die this way.

The good news is that school students are smoking at rates three times less than 30 years ago, with alcohol consumption also reducing in this age group.

Mental health remains a challenge for young people, with a recent study showing one in five young people aged 18–24 experienced high or very high levels of psychological distress.

As we have learnt in the previous chapters, it is difficult to get on top of our physical health when we are not coping psychologically. It is important young people are supported to start and maintain healthy habits around diet, exercise, sleep and coping strategies while they are physically in the 'prime of their life' to help prevent the spiral of lifestyle-related disease.

OLDER PEOPLE

As we get older, the likelihood and severity of illness and disability increases. Risk factors accumulate, and our bodies break down. For example, almost 60% of cancers develop after a person reaches the age of 65 years. The prevalence of dementia increases from 3% at age 65–74, to 30% from age 85.

Social connection becomes more important as a person gets older and leaves the workforce, both for emotional health but also for welfare checks. Hospital trauma services treat more older people for serious injuries sustained from falls than they see car crash patients.

Women's risk factors and diseases

Women are not only more likely to be a care-giver for someone with a chronic illness, they are also at higher risk of some conditions, especially once they reach menopause.

Symptoms for a range of common conditions and illnesses can be different for women than they are for men. This can often result in delayed diagnosis and treatment.

WOMEN AND HEART DISEASE

Heart disease kills almost three times as many women as breast cancer. Every day, 11 Australian women die from a heart attack. However, women are less likely to experience the classic chest pain symptoms than men. Consequently, they are less likely to call for an ambulance if they are

experiencing a heart attack, as most women don't
know that jaw, shoulder, neck or back pain can be
symptoms.

Women are more likely to have diagnostic tests
that are not conclusively positive or negative, and
they are less likely to be recommended advanced
treatments like bypass surgery or angioplasty.
Later in life they are more likely than men to
develop heart failure.

WOMEN AND DIABETES

Women can suffer different symptoms of both
type 1 and type 2 diabetes, such as urinary tract
infections and vaginal yeast infections. Women
with diabetes have higher risk of blindness,
depression and heart disease than men. Premen-
opausal women are generally protected from
cardiovascular disease but this protection is
lost if they have diabetes. In these cases,
they have the same risk as men.

WOMEN AND OTHER DISEASES

High blood pressure and cholesterol are
uncommon in women until they hit menopause.
Around this time, a woman's prevalence for

these conditions catches up to men, as she loses
the protection supplied by estrogen.

Women are also at greater risk of osteoporosis,
and depression is twice as prevalent in women
as men.

Two-thirds of Australians with dementia are
women, with the highest prevalence in those aged
over 85 years. This is a major health challenge of
this century and is the focus of much promis-
ing research. There are rare genetic causes but for
most of us, keeping fit in body and mind, and in
control of the risk factors (such as those described
in chapter 4) is good insurance against dementia
later in life.

Men's risk factors and diseases

Australian men are more likely than women to suffer serious health problems. Yet they visit a doctor
less often, and usually delay seeing a doctor until a
complaint is in advanced stages. Men have almost
twice the chance of an avoidable death due to injury,
illness or where early treatment could have applied.

Looking at conditions that affect both the sexes,
men are more likely to die from suicide (78% of
such deaths are in males), as well as trachea and
lung cancer.

More than half of deaths from coronary heart
disease, colon and rectum cancer, blood cancers and chronic respiratory diseases (including
chronic bronchitis, emphysema, and asthma)
are experienced by men.

Overall, more men develop and die from
cancer. In Victoria, the ratio is 114 men to 100
women. These figures are mainly from tobacco-
related cancers.

Every day, 98 Australian men will have a heart
attack, and 14 of these men will die. Coronary
heart disease, triggered by fatty deposits clog-
ging up the arteries, is typically the cause of heart
attacks. This is something that is largely preventable with a healthy lifestyle.

New studies are showing that even minor erec-
tion difficulties can be indicators for heart disease.
There are many causes of erectile dysfunction.
For these reasons, erectile difficulties should be
discussed with your doctor

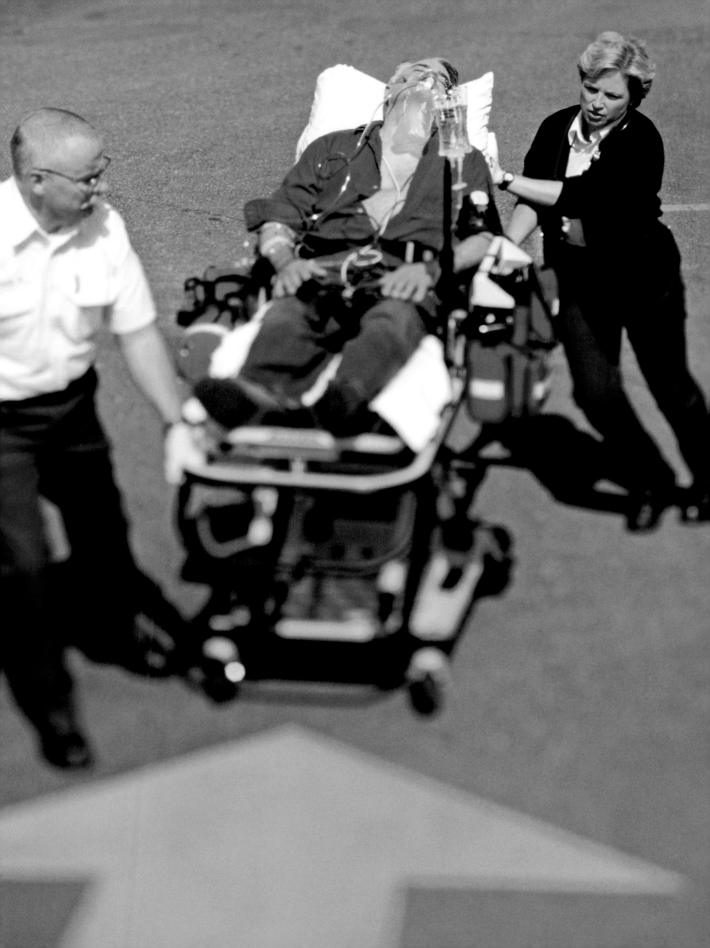

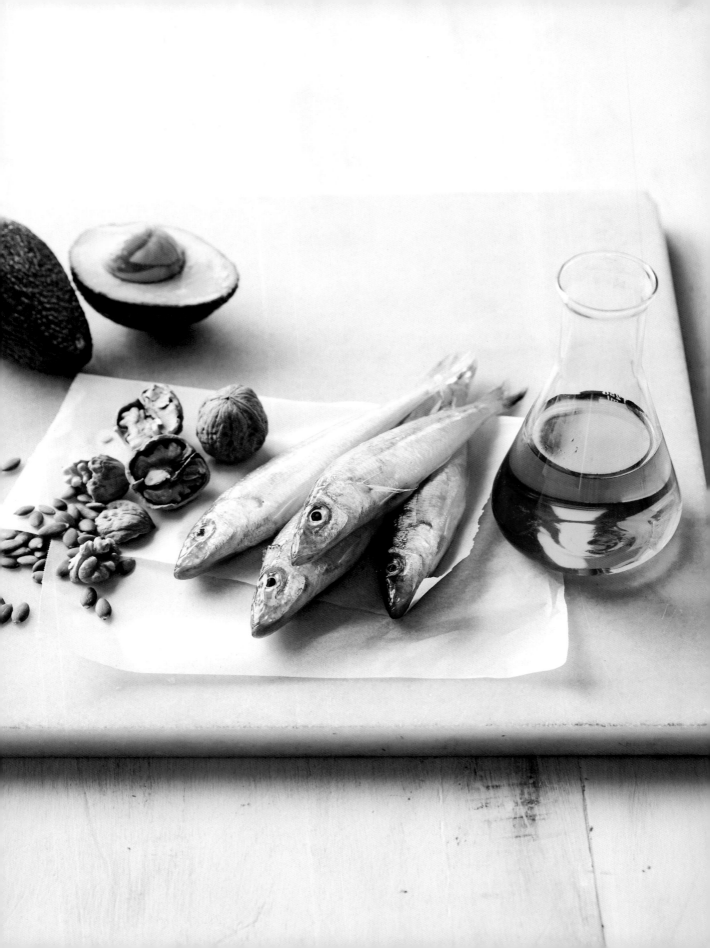

5

THE IMPORTANCE OF PREVENTION

Maintaining good health is everyone's responsibility. Individuals, families, schools, businesses and policy makers – we all have a role to play.

Government, at all levels, plays a major part in optimising our health. They do this through childhood immunisation programs, restricting the sale of tobacco and providing equitable access to health services. This focus on good health is strengthened by legislating to have nutritional panels on food labels, providing sport and recreation facilities in our neighbourhoods, and funding hospital beds. It is our responsibility to make use of these services.

As a community, we could all do more. There is still a disproportionate amount of the health budget spent on cures rather than on proven prevention strategies.

Our experience with reducing tobacco smoking rates, which have come down from about 50% of the adult population a few decades ago to just over 13% today, is that the measures need to be consistent and multi-faceted. Some of the changes in smoking rates were due to taxation, some to public awareness campaigns, and some due to legislation making it more difficult to smoke in public.

The same approach is needed to help reduce obesity-related chronic disease in the community. No single measure will work. However, we cannot leave this to government alone. People need to work together. The education system and local government can contribute, as can employers and town planners.

There is a clear link between socio-economic disadvantage and poor health. Some Australians can expect to live on average up to seven years longer due to factors such as wellbeing and preventable deaths. There is a 10-year difference in life expectancy between Indigenous and non-Indigenous Australians. And even in more privileged households, there remain challenges in making healthy choices.

But ultimately, each person needs to take ownership for their lifestyle. This is a lifelong process.

We need to take the time to learn about the risk factors we carry, and understand what can be done to prevent these from tipping us into disease. We need to work with our doctor on an action plan, whether this be lifestyle change, medications or surgery, which will maintain our health and longevity.

The cost of poor health

Anyone who has waited months, or even years, for an elective surgery procedure at a public hospital, or spent time on a trolley in the emergency department waiting for a bed, will understand the frustration of limited resources in our acute health system.

There are over 500,000 avoidable hospital admissions in Australia each year. The more people partaking in unhealthy lifestyles that result in hospital treatment, the fewer health resources that are left for others.

The effect of poor lifestyle choices

The World Health Organization estimates that up to 80% of all heart disease, stroke and type 2 diabetes, and up to 40% of all cancers, could potentially be avoided through preventive health interventions. Around 37,000 Australian cancer cases could be prevented each year largely through lifestyle changes.

Unhealthy diets account for about 10% of Australia's total disease burden, followed closely by high body mass and smoking. If current trends continue, three-quarters of Australians will be overweight or obese by 2050.

Prevention starts with the basics. More than a third of the total kilojoules we consume come from discretionary foods – foods that don't fit into the major five food groups. Just 7% of adults eat enough vegetables. Less than half the adult population consume the daily recommended fruit servings.

Smoking

In Australia it has been estimated that tobacco smoking is responsible for over 1500 deaths each year, with hospital costs approaching $1 billion each year. Smoking rates have considerably reduced since the 1990s, but just over 13% of Australian adults overall and 42% of Indigenous people aged 15 and over, still smoke daily.

About 11% of Australian women smoke at some stage during their pregnancy, with rates higher among disadvantaged and Indigenous women. Passive smoking may be just as dangerous as direct smoking. Smoking during pregnancy can only be bad for the baby.

Making healthy changes later in life is better than never. Studies show that quitting smoking before the age of 40 can help you avoid 90% of the health risks associated with the habit in later life.

Health promotion campaigns have looked at how every cigarette you *don't* smoke is doing you good. Within six hours of butting out, your blood pressure decreases. Within two to five years, a woman's risk of cervical cancer is the same as someone who has never smoked. After 15 years, an ex-smoker's chance of heart attack and stroke is close to that of someone who has never smoked.

It is easier, cheaper and less traumatic to act early rather than endure months in hospital following an acute medical event.

Your family medical history

Every adult should know their blood pressure and cholesterol, blood fats and glucose. Everyone should endeavour to know their family medical history. Be inquisitive and ask questions about your family. Why did all your father's brothers die in their 50s? Do your mother, aunts and grandmother have a history of cancer? Type 2 diabetes, high cholesterol, mental illness and some cancers are among the many serious conditions that have genetic links, which may put you at increased risk.

Chapter 6 will explain the different tests and self-examinations available, the merits and disadvantages of these, and how often each test should be done.

Separating facts from myths

With so much conflicting health advice in the media it can be hard to know what to believe and what to do. We believe the best approach is one based on evidence. The following table will help you sort out the facts from the myths.

Common health myths

MYTH: I should avoid foods high in **cholesterol** to keep my blood cholesterol down.

FACT: Cholesterol is found only in animal-sourced foods, with higher sources including eggs, prawns, liver, meat and dairy products. But dietary cholesterol has only a modest impact on raising low density lipoprotein LDL 'bad' cholesterol. Saturated and trans fat are the real culprit.

Choosing low or no-fat dairy products, choosing lean meats or removing excess fat and skin from meats, reducing the amount of takeaway food and bakery products you consume, as well as plant-based saturated fats such as coconut and palm oil products, are a simple way of cutting the amount of unhealthy fats in your diet. Use olive oil or foods labelled 'polyunsaturated' or 'mono-unsaturated' instead.

MYTH: High blood pressure (hypertension) is caused by high stress levels.

FACT: Blood pressure may rise temporarily when you become stressed, however stress has not been proven to always cause ongoing high blood pressure. Our bodies respond to stressful situations by releasing stress hormones, adrenaline and cortisol, into the blood stream. It causes our heart to beat faster and our blood vessels to constrict to preserve blood flow to vital organs, as we prepare for our 'fight or flight' response. When the situation resolves, our blood pressure returns to a normal level.

Although stress doesn't always cause heart disease, managing stress is important for your overall wellness. In chapter 8, we look at strategies to help you manage stress.

MYTH: I should avoid all types of **fat** as part of a healthy diet.

FACT: Fats are an important part of a healthy balanced diet and you should not exclude them. They help your body absorb vitamins, are a useful source of energy and provide essential fatty acids your body cannot make. Instead of cutting all fat from your diet, replace saturated and trans fats (found in fried fast foods and bakery products) and replace them with polyunsaturated and monounsaturated fats.

Use vegetable or seed oils instead of coconut or palm oils. Include oily fish such as sardines, tuna or salmon, eggs and nuts in your diet regularly. Bulk out or replace some meat-heavy meals with beans or legumes.

The Heart Foundation recommends limiting the amount of saturated fat that you eat to less than 7% of your total daily kilojoules.

MYTH: Taking **fish oil supplements** is the best way I can reduce my risk of diabetes or heart disease.

FACT: Fish oil is a $200m market in Australia, with a quarter of adults taking these supplements daily in the hope of warding off heart disease and arthritis, boosting brain power, and protecting themselves against diabetes and Alzheimer's disease. Many studies contradict each other over the benefits of omega-3 fatty acids taken as supplements. We must consume omega-3s from an external source, as our bodies cannot produce them. But nutrition experts agree that eating fish and seeds regularly seems to be a better strategy than taking supplements.

Foods that are rich in the two main types of omega-3s include fatty fish like salmon, mackerel, and sardines. Eating two unbattered fish meals each week is recommended. Plant-based sources such as walnuts, canola oil, flaxseeds/linseeds, chia seeds and pumpkin seeds are heavy in another type of omega-3, which the body can convert for useful purposes.

MYTH: The latest fad **diet** will work for me.

FACT: Most popular or fad diets work for a while as they restrict total kilojoule intake.

But these popular fad diets see people miss out on vital nutrients. Omit all fats from your diet and you exclude foods like avocado, olive oil and nuts that have proven health benefits. Eliminate carbs and you miss out on the health gains from milk, legumes, fruit, yoghurt and whole grains.

The body will fight this initial weight change, and eventually most people go back to their original weight. The most important aspect about healthy eating is that you find a plan or ethos you enjoy and that is realistic to follow over the long term.

MYTH: I am '**big boned'**. I can't help being overweight.

FACT: Big bones in the context of weight gain are a myth. Yes, people have different size frames, but most of our weight is carried in soft tissue such as muscle, fatty tissue and organs.

MYTH: Taking the **prescribed medication** is the only thing I need to do to control my blood pressure/cholesterol/diabetes.

FACT: Your doctor may decide that prescription medication for your chronic condition is needed in addition to lifestyle changes. Many people don't reap the benefits of these therapies, as about half of patients don't take medication as prescribed. Over time, these medications can help stabilise the physiological processes putting you at risk of poor health and other disease.

But healthy lifestyle changes are vital for the overall health benefits we have discussed earlier. They may also help some people avoid or reduce their reliance on medications. This is true for type 2 diabetes, those with high blood pressure and those with high cholesterol.

MYTH: There is no point bothering about **exercise or healthy eating**. We are all going to die one day.

FACT: You will die of something. But you need not die prematurely from something preventable or suffer with illness and disability. When you make healthy changes to your life, other people are affected as well. An early death is something that also affects your family and friends who would be left to cope with having you taken from their lives too soon.

Each year, almost 50,000 Australians die prematurely before the age of 75. Half of these deaths are considered potentially avoidable through health interventions. Coronary heart disease, lung cancer and suicide are the most common cause of premature death.

We aren't here for long. We get one shot at life. A healthy lifestyle gives you the best chance of having as many healthy years as possible – free from mobility problems, pain and with the cognitive competence – to achieve all you want to in life.

MYTH: I need to take **dietary supplements** to keep healthy.

FACT: Pharmaceutical companies spend millions of dollars on advertisements marketing supplements to maintain a healthy lifestyle. But vitamins aren't medication and they aren't the miracle cure. In fact, some can be toxic at high levels, such as B6 and vitamin A. It is best to get your vitamins from eating a healthy diet.

There is no evidence that vitamin C prevents the cold or flu, no proof that vitamin E prevents heart disease or that vitamin A cures cancer.

There are a few people who may benefit from added supplements, including women who are pregnant or breastfeeding, alcoholics and drug addicts, vegetarians, the elderly or those with malabsorption problems (such as coeliac disease or cystic fibrosis).

Consult your doctor for advice on whether you need supplements.

MYTH: If I **quit smoking I'm going to gain weight,** so it's healthier for me to stick with the cigarettes.

FACT: Quitting smoking is not easy. The nicotine in cigarettes that makes them addictive, and the earlier you start smoking in life the harder it is to butt out. Quitting takes practice. It often takes a number of attempts to quit for good.

Most smokers put on weight when they quit, with an average weight gain of about 5 kg in the first year. Many smokers experience increased hunger as part of withdrawal or they can substitute treat foods for cigarettes. Nicotine speeds up the metabolism, so ex-smokers no longer have this added support.

But research shows in the long-term, the average weight of ex-smokers is the same as those who have never started the habit. Ultimately, carrying a few extra kilos is far healthier than continuing to smoke.

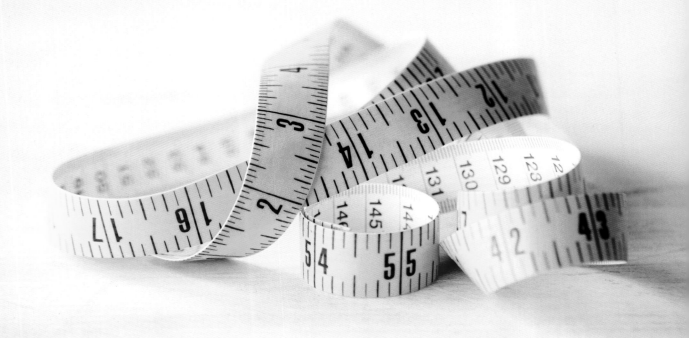

6

MONITORING, SCREENING AND DETECTION OF RISK FACTORS

It is important to follow the very best evidence and views held by health experts in regard to prevention testing. While medical tests used appropriately can save lives, when done by the wrong person or in the wrong way they have the potential to cause harm. You might be surprised to know that some common tests are not recommended for general screening by international specialists. Others are so useful they are mandated by governments.

No medical test is perfect. All tests carry the chance of either missing a problem or detecting something that is not really there. A person has a lower probability of having a particular problem if the disease is rare, or it is rarely experienced by their age group. This is true even if the test returns a positive result. This caveat applies to all screening tests and for this reason they must be used with care. It is tempting to say you want the most advanced and sophisticated tests available, no matter what cost. However, a stepwise approach, starting with the simplest evaluation and building up to more complicated testing when there are clues that something is not quite right, is a much better approach in most cases.

What checks should I do?

In this chapter, we start with checks you can do yourself. Putting this together with things you already know about yourself – such as your family history, smoking or drinking habits – will put you well on the way to deciding what is important to follow up with your doctor. We follow this up with a section on relatively simple testing that can be done on a routine visit to your doctor. Finally, we outline some of the more complex tests that you might encounter.

Self-checks

WEIGHT AND WAIST GIRTH CHECKS

Overweight and obesity are risk factors for many conditions such as type 2 diabetes, heart disease and stroke.

Regardless of your height and build, waist circumference – the measurement taken between the hip bone and lower rib – should be under 94 centimetres for men and under 80 centimetres for women to reduce the risk of disease. You are at a greatly increased risk if your waist circumference is more than 102 centimetres (for men) and 88 centimetres (for women).

Knowing your body mass index (BMI) is another good indicator of whether you are of healthy weight. The disadvantage of using BMI is that it doesn't differentiate between body fat and muscle mass, and doesn't account for age, gender or ethnicity. For example, a short, muscular person might have a high BMI due to their extra muscle weight, but they are not overweight or obese. However, BMI remains useful as a general guide, and is a good place to start considering if you are in your healthy weight range.

As the table below shows, there are different levels recommended to separate healthy weight ranges from being overweight and obese in different populations.

To calculate your BMI, divide your weight (kilograms) by the square of your height (meters). Search for 'BMI calculator' online to find one of many sites that will do this for you. The table below will help you gauge whether you would benefit from losing weight.

Pregnancy and weight gain

Steady weight gain during pregnancy is healthy and normal, but excess weight gain is harmful to both mother and baby. Mothers-to-be don't need to 'eat for two'. New Australian research suggests that metabolic changes in pregnancy allow women to conserve more energy and extract more kilojoules from food so they do not need to eat more.

The following table shows the recommended weight gain during pregnancy.

In the following chapters, you will learn about what diet, exercise and lifestyle changes can help you lose or maintain your weight.

PRE-CONCEPTION BMI	RECOMMENDED TOTAL WEIGHT GAIN
Under 18.5	12.5–18 kg
18.5–24.9	11.5–16 kg
25–29.9	7–11.5 kg
Over 30	5–9 kg

Pregnancy is not the time for diets or extreme exercise plans. If you have put on more weight than you should while pregnant, talk to your doctor.

BREAST SELF-EXAMINATION

More than half of breast cancers are diagnosed after investigation of a breast change found by the woman or her doctor. There is no evidence that one type of self-examination technique is more effective than another in terms of reducing mortality. The important thing is that women are aware of the normal feel and look of their breasts, and seek medical advice immediately if they do find abnormalities.

Women should use their fingers to check for lumps across the entire breast and armpit area – from the collarbone to below the bra line – looking for any thickening, hard knots or bumps. They should also look for any changes in shape, swelling, dimpling of the skin, or changes in the nipples such as puckering or discharge. Some changes may be benign so don't be alarmed but do see your doctor. Although it is rare, men can also get breast cancer and should be alert to any changes, especially lumps around the nipple.

BMI RANGE	WHITE AUSTRALIANS	INDIGENOUS AUSTRALIANS	ASIANS	MAORIS AND PACIFIC ISLANDERS
HEALTHY	20–25	18.6–23	18.6–23	18.5–26
OVERWEIGHT	26–30	23–27.4	23–27.4	26–32
OBESE	Over 30	Over 25	Over 27.5	Over 32

SKIN CHECKS

Melanomas can become life-threatening in as little as six weeks, but skin cancer can typically be treated if found early. Most melanomas are found by patients or their partners.

It is important to become familiar with your skin to know what is normal – whether they be spots, blemishes, moles or freckles – and not just on areas that are exposed to the sun. If you notice changes, see your doctor.

Look for:
- crusty, non-healing sores
- small lumps that are red, pale or pearl-coloured
- new spots, freckles or moles that change colour, thickness or shape over weeks to months (especially those that are dark brown to black, red or blue–black).

Remember to ask someone to help check difficult-to-reach areas such as your back, scalp and back of the neck.

People at high risk for skin cancer include those with:
- fair skin, freckles, light eye colour, light or red hair colour
- increased numbers of unusual moles
- depressed immune systems
- a family history of melanoma among immediate family members
- previous melanoma or non-melanoma skin cancers.

Australian clinical practice guidelines recommend people at high-risk should undergo regular checks by a doctor, including a full-body examination, every 3–12 months.

TYPE 2 DIABETES

The Australian Type 2 Diabetes Risk Assessment Tool (AUSDRISK) was developed by Baker IDI Heart and Diabetes Institute on behalf of and for federal, state and territory governments as a calculator of your risk of disease in the next five years. To use the tool on the following page, simply answer the questions and add up your score to see your results. If you find that you are at intermediate or high risk of developing type 2 diabetes, see your doctor to discuss your results further.

The Australian Type 2 Diabetes Risk Assessment Tool (AUSDRISK)

Calculate your risk

1.	**Your age group**	**Under 35 years**	☐ [0 points]
		35–44 years	☐ [2 points]
		45–54 years	☐ [4 points]
		55–64 years	☐ [6 points]
		65 years or over	☐ [8 points]
2.	**Your gender**	**Female**	☐ [0 points]
		Male	☐ [3 points]
3a.	**Are you of Aboriginal, Torres Strait Islander, Pacific Islander or Maori descent?**	**No**	☐ [0 points]
		Yes	☐ [2 points]
3b.	**Where were you born?**	**Australia**	☐ [0 points]
		Asia (including the Indian sub-continent), **Middle East**, **North Africa**, **Southern Europe**	☐ [2 points]
		Other	☐ [0 points]
4.	**Have either of your parents, or any of your brothers or sisters been diagnosed with diabetes (type 1 or type 2)?**	**No**	☐ [0 points]
		Yes	☐ [3 points]
5.	**Have you ever been found to have high blood glucose (sugar) (for example, in a health examination, during an illness, during pregnancy)?**	**No**	☐ [0 points]
		Yes	☐ [6 points]
6.	**Are you currently taking medication for high blood pressure?**	**No**	☐ [0 points]
		Yes	☐ [2 points]
7.	**Do you currently smoke cigarettes or any other tobacco products on a daily basis?**	**No**	☐ [0 points]
		Yes	☐ [2 points]
8.	**How often do you eat vegetables or fruit?**	**Every day**	☐ [0 points]
		Not every day	☐ [1 point]
9.	**On average, would you say you do at least 2.5 hours of physical activity per week (for example, 30 minutes a day on 5 or more days a week)?**	**Yes**	☐ [0 points]
		No	☐ [2 points]

10. What is your waist measurement taken below the ribs (usually at the level of the navel, and while standing)

The correct place to measure your waist is halfway between your lowest rib and the top of your hipbone, roughly in line with your navel. Measure directly against your skin, breathe out normally, make sure the tape is snug, without compressing the skin. Make a note of your waist measurement and score as below.

A. For those of Asian or Aboriginal or Torres Strait Islander descent:

Men
- **a.** Less than 90 cm ☐ [0 points]
- **b.** 90 – 100 cm ☐ [4 points]
- **c.** More than 100 cm ☐ [7 points]

Women
- **a.** Less than 80 cm ☐ [0 points]
- **b.** 80–90 cm ☐ [4 points]
- **c.** More than 90 cm ☐ [7 points]

B. For all others (i.e. not of Asian or Aboriginal or Torres Strait Islander descent:)

Men
- **a.** Less than 102 cm ☐ [0 points]
- **b.** 102–110 cm ☐ [4 points]
- **c.** More than 110 cm ☐ [7 points]

Women
- **a.** Less than 88 cm ☐ [0 points]
- **b.** 88–100 cm ☐ [4 points]
- **c.** More than 100 cm ☐ [7 points]

Check your total score* against the three possible point ranges below

- **5 or less: Low risk**. If you scored 5 or less, you are at low risk of developing type 2 diabetes within 5 years.
- **6–11: Intermediate risk**. If you scored 6–11 you are at intermediate risk of developing type 2 diabetes within 5 years. Take this form to your doctor to discuss your individual risk and ways to improve your lifestyle.
- **12 or more: High risk**. If you scored 12 or more you are at high risk of developing type 2 diabetes within 5 years, or you may have undiagnosed type 2 diabetes. For scores of 12–15, approximately one person in 14 will develop diabetes. For scores of 16–19, approximately one person in 7 will develop diabetes. For scores of 20 and above, approximately one person in 3 will develop diabetes. Ask your doctor about having a fasting blood glucose test. Act now to prevent type 2 diabetes.

*The overall score may overestimate the risk of diabetes in those aged less than 25 years.

Note: This diabetes risk assessment tool is copyright belonging to the Commonwealth of Australia and was designed for the Australian population, with risk scores calculated and validated based upon the results of the participants in the Australian Diabetes, Obesity and Lifestyle Study (AusDiab). Consequently, the results are not reliable or suitable for use in non-Australian populations.

Simple medical tests

The test in this section are simple tests that can be performed by your doctor.

BLOOD PRESSURE

Blood pressure, the force of blood in the arteries as it is pumped around the body, is typically measured by strapping an inflatable pressure cuff around your upper arm.

Blood pressure is recorded as two numbers, such as 120/80. The larger number, called systolic blood pressure, is the pressure in the arteries as the heart pumps out blood with each beat. The lower number, called diastolic blood pressure, specifies the pressure as the heart relaxes before the next beat.

What do the results from a blood pressure reading mean?

There is no concrete definition for blood pressure, but as a guide:
- normal blood pressure: generally less than 120/80 mmHg
- normal to high blood pressure: between 120/80 and 140/90 mmHg
- high blood pressure: 140/90 mmHg or higher
- very high: 180/110 mmHg or higher.

Blood pressure doesn't stay the same. It changes in response to different bodily functions throughout the day. Your doctor will typically measure your blood pressure a number of times over different days to check if you have high blood pressure. They may advise you to do a 24-hour test, or get you to measure your own blood pressure at home to confirm the diagnosis.

BLOOD GLUCOSE

A blood glucose test measures the amount of a sugar, called glucose, in the bloodstream. This blood test can either be done as a 'fasting' test – performed when you have not eaten for eight hours – or a 'random' test at any time either side of meals. If the results are high, then type 2 diabetes is likely.

If results are borderline, you may need to undergo an oral glucose tolerance test before a diagnosis can be confirmed. This involves blood samples being taken before and after drinking a glucose drink. In someone with diabetes, their blood glucose levels rise rapidly after consuming the glucose and remain higher afterwards.

CHOLESTEROL

A blood test is used to measure the levels of two types of cholesterol in the blood – high density lipoprotein (HDL) and low density lipoprotein (LDL) – as well as levels of triglycerides, and the overall amount of cholesterol. You usually need to fast for 9–12 hours before the test.

Your risk will be calculated by your doctor, who will also consider other risk factors such as age, family history, smoking and high blood pressure.

It is recommended that your cholesterol level be no higher than 5.5 mmol per litre if you have no other risk factors. If there are other cardiovascular risk factors (such as smoking, high blood pressure or pre-existing heart disease), the LDL levels would ideally be less than 2 mmol per litre.

Absolute risk

Absolute risk is a method of combining information on a number of risk factors into a single figure. This chart provides a statistical assessment of the likelihood of a major cardiovascular event, such as heart attack or stroke, happening to you within a given time period, usually five or 10 years.

The Australian cardiovascular risk charts (for people without diabetes)

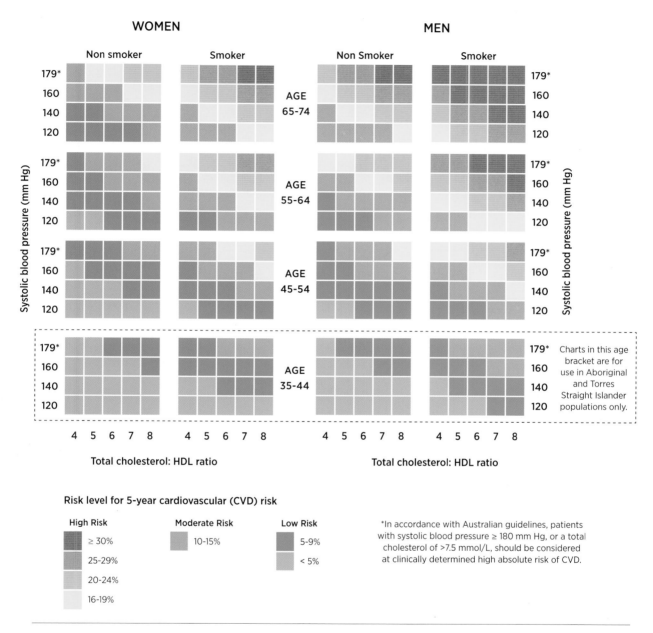

Risk level for 5-year cardiovascular (CVD) risk

High Risk	Moderate Risk	Low Risk
≥ 30%	10-15%	5-9%
25-29%		< 5%
20-24%		
16-19%		

*In accordance with Australian guidelines, patients with systolic blood pressure ≥ 180 mm Hg, or a total cholesterol of >7.5 mmol/L, should be considered at clinically determined high absolute risk of CVD.

Source: National Vascular Disease Prevention Alliance (2009). Absolute cardiovascular disease risk assessment: Quick reference guide for health professionals.

This chart, developed by the National Vascular Disease Prevention Alliance, uses your gender, age, diabetes status, smoking history, blood pressure and cholesterol level to calculate your risk of experiencing a major cardiovascular event in the next five years. People in the red zone have at least a 30% risk of a major event in five years, and need to take preventive action urgently. Those in the light green zone have a five-year risk of less than 5%. This does not mean they can rest easy. A one in 20 chance in five years might develop into a one in 10 chance in 10 years or more if someone lets themselves go health wise, but it does suggest there is time to work on ageing healthily.

Absolute risk

As we know, there are multiple factors such as blood pressure, smoking, blood fats and diabetes that contribute to the risk we have for heart disease and we need a way of putting all the information together in a single figure. This is called absolute risk. Absolute risk is also used as a way of putting a number to somebody's risk of having an event such as a heart attack over a specified time period. For example; 'You have a 2% chance of a heart attack or death in the next five years'.

Relative risk

Relative risk is the probability of a similar thing happening to a person in comparison to others of the same age, gender, etc. This is calculated from large populations where possible risk factors were measured at the beginning, and participants were followed for a long time to count deaths and major health outcomes.

Risk factors that are subsequently found statistically to predict an outcome are fitted to an equation. This equation can then be used to develop charts or computer programs where you input your information to predict your risk, usually over the next five or 10 years. It is important to remember this is a statistical probability, not a guarantee.

Guidelines for absolute risk

In Australia, there is a national guideline for the measurement of absolute risk (see www.heart-foundation.org.au) and it is recommended that everybody over the age of 45 should have this measured.

This is particularly helpful for people who are at the upper end of the normal range for risk factors such as cholesterol or blood pressure. While no single factor may put them into a high risk area, the combination of factors when fed into a risk calculator does, and points the way for more active intervention. The major risk factor for most common conditions, including most cancers and cardiovascular disease, is age. There are many risk calculators available online for a range of different chronic diseases. See Resources (page 298) for more information.

The concept of reduction in absolute risk is a very important one when you are assessing the importance of a media breakthrough on health. Often in the media we see stories about health breakthroughs but remember that statistics can be misleading. A new medicine that reduces death rates from two-in-a-million to one-in-a-million can be reported in the same way as a 50% reduction from one-in-ten to one-in-five. The relative reduction in risk expressed this way is the same, but unless you are that one in a million it is the change in absolute numbers that is more important in practical terms.

One advantage of measuring absolute risk is that it identifies the potential for high risk due to a mild elevation of a number of risk factors, where none alone are sufficiently abnormal to raise the alarm.

Many people have a pattern like this. This cumulative pattern accounts for a large number of people who seemingly have a heart attack that comes from nowhere.

There are many other absolute risk charts and calculators available. Most of these include the same risk factors but it's important to note that they provide an average figure for an average person, and we all know how rare they are! Also, all of the charts and calculators tend to underestimate risk in certain populations including Indigenous people, and those with diabetes, chronic kidney disease or major psychiatric disorders.

Bowel cancer can develop without symptoms, and exist for several years before spreading elsewhere in the body. Pre-cancerous polyps that grow in the bowel can cause miniscule amounts of blood, often invisible, to leach out and pass into faeces. These polyps (adenomas) can grow into an advanced cancer in 10 years. Australia has one of the highest rates of bowel cancer in the world.

The bowel cancer screening test called the faecal immunochemical test (FIT) or immunochemical faecal occult blood test (iFOBT) can pick up these small amounts of blood in bowel movements. Ask your doctor or pharmacist if you are eligible for a free testing kit to be mailed to your home.

The test is simple. You put a small sample of toilet water or stool on the testing card and post it to the laboratory. The test is recommended to be done every two years for those over the age of 50.

Bowel cancer is one of only three cancers for which population-based screening is recommended. The Federal Government will continue to roll-out its National Bowel Cancer Screening Program until everyone over the age of 50 is screened by 2019, with the aim of having every Australian adult aged over 50 having the test every one to two years at home.

More complex tests

CORONARY DISEASE

Testing for coronary disease starts with you and what you know. Do you have a family history of heart disease – particularly in parents, uncles, aunts or siblings occurring before the age of 55? Do you smoke? Are you overweight? Do you have high absolute risk when your blood pressure, cholesterol and other risk factors are measured?

If you answer 'yes' to these types of questions, it will be time to discuss these factors with your doctor. They will be able to schedule more complex coronary disease testing.

Electrocardiogram

The simplest direct test for heart disease is an electrocardiogram (ECG or EKG), which records the pattern of electrical activity of the heart. This can be very useful if there is an abnormality. However, many people – even some with severe heart conditions – can have a normal electrocardiogram. There are also many false positives that are normal variations in a healthy person that mimic a cardiac problem. For this reason, we do not recommend routine screening of the general population with this test. It does make sense however for certain groups, such as those with risk factors that put them into a very high-risk category, or in certain occupational groups (such as airline pilots or long distance transport drivers) where the consequences of an underlying heart problem could be catastrophic.

If there appears to be a high risk of coronary disease, the next step to consider is recording the electrocardiogram and perhaps capturing images of the heart using ultrasound or nuclear medicine techniques during exercise. These are known as an exercise tolerance test (ETT) or an exercise electrocardiogram (ECG). Quite often, the heart is able to function normally at rest, but the first symptoms and changes in these tests occur when exercise demands more oxygen supply to the heart. This test can be very revealing.

Coronary angiogram

If the results so far have raised a reasonable suspicion that you might have heart disease, you may be referred to a cardiologist for a coronary angiogram. A traditional coronary angiogram involves a day in hospital. A catheter will be inserted into your artery through the groin or arm and threaded through blood vessels to the heart. Dye will be injected through the catheter (a tube), and X-ray images of the heart will be taken to find blockages and areas of narrowing in the arteries.

Angioplasty

If treatment is needed to improve blood flow to the heart, a procedure called an angioplasty can be performed. This is an extra part of the coronary angiogram procedure where a balloon in the end of the catheter is blown up to stretch the narrowing in the arteries. Often a small inert device called a stent is inserted at the point that was narrowed before stretching and used to keep the narrowing from recurring.

It is not always necessary to go as far as a coronary angiogram, however. With a computed tomography (CT) angiogram, no catheter needs to be inserted into the groin. Instead, the dye is injected through an intravenous line in the hand or arm. If treatment is needed, this would have to occur in a separate procedure. A CT angiogram is very accurate and very reassuring if the results are completely normal. It is less clear how useful it is over and above simpler tests if it seems to reveal a problem. Like all the tests described in this section, it should not be used wholesale in the general healthy community.

None of these tests will tell whether a given narrowing is likely to be the cause of major events down the track or remain stable, causing a little angina.

BONE DENSITY

A bone density test, or bone mass measurement, is used to determine bone strength and identify osteoporosis or the milder form of osteopaenia, which increase the risk of future bone fractures.

Both men and women lose bone mass as they age. Women, however, are at higher risk of developing osteoporosis, as the sudden reduction in estrogen levels at menopause sees bones lose calcium and other minerals faster.

You are more at risk of osteoporosis if you have:
- an immediate family member who has been diagnosed, or has broken a bone from a minor fall
- low vitamin D levels
- low calcium intake or
- some health conditions such as early menopause, chronic disease (such as rheumatoid arthritis) or chronic liver or kidney disease.

Some medications such as corticosteroids, some antidepressants, and medications for cancer can also affect your bone density.

Your doctor will assess your risk before referring you to a scan.

X-ray and ultrasound are the most common ways to measure bone density. It is a painless procedure, and you remain fully clothed for your scan.

Other bone density tests include:
- dual energy x-ray absorptiometry (DEXA): a fast and highly accurate way to measure bone density in the spine, hip, forearm and the total body
- single energy x-ray absorptiometry: the body part to be tested, typically the heel or forearm, is wrapped in tissue-like material or placed in water.

There is also a test called a heel ultrasound. However, Osteoporosis Australia doesn't recommend this as a standard test.

COLONOSCOPY

A sigmoidoscopy is a screening test to look inside the rectum and further up into the lower part of the colon where half of all bowel cancers and advanced adenomas grow.

A colonoscope is similar to a flexible sigmoidoscope, but much longer and can look at the entire length of the large bowel. It also allows biopsies to be taken and polyps to be removed.

Colonoscopy is the recommended follow-up test for those with positive findings from the immunochemical faecal occult blood test (iFOBT) or screening sigmoidoscopy. It is also advised as the main surveillance tool for those with an increased cancer risk.

Despite it being highly effective at detecting cancers, colonoscopy is not recommended as the main screening tool for the general population given its cost, invasive nature, use of anesthesia and strict bowel preparation.

CERVICAL SCREENING

A primary human papillomavirus (HPV) test every five years is replacing the two-year Pap test for cervical screening. Essentially it will be the same experience for the woman, as the cells are removed from the cervix with a plastic brush in the same way. But the new test detects the HPV infection, which is the first step to developing cervical cancer. Ongoing infections over years, often over at least a decade, can cause abnormal cell changes that can lead to cancer.

Pap tests, which have halved the incidence and deaths from cervical cancer, also detect abnormal cell change. But the new test picks up persistent HPV infection, and coupled with the national roll-out of HPV vaccine for young women and men will further reduce rates of cervical cancer by 15%.

PROSTATE SPECIFIC ANTIGEN

Screening asymptomatic men with the prostate specific antigen (PSA) test to find early cancers remains controversial. Prostate cancer is the second most common cancer in Australia and leading cancer in men.

The PSA blood test is useful. It can pick up the level of this protein, often elevated in men with prostate cancer, and detect cancers earlier. In the 1990s, the survival rate was 60%. This has now increased to about 94%.

On the flip side, the PSA test can also find cancers that would cause no harm to the man in his lifetime. This is particularly true for elderly men. This can subject men to an intensive regimen of surgery, radiotherapy and hormone treatments, which can cause significant side effects such as urinary incontinence and impotence.

But there is no way to know what cancers will cause harm and what cancers men will die with, never knowing they carried them. A number of benign conditions can also cause PSA levels to rise.

Consequently, Australian authorities don't recommend PSA testing as a population-based screening tool. Testing protocols have improved. Globally, PSA is now being offered on an individual basis to men with a family history and who are aged 50–70 years.

When an early cancer is found these days, it is more common to manage men more cautiously than in the past, adopting a surveillance approach before committing to treatment.

MAMMOGRAMS

Mammograms are an x-ray investigation of the breast, and they aim to detect a cancer while it is small and has not spread beyond the breast.

Women aged between 50–74 years are invited to undergo free mammograms every two years through the national screening program, Breast-Screen Australia. Women in this target age group receive a letter from BreastScreen every two years reminding them they are due for a mammogram. Increasing age is one of the biggest risk factors, with more than three-quarters of Australian cases found in women aged over 50. Women in their 40s and those who are over 74 can also have free screenings, but they are not sent reminder letters.

Early detection and treatment can greatly increase the chance of survival from breast cancer. But just as with prostate cancer testing in men, testing women with no symptoms, family history or gene mutations leads to over-diagnosis and the discovery and treatment of cancers that may never go on to cause harm. Currently, there is no way of knowing whether cancers will ever become symptomatic in the patient's lifetime.

The risk of false negative results decreases with age, and are least common in the highest-risk group of women aged 40–69 years. For women in their 40s, there is mixed evidence about the effectiveness of screening versus the harms, so mammograms are not recommended for this group.

Women of all ages who are at increased risk of developing breast cancer should develop a personalised surveillance program with their doctor.

PART 2

THE PATH TO
GOOD HEALTH

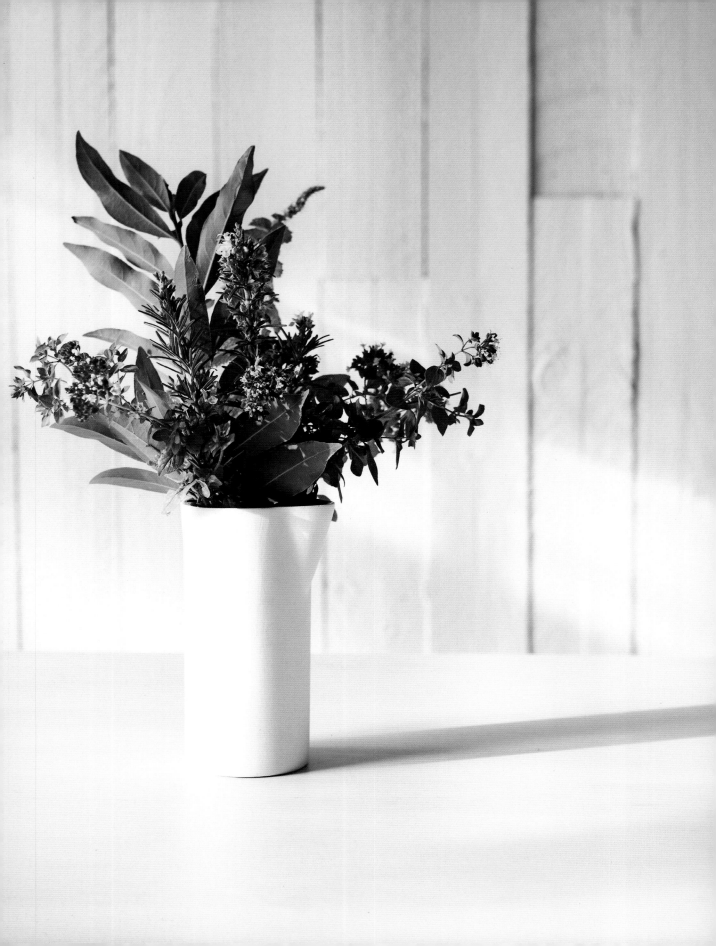

Wellness Action Plan

Over the last six chapters, we have discussed the concepts of 'wellbeing' and why it is important. We have seen what we need to be mindful of at different life stages to achieve long-lasting wellbeing, and we have begun to demystify risk factors and diseases.

In this section, we present the Wellness Action Plan. This shows what you as an individual can do to help increase your wellbeing. The plan is designed to help you make a series of straight-forward, long-lasting changes to improve your overall health and wellbeing. It covers six major categories: decreasing your risk factors, getting good quality sleep, moderating your alcohol and drug intake, improving your mental health and wellbeing, developing a physically active lifestyle and eating healthily.

It is, however, important to remember that no person acts in isolation. There are external environmental and social factors which affect us all and our wellbeing. However, by taking charge of the factors that are within our control, we can all begin to improve – and hopefully maximise – our wellbeing. By presenting you with the advice and suggestions in the following chapters, we hope to empower you on your quest for wellness.

To use the plan, start by ticking 'no' or 'yes' to the questions in each category in the following table. This will help you identify where you need to start taking some action. Then, in the 'Tips for success' column, we direct you to where you will find more information in this book – including meal plans, recipes and checklists – that will help you put your plan into action.

Remember, though, it's not a race. We want you to make changes that last a lifetime – and that is going to take some time. If you are feeling over-whelmed, or have a lot to change in a number of categories – choose one category and concentrate on getting to 'yes' in all of its sections before moving on to the next one. You might like to talk to your GP about where a good starting point for you might be.

Be aware that some of the activities might only need to be done once, or are simple and easy to do – such as completing your family medical history. Others – like giving up smoking or being in a healthy weight range – are more complicated and will take some time to achieve.

Then, come back in three months' time (and then at six months) and answer the questions again. Ideally, your answers will be moving from 'no' to mostly 'yes'. You will be able to track your progress, and the areas that you still need to work on.

By adopting the principles summarised in this list, you will be creating a health and wellbeing lifestyle that will keep you happier, healthier and active for longer.

These six aspects of wellbeing lead to an optimal and long-lasting lifestyle

WELLNESS ACTIONS	CHECKING YOUR PROGRESS			TIPS FOR SUCCESS
DECREASING YOUR RISK FACTORS				
Are you in the healthy weight range for your age and gender?	Now After 3 months After 6 months	☐ No ☐ No ☐ No	☐ Yes ☐ Yes ☐ Yes	• See page 42 for information on what weight range is healthy for you. • See page 66 for information on how you can reduce weight and move into your healthy weight range. • See our meal plans on pages 104–119 for information on how to put a healthy nutritious eating plan into action.
Are you up-to-date with your regular health checks?	Now After 3 months After 6 months	☐ No ☐ No ☐ No	☐ Yes ☐ Yes ☐ Yes	• See page 41–51 for information on the health checks you need to keep up-to-date with.
Are you a non-smoker?	Now After 3 months After 6 months	☐ No ☐ No ☐ No	☐ Yes ☐ Yes ☐ Yes	• See page 16 for information on giving up smoking.
Have you developed a close working relationship with your GP?	Now After 3 months After 6 months	☐ No ☐ No ☐ No	☐ Yes ☐ Yes ☐ Yes	• See pages 46–51 , 73 on how to develop a good relationship with your GP.
Have you completed your family medical history and shared it with your GP?	Now After 3 months After 6 months	☐ No ☐ No ☐ No	☐ Yes ☐ Yes ☐ Yes	• See page 36 on how to complete your family medical history.
EATING HEALTHILY				
Do you and your family regularly follow the Australian Guide to Healthy Eating?	Now After 3 months After 6 months	☐ No ☐ No ☐ No	☐ Yes ☐ Yes ☐ Yes	• See pages 87–8 for information on following the Australian Guide to Healthy Eating. • See our meal plans on pages 104–119 for information on how to put the Australian Guide to Healthy Eating into action.
Do you eat – and shop for - your food in a healthy and mindful manner?	Now After 3 months After 6 months	☐ No ☐ No ☐ No	☐ Yes ☐ Yes ☐ Yes	• See pages 96 for information on how to eat mindfully. • See pages 89–90 for information on shopping with a healthy and mindful manner.

WELLNESS ACTIONS	CHECKING YOUR PROGRESS			TIPS FOR SUCCESS
Are you serving food in the appropriate portion sizes?	Now	☐ No	☐ Yes	• See page 93 for information on appropriate portion sizes.
	After 3 months	☐ No	☐ Yes	
	After 6 months	☐ No	☐ Yes	
Do you limit your consumption of packaged and processed foods?	Now	☐ No	☐ Yes	• See pages 97–9 for information on how to reduce your consumption of packaged and processed foods.
	After 3 months	☐ No	☐ Yes	
	After 6 months	☐ No	☐ Yes	
Are you limiting treat or unhealthy foods to once a week?	Now	☐ No	☐ Yes	• See page 91 for information on limiting your treat foods.
	After 3 months	☐ No	☐ Yes	
	After 6 months	☐ No	☐ Yes	

DEVELOPING A PHYSICALLY ACTIVE LIFESTYLE

WELLNESS ACTIONS	CHECKING YOUR PROGRESS			TIPS FOR SUCCESS
Do you exercise for at least 30 minutes per day, 7 days per week?	Now	☐ No	☐ Yes	• See page 76 for information on how much exercise you need.
	After 3 months	☐ No	☐ Yes	
	After 6 months	☐ No	☐ Yes	
Have you chosen exercises or physical activities that are suitable for you?	Now	☐ No	☐ Yes	• See pages 77–8 for information on choosing the right exercise for you.
	After 3 months	☐ No	☐ Yes	
	After 6 months	☐ No	☐ Yes	
Have you set yourself some SMART exercise goals?	Now	☐ No	☐ Yes	• See page 80 for information on how to set SMART exercise goals.
	After 3 months	☐ No	☐ Yes	
	After 6 months	☐ No	☐ Yes	
Have you developed a 'whole day' exercise mindset and look for opportunities to move regularly during the day (such as taking the stairs instead of getting the lift)?	Now	☐ No	☐ Yes	• See page 64 for information on developing a 'whole day' attitude to exercise.
	After 3 months	☐ No	☐ Yes	
	After 6 months	☐ No	☐ Yes	
Do you get out of your chair every 30 minutes during the day and stand, stretch and/ or move around?	Now	☐ No	☐ Yes	• See page 64 for information about not being sedentary during the day.
	After 3 months	☐ No	☐ Yes	
	After 6 months	☐ No	☐ Yes	

WELLNESS ACTIONS	CHECKING YOUR PROGRESS			TIPS FOR SUCCESS
IMPROVING YOUR MENTAL HEALTH AND WELLBEING				
Can you recognise the signs of when you need to seek help for your mental health, and do you know where to find that help?	Now After 3 months After 6 months	☐ No ☐ No ☐ No	☐ Yes ☐ Yes ☐ Yes	• See page 73 for information about recognising when you need help. • See page 73 for information about where to find help.
Do you have strategies to help you deal with your overall mental health and wellbeing, including the effects of stress in your life?	Now After 3 months After 6 months	☐ No ☐ No ☐ No	☐ Yes ☐ Yes ☐ Yes	• See pages 71–3 for information about developing strategies to improve your mental health and wellbeing. • See pages 69–70 for some information about coping with stress.
Have you developed some positive mental wellbeing techniques, such as mindfulness or relaxation practices?	Now After 3 months After 6 months	☐ No ☐ No ☐ No	☐ Yes ☐ Yes ☐ Yes	• See pages 71–3 for information about developing positive mental wellbeing techniques. • See page 71 for information about developing mindfulness. • See pages 62 and 71 for information about developing relaxation practices.
Do you regularly take time out to recharge your batteries?	Now After 3 months After 6 months	☐ No ☐ No ☐ No	☐ Yes ☐ Yes ☐ Yes	• See pages 66–7 for information about developing time out strategies.
Do you feel sad or have you lost interest in things you used to enjoy doing?	Now After 3 months After 6 months	☐ No ☐ No ☐ No	☐ Yes ☐ Yes ☐ Yes	• See page 73 for information about what you can do if you are feeling sad or have lost interest in things that you used to enjoy doing.
Do you feel anxious most of the time?	Now After 3 months After 6 months	☐ No ☐ No ☐ No	☐ Yes ☐ Yes ☐ Yes	• See pages 71–3 for information about what can be done to alleviate anxiety.
Do you regularly catch up with family, friends or colleagues?	Now After 3 months After 6 months	☐ No ☐ No ☐ No	☐ Yes ☐ Yes ☐ Yes	• See page 72 for information about the importance of remaining connected to family, friends and colleagues.
Do you have someone with whom you can regularly discuss intimate matters?	Now After 3 months After 6 months	☐ No ☐ No ☐ No	☐ Yes ☐ Yes ☐ Yes	• See page 72 for information about the importance of having a confidant.

WELLNESS ACTIONS	CHECKING YOUR PROGRESS			TIPS FOR SUCCESS
Do you make some time for yourself to do something you enjoy doing?	Now After 3 months After 6 months	☐ No ☐ No ☐ No	☐ Yes ☐ Yes ☐ Yes	• See page 71 for information about why self-care is important.

GETTING GOOD QUALITY SLEEP

Do you stick to regular sleep and wake times?	Now After 3 months After 6 months	☐ No ☐ No ☐ No	☐ Yes ☐ Yes ☐ Yes	• See page 62 for information on developing regular sleep and wake patterns.
Do you let natural light into your bedroom in the morning?	Now After 3 months After 6 months	☐ No ☐ No ☐ No	☐ Yes ☐ Yes ☐ Yes	• See pages 63 for information on the importance of natural light and its effect on your sleep patterns.
Have you removed electronic screens/devices from your bedroom?	Now After 3 months After 6 months	☐ No ☐ No ☐ No	☐ Yes ☐ Yes ☐ Yes	• See page 62 for information on how removing electronic screens and devices from your bedroom can improve the quality of your sleep.
Have you established, and regularly follow, your bedtime ritual?	Now After 3 months After 6 months	☐ No ☐ No ☐ No	☐ Yes ☐ Yes ☐ Yes	• See page 62 for information on how to develop a good bedtime ritual.
Do you avoid stimulants (like coffee and alcohol) before going to bed?	Now After 3 months After 6 months	☐ No ☐ No ☐ No	☐ Yes ☐ Yes ☐ Yes	• See page 62 for information on why avoiding stimulants before going to bed can improve the quality of your sleep.

MODERATING YOUR ALCOHOL AND DRUG INTAKE

Do you pace your alcohol drinking by alternating with non-alcoholic options?	Now After 3 months After 6 months	☐ No ☐ No ☐ No	☐ Yes ☐ Yes ☐ Yes	• See page 63 for information on alternating your alcohol and non-alcoholic drinks.
Do you avoid mixing energy drinks with alcohol?	Now After 3 months After 6 months	☐ No ☐ No ☐ No	☐ Yes ☐ Yes ☐ Yes	• See page 64 for information on the impact of mixing energy drinks with alcohol.
Do you drink two or less alcoholic drinks per day?	Now After 3 months After 6 months	☐ No ☐ No ☐ No	☐ Yes ☐ Yes ☐ Yes	• See page 63 for information about a 'standard drink'.
Do you avoid recreational drug use?	Now After 3 months After 6 months	☐ No ☐ No ☐ No	☐ Yes ☐ Yes ☐ Yes	• See page 63 for more information on the impacts of drug use.

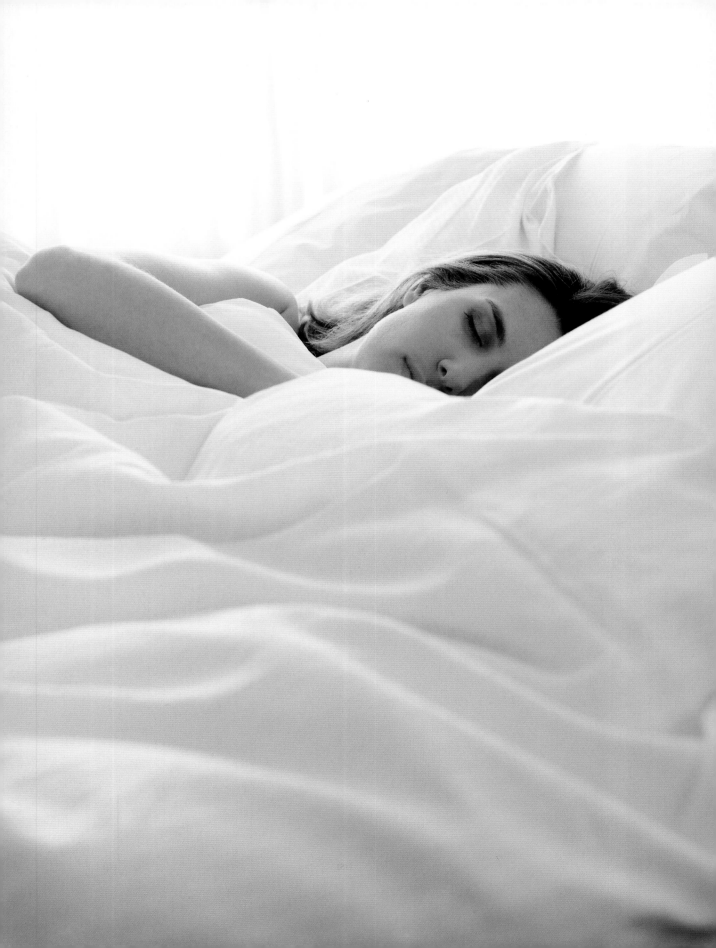

7

HABITS AND CHOICES

Technology has brought great convenience and ease to our modern lives. We can readily buy pre-made meals at the supermarket or takeaway shop. We can drive our car to the railway station before we catch the train. We can order our groceries online. We have machines that wash, clean, cook, dice and chop for us.

Despite these gains, modern conveniences also see us lose many opportunities to make healthy choices. They make it easy for us to be less physically active. We no longer have to create every meal with fresh ingredients from scratch. We also seem to have less face-to-face contact with our friends and family.

Many of us accept tiredness and stress as trade-offs for living our productive 21st century lives. We live in an era where our bosses and our friends expect us to be contactable at any hour. With technology blurring the times of the day once designated for work and home life, we are increasingly time-poor.

That's why the easy option – whether that's involving our diet, our physical activity levels, how we spend our leisure time and choices for managing our mental health – becomes our default option. It is easier in the short term to pop a pill, open a bottle, buy the pre-made meal, drive the car or sit on the couch.

But having an easy and convenient lifestyle isn't always the healthiest choice. Modern life has put barriers in our way in our quest for wellbeing, but there are ways we can work around these obstacles. The following sections are designed to help you make the best choice for your wellness. We saw in chapter 6 how risk factors can set us on the path to spiralling poor health. The reverse is also true – when we make the healthy choices, many aspects of our physical and mental health also improve.

Sleep

Sleep can be one of the first things to suffer when we are time-poor or stressed. But regular, good quality sleep is vital to our daily resilience, physical health and our long-term health. As we discussed in chapter 2, we are learning more about the vital role sleep plays in flushing toxins out from the brain as a daily 'reset'.

You may not be able to control when you fall asleep. But you can create the right conditions for getting the right amount of sleep recommended for adults. And yes, you've heard correctly – eight hours sleep a night is what the average adult body requires.

WORK WITH YOUR BODY CLOCK, NOT AGAINST IT

Our sleep–wake cycle is controlled by two processes. Shift work, all-nighters and international travel can play havoc with our body clock, the 24-hour circadian rhythm that regulates the timing of sleepiness and wakefulness. Sleep is also controlled by the sleep/wake homeostasis, an internal timer than builds up pressure and releases hormones based on how long we have been awake.

> Sticking to regular sleep and wake times – even on weekends – helps keep these two biological systems in check to produce quality sleep.

AVOID STIMULANTS BEFORE BED

Alcohol initially acts as a sedative to induce sleep. Before too long, however, it becomes a stimulant. It disturbs the rhythm of sleep patterns, causing restless sleep. Similarly, the nicotine in cigarettes can increase your heart rate, which makes falling asleep harder.

> Avoid using both alcohol and cigarettes in the few hours before bedtime.

REMOVE SCREENS FROM THE BEDROOM

The blue light from electronic screens – such as a mobile phone, a laptop, a TV or an iPad – mimic daylight. This, in turn, can hamper your body's production of the hormone melatonin. Because melatonin makes you feel sleepy, having these types of devices in your bedroom can mean you take longer to fall asleep (and you may also wake up more often during the night).

> Turn off your devices at least 30 minutes before going to bed. You can also adopt one of the relaxing bedtime rituals listed below.

ESTABLISH BEDTIME RITUALS

A bath followed by a bedtime story is used the world-over to help children get to sleep, but there is wisdom in this for adults, too. A relaxing ritual can help induce sleep by signalling to your body and brain that it is time to relax. A bedtime ritual can include taking a shower, reading a book, writing down reflections from the day or preparing a to-do list for tomorrow. You might also like to try a little light exercise like yoga or stretching.

> Choose a relaxing ritual and make it a bedtime habit. Your body will soon recognise the cue that it's time to go to sleep.

RELAX YOUR MIND

For some people, bedtime can be the period of the day where their mind is free to think, worry, ponder, agonise and stress. Making sure you are physically tired by getting your daily quota of exercise can help ensure you are sufficiently tired at night. Emptying your mind of worries by writing them down, as a reflection or game plan for the next day, can also be helpful.

> Try relaxation exercises at bedtime, such as focusing on the rise and fall of your breath, or clenching and unclenching each part of your body. These simple exercises can help reduce tension.

LET THE MORNING LIGHT IN

Our circadian biological clock is controlled by cells in the hypothalamus, the brain's 'control centre'. It responds to light and dark signals received through the eyes. When we are exposed to light in the morning, our eyes send signals to the relevant brain cells, triggering the release of hormones into our brain. Our body temperature also increases at this point, which is another trigger that helps us to wake up.

Opening the curtains in the morning to let the light in will help you feel less groggy when you first wake up.

Drugs and alcohol

Alcohol, in moderation, can form part of a healthy lifestyle that also includes exercise and healthy eating. However, many negative health consequences come from long-term regular use or single occasion use at risky levels. Long-term habitual alcohol consumption is linked to some cancers (mainly breast, bowel, cancers of the mouth and digestive system), heart disease, liver failure and acquired brain damage. Binge drinking – drinking more than four standard drinks in one sitting – increases the chance you'll put yourself in dangerous situations and be involved in violence, including domestic violence.

Some individuals also need to practice caution when it comes to alcohol consumption, even at low levels. For example, there is no known safe level of alcohol consumption during pregnancy.

When it comes to drug intake, some types can trigger the onset of a pre-existing mental illness such as schizophrenia, while others can cause drug-induced psychosis. Depression and anxiety is common among drug and alcohol users. People who abuse alcohol are up to six times greater risk of suicide than the general population. Cannabis users are up to 10 times more likely to die by their own hand.

The following tips are designed to help you drink moderately.

PACE YOURSELF WITH NON-ALCOHOLIC OPTIONS

Make your first drink a non-alcoholic one, and alternate one of these between your alcoholic drinks throughout the night.

DRINK SLOWLY

Put your glass out of arm's reach on a nearby table (while still keeping it within sight) or somewhere close where you need to reach out to get it. Removing it from your hand will see you avoid mindless sipping, and slow down your drinking.

GET TO KNOW A 'STANDARD DRINK'

A standard drink is 10 grams of alcohol, which is the amount the body can process in one hour. Factors such as your weight, age, what you have eaten that day and how tired you are can all affect how you process alcohol. An average 150 ml glass of wine is 1.5 standard drinks. A can of full-strength beer is 1.4 standard drinks. A can of spirits at 7% alcohol is 1.6–2.4 standard drinks.

DRINK TWO OR LESS ALCOHOLIC DRINKS PER DAY

Reduce the risk of harming your health over your lifetime by drinking no more than two standard drinks per day.

UNDERSTAND THE KILOJOULE CONTENT OF YOUR DRINK

You can easily accumulate a significant portion of your daily kilojoule allowance with 'liquid kilojoules' such as alcohol. Unlike the kilojoules you eat, those you drink are more likely to lead to weight gain because you are rarely likely to compensate for them at your next meal. A gin-and-tonic has more kilojoules than two chocolate biscuits. A glass of wine has more kilojoules than a scoop of ice-cream. A can of full-strength beer has a similar kilojoule content to a slice of pizza.

Few people would eat a whole packet of Tim Tams in one sitting, and yet quite a few people would drink four rum-and-cola cans in one session without hesitation.

AVOID MIXING ENERGY DRINKS WITH ALCOHOL

Consumption of these type of drinks can lead to 'wide-awake drunkenness', where the caffeine or stimulant masks the feeling of drunkenness without reducing the alcohol-related impairment. You are more likely to binge drink or engage in dangerous behaviours if you feel less drunk than you really are. Energy drinks are also linked to heart palpitations and disturbed sleep.

Sedentary lifestyle

We live in sedentary times. We drive or sit on public transport to get to work, where we sit largely uninterrupted for the next eight hours. We sit some more on the way home, only to plonk in front of the TV or computer to unwind at night. Our groceries can be home delivered, and we can send a text message to a neighbour instead of walking down the street to talk to them.

Research by Baker IDI and others has shown that we need to consider excessive sitting as a serious health hazard. Sitting for long periods of time causes your metabolism to slow down. Then, because your energy expenditure is low, the breakdown of sugar and fat in your body is also reduced. If you are mostly sedentary, you stop relying on your postural muscles, which support your spine, chest and legs. There is evidence that this leads to reduced glucose uptake and a shut-down of the processes that influence cholesterol production.

We all need to move our bodies more. Even if you are largely desk-bound during the day, there are ways you can include more incidental movement into your day to improve your health.

ADOPT A 'WHOLE DAY' APPROACH TO PHYSICAL ACTIVITY

Think beyond the one hour a day you walk the dog or spend at the gym. While this time is helping you make health gains to benefit your muscles and cardiovascular fitness, it doesn't fully negate the remaining hours of your day that are largely spent sedentary. Take every opportunity to move during the day.

INCLUDE EXERCISE IN YOUR DAILY COMMUTE

Ride, walk or jog to work or school. If you can't do the entire journey, park further away from the office or get off the bus or train a few stops early and walk the last part of your journey.

STAND, STRETCH AND MOVE

Stand and walk over to a colleague who is nearby instead of using email. Make your phone calls while going for a walk. Take the stairs instead of the lift. Get active in your lunch break with a fitness class, or go for a walk, run or swim. Get up from your desk every 30 minutes. In addition to improving your long-term fitness, you will feel less stiff and enjoy a burst of energy.

HOW OFTEN DO WE NEED TO MOVE?

When we sit, our muscles are effectively asleep. By getting up and moving throughout the day, we are contracting our muscles, which appears to be beneficial to our body's metabolic processes. Recent studies by Baker IDI suggest we need to get out of our chairs every 30 minutes. To help you do this, Baker IDI has developed Rise & Recharge, a smartphone app (see below) to help track and change sedentary behaviour. The app is available to download for free on Apple and Android platforms.

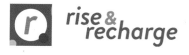

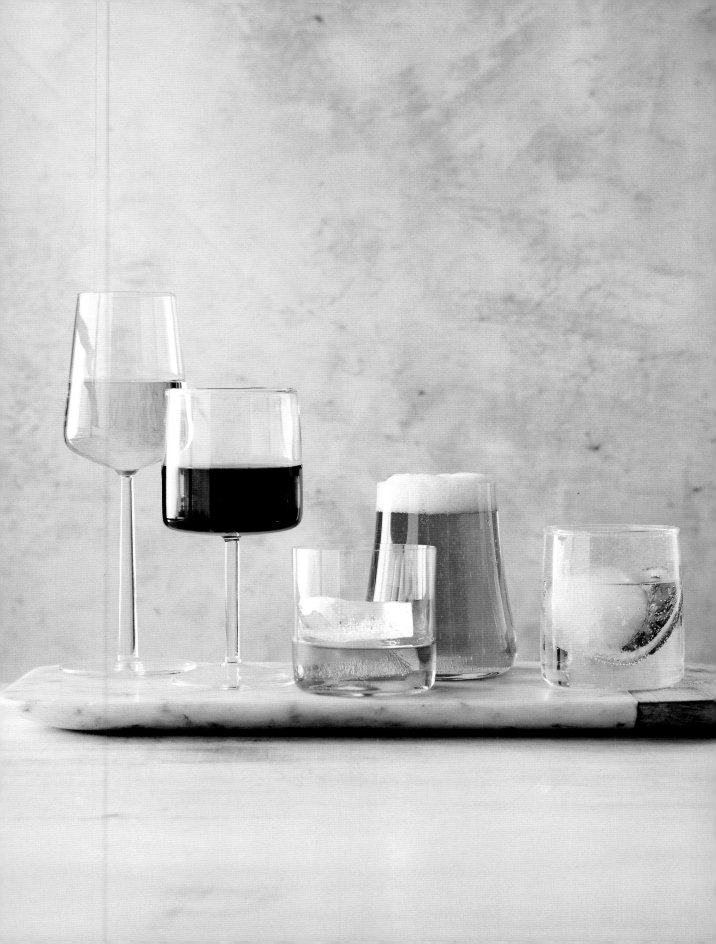

Nutrition

Home-cooked meals are best for our health and wallet. We can control exactly how much salt, sugar and fat goes into our meals, while loading up on extra vegetables, legumes and fruits. But fast food, takeaway and pre-prepared meals from supermarkets remain popular choices largely for their convenience.

WATCH YOUR PORTION SIZES

Fast food outlets thrive on offering 'upsized' meals by making it more cost effective to go big. Typically, these meals are larger servings than we would dish up for ourselves at home. Choose small sizes of meals, or only 'upsize' the healthier component (such as the side salad). Share a meal with your dining companion. Watch your portion size – you only need to eat a serving of protein that is as big as the palm of your hand.

KEEP A FOOD DIARY

A healthy diet contains a variety of foods, but many people are unaware they are not getting the range of nutrients they need. By writing down what you ate each day over a week, you can assess whether you are eating as well as you think you are and look for ways to squeeze in extra nutrition such as a piece of fruit, nuts or vegetables. You might find you are eating bread as toast for breakfast, in a lunchtime sandwich and again with a casserole at dinner. To add some variety and make some important nutritional gains, swap the toast at breakfast for an omelette or porridge, or have a side salad instead of bread at dinner. Did you realise you had six cups of coffee – with six teaspoons of sugar – throughout the day? Did you know you had no alcohol-free days this week? Are you getting your five serves of vegetables? Writing down what you are eating makes you accountable.

EAT NATURAL FOOD

'If it's made from a plant, eat it. If it was made in a factory, don't eat it.' This phrase is a reminder that the more natural state our food is in, the better it is for us. Look at the ingredient list on any packet off the supermarket shelf and chances are you'll find at least a couple of inclusions that you can't pronounce, let alone understand. Our food is largely stored in plastic. It also often contains many artificial colours, additives, preservatives and flavour enhancers. These keep foods from spoiling, and ensure foods have the colour and texture that consumers demand. But fresh and unprocessed, from whatever food group, is best. Eat as much as food as possible from the aisles along the outer edges of the supermarket – including the produce, meat, eggs and the dairy fridge – and less from the inside shelves and you will be making healthier choices.

COMPARE KILOJOULES

Many fast food outlets have the kilojoule content of items prominently displayed as part of the in-store menu. Some outlets also have nutrition calculators on their websites. Compare the kilojoule contents of the various menu choices and make a habit of opting for the healthier choice. You can readily see how adding extras to meals (such as cheese, extra meat or sour cream) and ordering sides (such as hot chips) quickly ups the kilojoule content of your meal.

Taking some time out

For all the convenience and energy saving advances that modern technology has brought us, it has also loaded us with lofty expectations and blurred borders.

Technology has allowed us to be contactable by our bosses and friends at any hour, anywhere. Parents are often juggling work commitments as well as caring for their children (or juggling child-care schedules). Young people have after-school schedules packed with classes and study tutorials. Adults check and send work emails after hours, including in bed. Our leisure time is not as sacred as it was. Weekend work, or taking work home, is a common occurrence in many households.

When we are stressed, we don't sleep well. We're left emotionally depleted and physically run down. This can trigger more stress, as we're not up to meeting the obligations we need to at work, home and with friends. Anxiety and depression can ensue.

It's easy to say we need to slow down and stop stressing. But many of us don't have the luxury to make radical changes to our week. That's not to say we cannot make healthier choices each day, taking smaller options to take time out, to reduce the impact of stress. First we must recognise the cues that signal we are becoming stressed, and practice ways to dampen this response. Our bodies, our mood and our mental health will thank us for it.

The following tips will help you take some precious time out from your busy life.

LIFE HACKS

Search the internet for 'life hacks' and you'll find hundreds of quick practical tips to make everyday life a little easier; from home storage and fix-it-jobs, cooking tips, health care and technology. Use these ideas to make the most of each chore or obligation you have during the day. For example, combine a trip to the park with the kids with your workout, using seats for step-ups and dips, and monkey bars for knee tucks and chin ups. Make phone calls to friends or family when you are watering the garden. Bake a tray of roasted vegetables if you are using the oven for dinner that night. The vegetables can be used in a salad or risotto the next day. Look for every opportunity to double up your activities to save time.

LEARN TO SAY NO

Saying 'no' to others means saying 'yes' to you. Many of us feel obliged to say 'yes' to whatever is asked of us. We don't want to disappoint other people, or we are scared that saying 'no' now will lead to us missing out on a greater opportunity down the track. Consequently, we find ourselves stretched, over-committed and exhausted. Setting boundaries is healthy, and so is saying 'no' to opportunities and people that will lead you down the path to poor health.

PRACTICE RELAXATION RESPONSES

When we are stressed, our breathing patterns can change as the 'fight or flight' reaction is activated. When we are stressed, we start to take short and shallow breaths through our mouth. The usual way we breathe when we are relaxed is through the nose, evenly and calmly. Remember to consciously breathe through your nose in a controlled way if you feel your breathing pattern escalating. Some people find that practising mediation, yoga or tai chi can help them be calm and relaxed.

TAKE A BREAK FROM TECHNOLOGY

The internet can be important in providing ways to save time, which can help reduce feelings of being overwhelmed, but it is equally important to unplug. Take out the headphones while you're walking. Resist the urge to watch videos on your phone on the train ride to work. Turn off the radio in the car. This gives us the chance to be with our thoughts, instead of mindlessly filling our brain and senses with more noise and stimulation. This can be productive thinking or reflective time. It can help us look around and appreciate our environment.

GET ACTIVE

The benefits of exercise for both our physical and mental health are indisputable. Exercise releases the feel-good endorphins, the neurotransmitters from the brain that help reduce our perception of pain and relieve anxiety. Whether you take part in stretching and flexibility-based exercise, team sports or vigorous exertion, our bodies were born to move. These precious endorphins will be released, whatever the activity. The benefit of exercise can also be as it serves as a 'time out' or type of meditation. It forces us to switch off and concentrate on breathing, our technique or opponent, while shutting out the stressors from daily life. Find an activity you enjoy, or do it with a friend so exercise doesn't just become another chore to add begrudgingly to your daily to-do list.

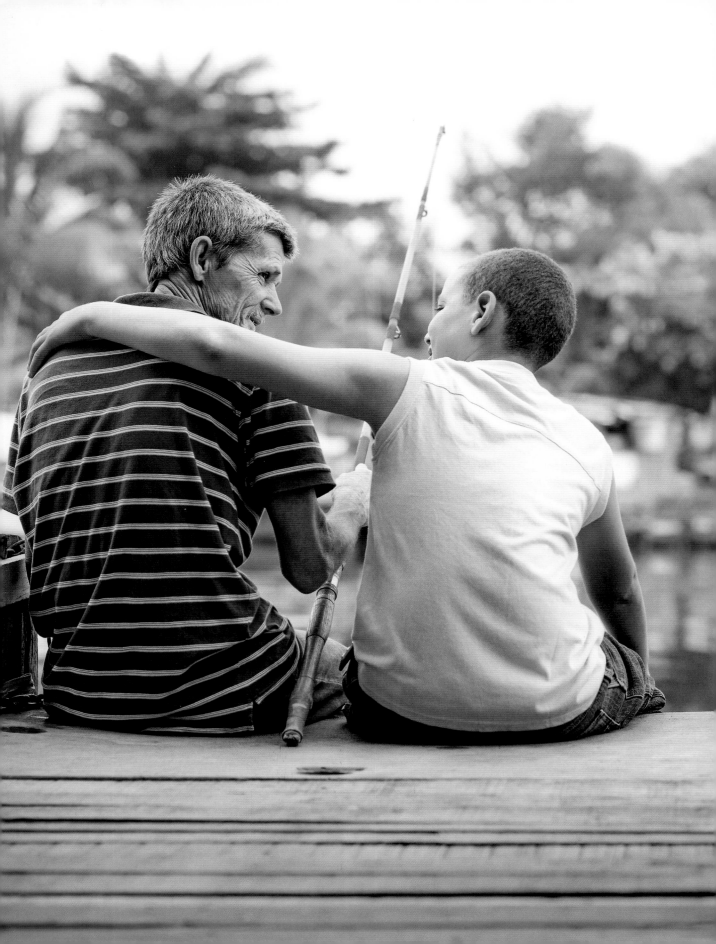

8

MENTAL HEALTH AND WELLBEING

Our sense of wellbeing is strongly linked to our mental state. Even in the presence of physical disease, a positive frame of mind can help us cope and deal with pain and discomfort and also lessen the duration and severity of illness. Being mentally healthy, however, is not merely enjoying the absence of mental illness. Rather, it refers to a holistic pursuit of complete health which ultimately strengthens our own resources and capacities for wellbeing.

A modern view of wellbeing

In traditional medical practice, we try to make people well by eliminating disease. However, this way of defining 'wellbeing' often overlooks the gains we can make if we also seek to improve a person's overall physical and mental health. By taking a mind–body–spirit approach, we can do more than merely avoid disease – we can actively improve overall health and sense of vitality.

The vitality an individual projects is perhaps the best indicator of a person's overall levels of health and wellbeing. Although an individual

might be free from physical disease, lacking a sense of motivation, optimism and wonder about life can leave them feeling ill at ease and uncomfortable with themselves, others or the world around them.

In the following sections, we are going to discuss mental health issues, such as stress, anxiety and depression, and the effects these can have on overall health and sense of wellbeing. We then offer some strategies to improve mental wellbeing.

A question of stress

Stress is a part of life and living. Even when only transient, it is uncomfortable and likely to dictate the tone of our day. However, when stress becomes disproportionate and sustained, it can turn to distress and negatively impact our sense of mental and physical comfort. Our nervous system is directly affected by stress and it is primed to respond to it in an orchestrated manner where stress hormones are released to bring about physical responses, ranging from increased heart palpitations to changes in body temperature and muscle tone. Mental changes also occur with stress, making it harder to focus on tasks and increasing our physical vigilance

Whenever we react to stress, the body's natural alarm response is activated, giving rise to the 'fight or flight' response. This primitive response, which has evolved over time, is our in-built survival mechanism which allows us to respond to perceived threats automatically by prompting hormonal changes that create physical responses designed to help us defend ourselves by fighting the threat or fleeing to safety. In the modern world, everyday events can be misinterpreted as significant threats, so for some, running late for work in the morning and visualising an angry boss can have the same physiological response as our ancestors had when they were being chased by a sabre-toothed tiger.

Repeated exposure to perceived stress can promote detrimental effects on the body. Research has shown that constant levels of high stress can cause brain changes which may contribute to the development of anxiety and depression. Physiologically, stress has been shown to promote high blood pressure, type 2 diabetes and vascular disorders and possibly cancers. Stress can also promote unhealthy behaviours responsible for these conditions by causing people to consume more food, drink more alcohol, smoke more as well as sleep and exercise less.

REACTIONS TO STRESS

Experiencing a significant and sudden event can lead to a person feeling sad, worried, angry, confused, misunderstood and isolated. In some instances, when the perception or experience of stress is chronic, the body's natural restoring system might fail to activate efficiently. This can lead to a prolonged stress response. In this case, negative feelings can last beyond a few hours, days, weeks or even months. So, while it is important to understand that fear and sadness are a perfectly normal response to stress, if these feelings fail to improve (and even worsen over time and become more entrenched), the person might be dealing with the more serious issue of having developed a mental illness, such as depression or anxiety. The persisting release of stress hormones, even at low levels, can promote biological mechanisms which makes the person more concerned about the possibility of threat, thus keeping the body in a state of high alert. This can lead to people feeling physically as well as mentally tired, even when they are relaxing.

Disease and mental health

Serious diseases not only affect people physically: they also affect people psychologically and emotionally. Anxiety and depression are the most common psychological symptom experienced by people suffering from chronic conditions such as cancer and heart disease. These symptoms can directly trigger physiological responses and behavioural reactions. These, in turn, can lead to a person having difficulties in being motivated to stick to the good diet and exercise routines necessary to maintain good health. In turn, this worsens a person's prospects for good health in the future.

In this way, the impact of anxiety and depression on major disease appears to be both a contributing factor and an obstacle to recovery. Mood and expectations can also impact on a person's ability to return to work when they have recovered.

What is depression?

Depression is much more than just feeling sad, having low mood or being upset in response to life events – it is a serious and debilitating illness. When you have depression, you can find it hard to do and enjoy everyday things. You might not feel like looking after yourself, showering, cooking or doing any of your normal activities. Your sense of humour might be lost and you can feel more sensitive to things than you used to be. You cannot focus and concentrate on tasks and you might not feel like talking and spending time with friends or family. Depression is significantly associated with the sense of having no hope.

Depressed people also lose interest in things they used to enjoy, like exercising and being intimate with their partner. Indeed, depression can affect the quality of your relationships and your overall sense of self and wellbeing.

For depression to be present, all of these things need to be present continuously and consistently for at least two weeks. They also need to be impacting your usual level of functioning to a significant effect.

Depression has been identified as a direct risk factor for the onset of heart disease. This makes its impact on health equivalent to that of smoking or having high cholesterol. Major depression has been found to increase the risk of cardiac death in patients more than four-fold.

What is anxiety?

Perhaps no other condition defines the modern world as well as the experience of anxiety. Anxiety is the uncomfortable feeling of worrying about the future. In mild forms, it can be perceived as being preoccupied or having something on your mind. In extreme cases, it can be a crippling and exhausting condition which mentally tortures the sufferer and significantly impacts their ability to function.

Anxiety can manifest itself in many different forms ranging from mental anguish to physiological manifestations (such as a racing heart, shortness of breath and stomach discomfort). Anxiety can be specifically related to something like heights (known as 'acrophobia') or it can be a generalised experience (often known as a 'generalised anxiety disorder'). Anxiety can alter our behaviours too; it can turn us into perfectionists, it can make us perform rituals (such as constant handwashing) and it can make us feel unable to venture outside and leave our home (in extreme cases, this is known as 'agoraphobia').

Improving your mental wellbeing

Chronic stress has an adverse effect on our health and wellbeing. Fortunately, there are a number of behaviours which can assist us in improving our sense of vitality, mood and overall quality of life.

PRACTISE RELAXATION

The stress response can be counteracted by using a combination of approaches that elicits the relaxation response. Breathing relaxation serves to relax our muscles and improves the delivery of oxygen to the organs in our body. As our muscles relax, blood pressure lowers, endorphins are released and the body is detoxified more efficiently. Breathing exercises can also strengthen your lungs and heart, making them more resilient. To use this breathing relaxation, find a quiet moment and focus on the movement of your diaphragm (the area just below your stomach). Take a deep breath through your nose, filling your diaphragm with air and then gently and slowly exhale through your mouth with a long, drawn-out breath. Relax your body as you breathe out.
When feeling overwhelmed with stress or when confronted with a situation which is likely to trigger an angry response, try and visualise a soothing image (for example, a picture of nature) or a soothing word (such as PEACE, RELAX or BE STILL).

TAKE TIME TO EXPERIENCE THE LIFE YOU LIVE

This might be learning to practice mindfulness – which is the art of being in the here and now *non-judgementally*. Mindfulness can help us to recognise when we are rushing around, tensing up. Practise self-compassion and take a moment to yourself. Consciously slow down, breathe deeply, notice your thoughts but don't judge them and relax any tension away. Mindfulness is about reconnecting with the experience in which you are engaged, rather than experiencing life as a blur. Allowing yourself time to do things for you is an important aspect of leading a balanced life. It allows you to be loving and caring to others as much as you are to yourself. If you enjoy the feeling of exercising, make the time to go out for a walk or join a gym class. If you enjoy passive pastimes, like gardening or listening to music, make the time to do these as an exercise in self-care and self-kindness.

EXERCISE IN BOTH ACTIVE AND PASSIVE FORMS

Both types are essential. Active exercise is covered on page 77. Passive exercise, like stretching or yoga, means focusing on slow, rhythmic breathing and gentle movements – this activates the body's parasympathetic response and restores your body to a normal physiological rhythm.

MOVE AROUND AS MUCH AS YOU CAN

Move consistently during each day and at a comfortable pace for you, rather than trying to move in sporadic bursts (such as going for a run once a month).

KEEP IN TOUCH WITH FAMILY AND FRIENDS

Make the time to connect with your family and friends. If this is difficult, seek out and join groups that share your interests. Everyone can feel lonely from time to time, however research shows that chronic social isolation can physically harm your heart. Social isolation, along with depression, is the most significant psychological factor associated with heart disease and mortality. Loneliness has been linked to hardening of the arteries, inflammation and poor immune system response. It is also highly associated with hypertension and insomnia. People who experience social isolation suffer more illnesses and higher rates of mortality than people who identify a sense of social connectedness.

Research also shows that the quality of your social connections, having intimate, close personal relationships, is just as important (if not more) than just knowing you have people around you. Indeed, having someone you trust and confide in is essential in making us feel deeply connected and (to a point) supported and understood. Ideally, your confidant allows you to express yourself freely and without fear of judgement.

EAT A BALANCED DIET

Focus on adopting good, healthy habits (such as eating more fresh food and having smaller food portions) rather than focusing on following diet fads which can disrupt your metabolism and gut flora.

GET PLENTY OF SLEEP AT NIGHT

Sleep is more significant than simply getting some rest. Depriving someone of sleep has powerful adverse effects upon their mental health. In anxious and depressive states, a person's sleep is also usually disturbed. Lack of sleep can lead to activation of excitatory and inflammatory hormones which can affect our rate of breathing as well as our metabolism. For instance, it can affect insulin resistance and hyperglycaemia. In addition, lack of proper sleep affects memory and focus, which can create a disturbed frame of mind. For some tips on getting a good night's sleep, see page 62.

ABSTAIN FROM ARTIFICIAL FORMS OF 'HAPPINESS'

The use and abuse of alcohol and illicit drugs ultimately sabotages the acquisition of a naturally happy state. These substances can, at a physical level, cause significant damage to our nervous system. At a psychological level, they can erode our sense of self and the ability to feel and think normally. For some tips on using alcohol in moderation, see pages 63–64.

TAKE YOUR MEDICATIONS AS INDICATED

There is a worrying tendency for people to not take their medication properly. The statistics are sobering: only 50% of people undergoing long-term therapy for chronic illnesses adhere to taking their prescribed medicines. Approximately half of people prescribed statins will stop taking them within six months. Patients with hypertension who take their medicine less than 20% of the time are twice as likely to be hospitalised as those who take their medicine more than 80% of the time. There are various reasons why people will stop taking medication. It is important that patients trust their doctors to discuss these before stopping their medications.

LAUGHTER IS THE BEST MEDICINE

The ability to be able to laugh in the face of stress allows our mind to contemplate a problem from a different perspective. It makes us see a lighter side, a more positive option. As a bonus, laughter helps us to release feel-good endorphins.

DEVELOP A GOOD RAPPORT WITH YOUR DOCTOR

We know that when we hurt or feel physically unwell we usually go to the doctor, however, when our mood, overall level of energy and sense of vitality are affected, we are less likely to seek medical support. Make and keep regular medical appointments, and seek to build a good relationship with your regular doctor. This ensures that your health and any condition you may have are monitored and that any issues arising from your health or treatment can be addressed promptly. Your medical appointments also allow for a review of your progress, overall effectiveness of treatment and gives you the opportunity to discuss plans to enhance your wellbeing.

SEEK EMOTIONAL ENLIGHTENMENT

Activities such as reading self-help books, talking to mental health professionals or a life coach can enhance our understanding of ourselves and improve our sense of personal connection and quality of life. For some people, getting in touch with their spirituality can also provide a sense of personal completeness and wellbeing.

ADOPT A PET

The benefits of caring for a pet can be tremendous. Pets can provide people with a sense of connectedness. They can encourage you to exercise (most dogs need to go out for a daily walk). And, importantly, pets provide companionship.

Good mental health is about connecting with our daily moments as much as possible, it is seeking pleasurable things to do and pushing ourselves to learn new things that are good for us. It is also about bringing a sense of balance to the experience of stress – going out for a walk or listening to music, catching up with friends or cooking a healthy meal are all things we can do to improve our sense of wellbeing.

When to seek help

If you are experiencing any of the following symptoms for most of the day, most days of the week for at least two weeks, you ought to discuss the way you are feeling with your doctor:

- feeling sad and tearful
- feeling unmotivated
- losing interest in things you used to enjoy doing
- feeling constantly worried
- experiencing sleep problems – not sleeping, having trouble sleeping or sleeping too much
- losing your appetite
- eating too much
- losing or putting on too much weight.

Make long-lasting changes

The information in this chapter can only help you to improve your wellbeing if it leads to a consistent change in your daily behaviour. The first step to improve your wellbeing is to recognise you care enough about yourself to commit to and implement lasting change. A healthy mental state is one in which we create a very special balance between work, family and personal demands and a life that includes playfulness, spontaneity and sense of inner comfort that brings about an overall sense of wellbeing.

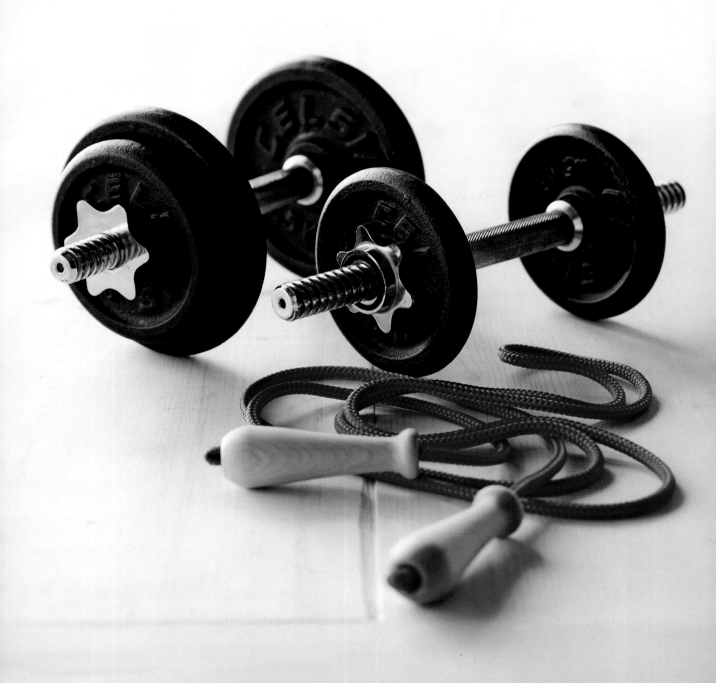

9

PHYSICAL ACTIVITY

Physical activity is an important part of any wellness program. It is the key to preventing most types of chronic disease. This is particularly true for heart disease, cancer and type 2 diabetes, where a moderate program of physical activity has been shown to save lives.

Physical activity will also improve your physical capacity, muscle and bone strength. It will lower blood pressure, especially in people with hypertension. It will also improve your metabolism by making the tissues more sensitive to insulin and preventing progression to established type 2 diabetes (if you are in the early stages). It can reduce blood glucose in those with more established type 2 diabetes. It can also improve your mental and emotional functioning. It can even bolster your productivity and relationships.

Regular aerobic exercise also provides three important sleep benefits. It helps you:

- fall asleep faster
- spend more time in deep sleep and
- wake less during the night.

In fact, exercise has been proposed as the only known way for healthy adults to boost the amount of deep sleep they get — and deep sleep is essential for your body to renew and repair itself.

Did you know?

If you sit for most of the day, just a few minutes of light exercise can help lower blood pressure for people with type 2 diabetes. A study conducted by Baker IDI in overweight and obese adults looked at the impact of three minutes of walking or simple resistance exercises, such as squats, every half hour. A light walking break resulted in an average 10-point drop in systolic blood pressure, while the resistance activities saw an average 12-point drop.

What physical activity can't do

Physical activity is an important part of any weight maintenance program, but it will not generally reduce body weight by itself. In part, this is because the number of kilojoules burned in 30 minutes of moderate exercise is easily overcome by having that an can of soft drink at some other time in the day.

If you are not reducing the kilojoules you consume despite exercising, your weight may not change. Internal changes are happening – the proportional size of your muscles are increasing and your fat levels are decreasing. Yet these positive changes may not be so obvious when you jump on the scales. Muscle burns more energy than fat, making it a crucial part of weight loss. Physical activity can also help redistribute fat around the body. It can help shift it from a less healthy distribution (mainly inside the abdominal cavity and around the organs) which is linked to metabolic and cardiovascular disease, to more 'subcutaneous' fat, the kind you can grab with your hand, in the lower body.

Physical activity alone will not lower your total blood cholesterol. This requires an associated improvement in nutrition (see chapter 10) or weight reduction. This does not mean that physical activity is not good for blood fats. A moderate program of regular physical activity will generally reduce blood triglycerides and a sustained high-level physical activity program will increase HDL, the 'good' cholesterol.

What is the right physical activity program for health?

The National Heart Foundation recommends 30 minutes of moderate leisure time activity each day. This is a reasonable and practical recommendation, though it is not presently met by more than two-thirds of the population.

There are many variations in the type of physical activity that people engage in. Some activities have been well studied for their health benefits and others have not. There are a few common messages in the research.

Some exercise is better than none

It seems that any physical activity is better than none at all. Our daily lives are increasingly structured towards us being sedentary. People who are not deliberately physically active in their leisure time and whose work is not physical are actually doing less than people who did a similar type of job years ago. For this reason, a lot of Baker IDI's work now focuses on the adverse health effects of being sedentary and implementing simple interventions (such as standing up regularly to break up deskwork). It is clear that the adverse effects on health of too much sitting are greater than can be explained simply by a lack of exercise. We will need to restructure our environment and our habits to address this.

The question of how much deliberate physical activity we should all do to maintain our health is not an easy one to answer. To some people, walking up a flight of stairs may be an unwelcome and uncomfortable workout. For others, who regularly love testing the limits of their physical capabilities, enough is never enough.

How much exercise is really enough?

As well as differences in our individual limitations, capabilities and aspirations, the amount of exercise required to achieve particular markers of health varies considerably. Some physiological factors are very sensitive to even small amounts of physical activity. Even a single 30 to 40-minute bout of exercise will improve the body's sensitivity to insulin and lower blood pressure for a few hours. On the other hand, if the objective of a physical activity program is to raise HDL, sustained high-level aerobic activities are required.

What is light, moderate or vigorous exercise?

Light exercise is the kind of physical activity that can be sustained for more than an hour. Moderate exercise can be sustained for at least 30 minutes, but not longer than an hour. Vigorous exercise cannot be pushed for longer than 30 minutes at a time.

The talk test is a good way to measure if you are exercising in the right zone for your goal. If you can talk and sing comfortably, you are moving at a low intensity. If you can talk but not sing, you are at a moderate intensity. If you struggle to get out more than a few words, you are at a vigorous level.

HEART RATE TARGETS

Targets for physical activity are commonly based on heart or pulse rates. Your heart rate increases proportionately to the intensity of the exercise you are doing. As you get fitter, the heart rate at a given level of exercise falls, as does your heart rate at rest. Charts and apps are available to provide a guide to the heart rate you should be aiming for, taking into account other important influences such as your age.

There is, however, large individual variability in heart rate changes in response to exercise among people of the same age. Remember these are average targets and your individual response may differ. Heart rate is also difficult to measure accurately during activity, especially by hand and even some of the special devices that measure this electronically can be misled by the movement of heavy exercise activities.

It is important that these are based on what the individual can do, and not an absolute recommendation for a particular or type or level of activity. In fact, as people engage in regular physical activity and become fitter, the amount they can sustain for a particular period will increase. The target will shift.

What exercise is right for you?

AEROBIC TRAINING

Experts recommend that 30 minutes of aerobic exercise – activities that make you 'huff and puff' – on most days will boost your cardiovascular health and help maintain your weight. It appears, however, that at least 60 minutes of moderate to high intensity exercise on most days is what is needed for weight loss. Aerobic activities such as power walking, jogging, cycling and swimming are good options. People who are starting exercise for the first time, after a long break or have contraindications from medical conditions making strenuous exercise unsustainable can look for ways to incorporate movement into their daily routine and build on this.

Moderate to vigorous exercise also boosts libido and performance. The Harvard Health Professionals Follow-Up Study found that men who exercised 30 minutes a day were 41% less likely than sedentary men to experience erectile dysfunction. Exercise helps women, too: in one study, 20 minutes of cycling boosted women's sexual arousal by 169%.

RESISTANCE TRAINING

Weight training should not be avoided if your goal is weight loss. With aerobic training, as soon as you step off the treadmill or swim your last lap, your heart rate decreases and your breathing returns to normal. But with resistance training, you continue to burn excess kilojoules for many hours after you put down the weights. Resistance training – whether using your body weight, free weights like dumb bells or weight machines – helps you tone up, and increase your strength and muscle mass. This can speed up your metabolism, and give you more balance and strength to better complete your daily activities.

Don't be put off if you don't know what to do at first. Most complex exercises can be broken down in easy steps or use basic equipment. For example, push-ups can be performed against a wall. Exercise equipment such as fit balls or resistance bands can be substituted for weights when you begin to give you more stability and confidence. Tap into the expertise of a personal trainer or exercise physiologist to develop a resistance program to meet your goals and abilities.

Beginner: Perform 1–3 sets of each exercise, with a weight you can lift for 8–15 repetitions. Rest for 1–2 minutes between each set. Complete exercises using largest muscle groups first. Complete workout 1–3 times a week (not on consecutive days) for 20–30 minutes.

Training for weight loss: Perform 1–3 sets of each exercise, with 6–20 repetitions using a weight less than 70% of your maximum effort for one lift. Rest for 1–2 minutes between each set. Alternate between body parts. Complete workout 1–3 times a week (not on consecutive days) for 20–30 minutes.

Training for strength: Perform 1–6 sets of each exercise, with 1–6 repetitions of a weight 80–100% of your maximum effort for one lift. Rest for 3–10 minutes. Complete the more complex movements first. Complete workout 2–4 times a week (not on consecutive days) for 45–60 minutes.

Training to build muscle: Perform 3–6 sets of each exercise, with 8–12 repetitions of a weight 75–90% of your maximum effort for one lift. Rest for 30 seconds–3 minutes. Complete the more complex movements first. Complete workout 3 times a week (not on consecutive days) for 30–60 minutes.

GROUP EXERCISES

There is evidence that people are likely to stay physically active when they are part of a group. Being part of a group adds a social dimension to the activity. It adds the kind of support and guidance that can only be provided by people having the same experience as you. There is an incentive to go along to an exercise session if you know you will be missed. You will try harder in the company of others in the group. Exercising with other people also gives you a benchmark to measure your strengths and weaknesses against, providing you the chance to grow and set yourself new challenges.

Set yourself some exercise goals

Whether you want to compete in a particular event, regularly climb those three flights of stairs at work or fit into a particular pair of pants, setting yourself some exercise goals will help you improve your physical capabilities. It will also help you to commit to and sustain being in an exercise program. Many people find it helpful to record what they do, whether they use an old-fashioned pen and notebook or a modern fitness-tracking device. If you have a particular health objective, such as lowering your blood pressure or improving your glucose control, home measurements can be very beneficial both in monitoring your progress and in empowering you to have greater control of your own health.

Exercising safely

Exercise plays a strong part in our ability to live healthy lives. Occasionally, however, we hear of the unfortunate sudden death of a competitive athlete during an event. Although the health benefits of being physically active are indisputable, these rare events do occur. Generally, it will be found that the athlete had an underlying health problem, although they may or may not have been aware of this.

Physical activity protects against heart disease. Classic risk factors such as high blood cholesterol, high blood pressure, tobacco smoking or type 1 and type 2 diabetes can negatively affect the heart. People with these conditions may need to take extra care with their exercise. However, even people with these conditions can carry out a program of regular physical activity. Indeed, exercise programs are a vital part of the medical management

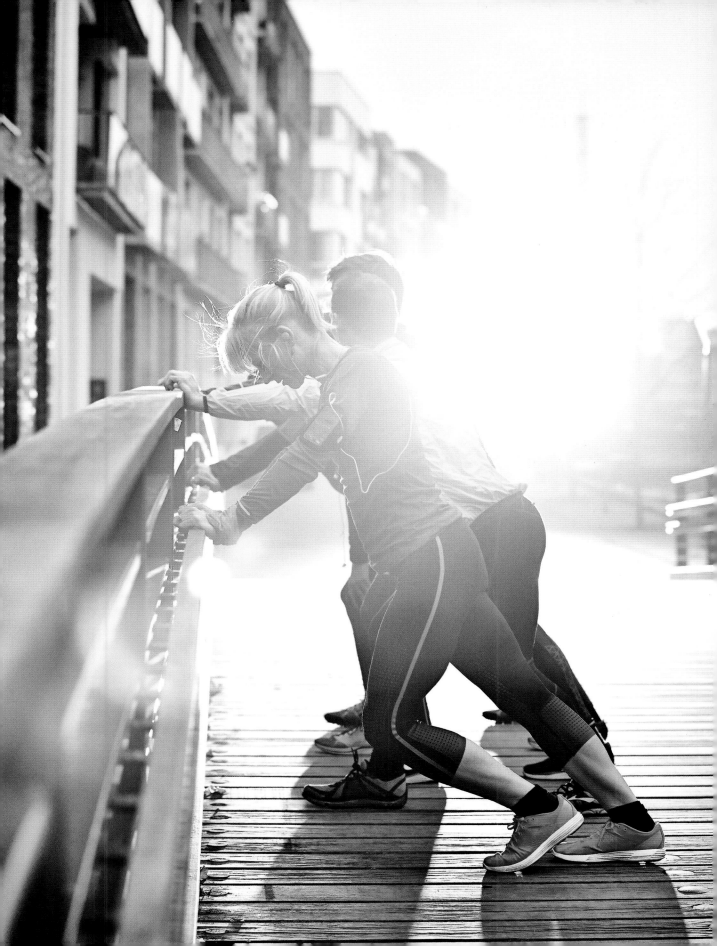

SMART goals have been shown to be an effective method for setting goals. They help identify what you need to do in order to achieve your goals. A SMART goal will be:

Specific **M**easurable **A**ttainable **R**elevant and **T**imely.

When you are setting your exercise goals, you think about what you want to achieve with your health, fitness and wellbeing in the context of how you are going to achieve it.

Specific goals

Make your goal detailed, not vague. The more specific your goal, the more awareness you have of how you can achieve it. For example, a goal might be: 'lose 5kg'. A SMART goal would be: 'lose 5kg over two months by walking for one hour each night after work, and swimming both days on the weekend.'

Measurable goals

Measurable goals allow you to know when you've reached your goal. Without a measurable component you don't know if you're on track or still have a lot of work to do. They can also serve as an extra motivator.

If your goal is to reduce your blood pressure to a certain reading, an effective SMART goal would be: 'Reduce my blood pressure to 130/80 in three months by participating in three gym sessions a week, and eating two serves of fruit daily and a salad with dinner.' There are four measurable aspects in this goal: a blood pressure measurement, a date that you will achieve this by, the number of gym sessions you will participate in and the number of serves of fruit and vegies you will eat each day.

Attainable goals

An attainable goal is one that you will be able to achieve. Even though you may want to lose 20 kg, you are not going to be able to do it in a single week. Your goal needs to be realistic, or else you are setting yourself up for failure. Breaking an ambitious goal into smaller short-term goals can help you stay on track. This will help ensure any lifestyle changes you make are safe, healthy and you can stick at them over the long-term.

Relevant goals

Your goals need to be relevant to you and your personal situation. Set yourself goals that you really want to achieve, and understand why you want to achieve them. Perhaps you had a close family member who became ill or died from a lifestyle-related disease that you want to avoid yourself. Instead of wanting to lose weight for the sake of it, think about if you want to look better for a particular occasion or feel more energetic when you play with your kids. Choose activities that you enjoy – if you don't like running, setting yourself the goal of running in a fun run is not going to keep you motivated.

Timely goal

Set yourself a deadline for completing your goal. It will help create a sense of urgency and accountability as you work towards your goal. It will also help you measure your achievements – will you get your blood pressure down by the set time? Do you perhaps have to change what you are doing in order to meet your goal? Have a timeline for completing your goal.

of people who have suffered a heart attack, and even in those with advanced heart failure.

Problems are more likely to arise in people who try to do too much too soon, in older people who are not aware of their risk factors, and people who are taking up a vigorous physical activity program.

Being safe with your exercise programs involves:

- starting at a low intensity of exercise and gradually building up to more vigorous forms
- if there is an interruption to your exercise program (for example, you have a viral infection or other illness or you have an extended break), it is best to restart your exercise at a lower level
- if you have been sedentary and are planning to take up an exercise program in middle-age, talk to your doctor before you start about whether any screening tests might be necessary
- if you have a family history of early cardiac death, talk to your doctor about any testing that should be done, especially if you are engaged in competitive exercise. In young people, this test may be as simple as a standard electrocardiogram (also known as an ECG or an EKG).

Many gyms require a medical clearance from your doctor before you can begin exercising, especially if you have a history of, or are at risk from, cardiovascular disease, both types of diabetes and some other chronic illnesses.

Is it safe to exercise after surgery?

For people who are recovering from surgery (such as knee reconstructions or hip replacements) or those who live in daily pain from chronic conditions such as arthritis or bursitis, exercise is crucial to strengthen the right muscles and ligaments to protect your long-term mobility and reduce pain. Tap into the expertise of a physiotherapist or exercise physiologist to develop an individual program to help improve these areas. Strengthening the quadriceps and hamstrings after

having a knee reconstruction is vital to ensuring you have a full and ongoing recovery. Studies have shown that regular moderate exercise for those with rheumatoid arthritis can reduce joint pain and stiffness, and increase mobility.

Should people with serious diseases still exercise?

The majority of cancer patients – despite being physically capable – typically stop exercising during treatment and return to lower activity levels afterwards. This is despite exercise being able to improve their mental health and their physical response to treatment, and reduce the likelihood of some cancers returning. It can also lessen their risk of the long-term co-morbidities they become more likely to develop such as high blood glucose, osteoporosis and cardiovascular disease. The benefits of exercise are there for everyone.

Exercise and cholesterol treatment

Statins, the most commonly used medicines for lowering cholesterol, are generally free of side-effects in most people. In a small proportion of people who take these drugs, statins can be associated with myositis or inflammation of the muscle. A person experiencing these symptoms experiences muscle pain. We all get muscle pain at some time in our lives, especially if we perform unfamiliar physical activity – so not all muscle pain experienced by people taking statins is due to myositis. If the pain is severe, protracted and unexplained, a blood test to measure muscle enzymes (such as creatine kinase) will usually provide a diagnosis. These enzymes are not generally present in significant amounts in the blood stream, but are elevated if there is muscle damage.

Myositis associated with statin therapy is generally reversible on stopping the drug. However, it is better to rest and take a break from your exercise program while recovery is taking place. People are prescribed statins for a reason – it is important not to forego the proven benefits of these drugs unnecessarily.

The benefits of rest

Building rest days into our regular exercise program can help us maintain a better balance between our personal, work and health goals. Elite athletes understand the importance of rest days to help their bodies recover, build muscle and repair. When we are enthusiastic about starting a new program or become tempted to push ourselves through fatigue and pain to get results, we risk becoming injured or losing motivation. Be sensible with exercise. We do need to continue challenging our bodies in order to make the weight loss and strength gains we desire, and avoid hitting a plateau when our bodies have become used with our routine. However, we also need to listen to our bodies and rest when we feel overly fatigued, sore and injured.

Do you need to take extra care with exercise?

Some people need to be a bit more careful about exercise and the types of exercise that they do.

Pregnancy
Women with uncomplicated pregnancies should continue their previous level of exercise after consulting their doctor. Engaging in regular weight-bearing exercise has been shown to improve maternal fitness, restrict weight gain without compromising foetal growth, and speed up postpartum recovery.

However, pregnant women should also listen to their bodies. Avoid heavy lifting and training in the heat. Avoid exercises on your back or stomach after the first trimester. This includes avoiding abdominal crunches while sitting on a fit ball for risk of causing rectus diastasis or abdominal muscle separation.

Hypertension
Regular aerobic exercise can reduce blood pressure at rest and during daily activities, as well as protecting against developing hypertension in the future.

However, people with hypertension should avoid extreme levels of strength training.

Coronary heart disease
Regular moderate intensity exercise has many benefits for clinically stable coronary heart disease patients. They should, however, avoid extreme levels of strength training. After a cardiac event such as a heart attack, a person can participate in at least two weeks of aerobic training before starting resistance training. After coronary artery bypass graft surgery, a person should avoid exercises that cause tension or pressure on the breastbone for the first three months. You can learn all about this and much more at a cardiac rehabilitation program, which everyone should attend after a heart attack or cardiac surgery.

Osteoporosis
Your risk of fractures is high if you have been diagnosed with low bone mass, so opt for low impact exercise such as low-moderate intensity aerobics or dancing, tai chi or stair climbing. These exercises will improve muscle strength and balance, which will help prevent falls. Heavy weight resistance training is not suitable, but moderate intensity – using a weight you can lift for at least 10 times before tiring – can help build muscle.

Exercise myths

MYTH: I need to drink sports drinks if I exercise.

FACT: For most active people, sports drinks are an unnecessary addition of salt, sugar and kilojoules. Water is absorbed almost as quickly (and is much cheaper) than energy drinks. Most of us already get too much salt in our diet, so our typical food intake should be adequate to replace any electrolyte loss. Sports drinks, however, could be useful if you are performing strenuous exercise for more than an hour in the heat.

MYTH: Doing sit-ups will get rid of stomach fat, and squats will help me lose fat on my thighs.

FACT: You can't spot train to remove fat from a particular area. When we lose fat, we lose it in a generalised way. Targeted exercises like sit-ups and squats will strengthen the muscles in those areas, but won't make those body parts look any more toned if you don't also remove the fat covering them.

MYTH: I need to feel pain while exercising to get any benefit.

FACT: Exercise can be uncomfortable, especially when you are working at higher intensity levels or restarting after a long break. Exercise can 'hurt' in the sense that you feel your muscles burn and fatigue, your heart beat furiously and your lungs are working hard. But any sharp pain during or straight after exercise can signal injury. If you feel pain, stop exercising immediately, and switch to working other body parts if possible. If you're in great pain the next day, you may have been exercising too long or too hard. Reduce your workout the next time, to see if that improves before slowly increasing your effort.
Be particularly alert to discomfort or heaviness in the centre of your chest. This may go up to the neck or down the arm at a regular point in your workout and goes when you rest. This can be angina, a marker of coronary heart disease, and is a sign to check in with your doctor. If the pain lasts more than a few minutes and does not settle with rest, it could be the beginning of a heart attack. Call triple zero (000) for assistance.

MYTH: Women should avoid lifting weights because they'll end up looking like Arnold Schwarzenegger.

FACT: Many women shy away from using weights as part of their exercise regime for fear of 'bulking up' or looking masculine. They are missing out on the benefits of increased metabolism, toning and increased bone mass. Women don't have anywhere as much testosterone as men. Toning is what happens in women when they develop muscles and lose fat. Without hard-core daily training and a whole lot of supplements, the average woman involved in regular weight training will never physically look like Arnie.

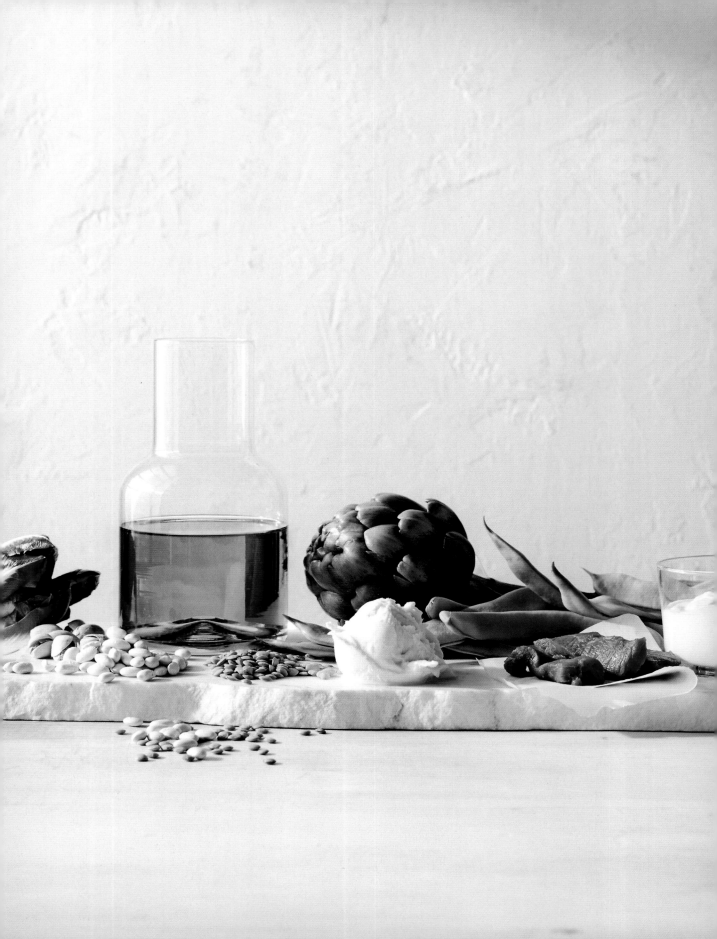

10

HEALTHY EATING

This chapter contains detailed information that summarises the 'best practice' for a healthy pattern of eating. You will notice that the ideas in this book do not always agree with what you may have read elsewhere or seen on television. There are, of course, different beliefs about what is best for us. It is important to understand that the evidence about nutrition and health evolves all the time. What we at Baker IDI are presenting here represents where mainstream nutrition finds itself today.

How is this information collected?

You may be interested in how such information is collected and interpreted. Most of it comes from studying large populations over lengthy periods of time. Having carefully collected information from the participants on their eating patterns at the beginning and during the study period, it has been possible to identify 'healthy' and 'unhealthy' patterns that either protect or accelerate diseases such as heart attacks, type 2 diabetes and cancer. Interestingly, almost all the studies agree. Healthy eating patterns include vegetables (including legumes), whole grain cereals, fruit, fish, nuts,

lean meat (including poultry), low-fat dairy and monounsaturated (olive) and polyunsaturated oils. The unhealthy eating patterns include fried foods, excess takeaway foods, excess soft drinks and high meat consumption.

This has given rise to cultural patterns of eating. Some – but not all – Mediterranean countries have a pattern resembling the 'healthy' diet. Asian patterns of eating, although quite different from Mediterranean ones, also have protective features (although they do feature a high salt content).

The details from these findings can be honed further. Total fat is not necessarily associated with chronic disease, except through obesity. However, almost all the studies show that polyunsaturated oils are protective against heart attack. Harmful trans fats from hydrogenating oils have virtually disappeared from the Australian scene. While trans fats are also found in ruminant fats (beef/ lamb meat and cow/ sheep full-fat dairy products and butter), the amounts typically eaten are small when people choose lean meats and low-fat dairy products.

Carbohydrates that are rich in fibre and have a low glycaemic index also appear protective against heart attack. So adopting a low-carb approach should apply only to restricting highly refined carbohydrates. Eating moderate amounts of whole grains is always in the pattern of protective diets. The type of grain moves with fashions: 'old' grains versus 'new' grains are probably much the same.

Dairy foods, especially if it is of the reduced fat variety and fermented (like yoghurt), may be linked to lower rates of diabetes.

About one in five people are 'salt sensitive' in terms of it potentially raising their blood pressure. This should be taken into account if there is a family history of high blood pressure.

Plant foods are rich in the antioxidants called flavonoids or polyphenols (there are a few thousand varieties). Some of these may be protective against heart attack and diabetes. Berries, apples, onions and garlic, citrus, soybean, beetroot, green tea and cocoa are among many foods rich in flavonoids and polyphenols. However, processing foods often destroys the antioxidant capacity for example, raw cocoa is very high in polyphenols, yet the heat-treating of cocoa in the production of chocolate substantially lowers these compounds and the amounts in chocolate (even dark chocolate) are quite low. It is generally agreed that a diet containing adequate vegetables and fruit contains all the antioxidants that we need.

For healthy people, eating one egg a day on average appears harmless and does not contribute to heart disease.

Legumes are great food. But for some people, especially those with irritable bowel syndrome, legumes might be difficult to tolerate.

The link between processed meats and bowel cancer has been around for some time; probably due to the processing and preservatives. However, any link between moderate consumption of lean meat and bowel cancer is far from established.

Eating at least two portions of fish a week is clearly protective against heart attack. Fish oil supplements, however, are less likely to provide protection.

Moderate alcohol consumption is also often in healthy eating patterns. Here the emphasis is very much on moderation. The national alcohol guidelines recommend the consumption of no more than two standard drinks per day for men and women.

What should we be eating?

Many people have spent the past 30–40 years attempting to follow the low-fat dietary prescription of the 1970s and 1980s. The main reason the 'eat less fat' message was used was to reduce saturated fat intake. However, this message also meant people cut out what we now know are healthy plant-based fats (including olive oil and nuts). The food supply chain has also changed over this time, with many low-fat (but highly processed) foods adding refined sugars or starches to mimic the taste and mouth feel of their higher fat counterparts. Choosing low-fat foods did not necessarily lead people to choose healthier foods, especially when portion sizes continued to increase.

A focus on blaming one set of foods – be it fat, sugars, or refined carbohydrates – for our current lifestyle disease 'epidemic' moves the focus away from what healthy eating looks like. To maintain health and wellbeing, people should choose a healthy, whole food balanced diet.

In the next section, we will explore what a healthy, balanced eating plan looks like.

An eating plan for health and wellbeing

The healthiest and longest-lived communities have dietary patterns that we can copy to give us the same health benefits. One traditional dietary pattern stands out for reducing chronic disease risk: the Mediterranean diet.

The Mediterranean diet is characterised by:
· being low in processed foods
· being high in vegetable intake
· including moderate amounts of carbohydrate, mainly from legumes and small amounts of whole grains
· including moderate amounts of protein, mainly from free-range eggs and seafood, but also including small amounts of red meat and chicken
· including moderate amounts of fruit
· including moderate amounts of nuts
· including small amounts of yoghurt and cheese.

The *Australian Guide to Healthy Eating* is a set of guidelines put out by the Australian Government. They are based on scientific evidence and up-to-date research, and aim to help people develop healthy eating patterns, with a focus on eating a balanced intake of mainly unprocessed whole foods.

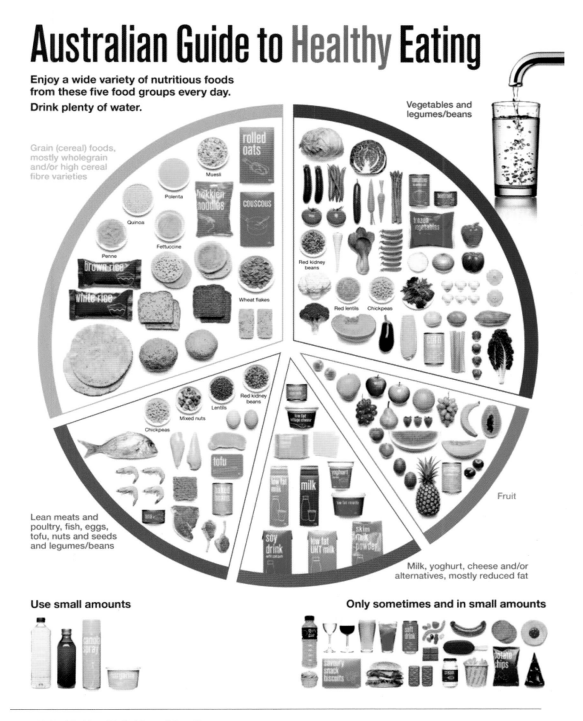

Australian Guide to Healthy Eating

Enjoy a wide variety of nutritious foods from these five food groups every day.

Drink plenty of water.

Grain (cereal) foods, mostly wholegrain and/or high cereal fibre varieties

Vegetables and legumes/beans

Lean meats and poultry, fish, eggs, tofu, nuts and seeds and legumes/beans

Fruit

Milk, yoghurt, cheese and/or alternatives, mostly reduced fat

Use small amounts

Only sometimes and in small amounts

Source: National Health and Medical Research Council

What does the Australian Guide to Healthy Eating look like in practice?

The recommended number of serves of each of the food groups depends on your gender, age and activity levels. Check out www.eatforhealth.gov.au/eat-health-calculators to work out how many serves you should be having for good health. The table below shows the **Recommended average daily food intake for a 35-year-old woman (F) or man (M)**.

FOOD GROUP	DAILY SERVES	
	F	M
Vegetables and legumes/beans	5	6
Fruit	2	2
Grain (cereal) foods, mostly wholegrain and/or high cereal fibre varieties	6	6
Lean meat and poultry, fish, eggs, tofu, nuts and seeds and legumes/beans	2.5	3
Milk, yoghurt, cheese and/or alternatives (mostly reduced fat)	2.5	2.5
Approx number of additional serves from the five food groups or fats/oils/spreads or discretionary choices *	0-2.5	0-3

* includes an allowance for unsaturated spreads or oils, nuts or seeds

Source: National Health and Medical Research Council

For a **35-year-old woman**, over a whole day, this could include:
- two slices of toast with tomato and avocado (2 serves grains, 1 serve vegetables)
- one skim latte (1 serve dairy)
- one serve of quinoa salad (1 cup quinoa = 2 serves grains, 2 cups salad = 2 serves vegetables) with chicken (85g = 1 serve lean meat)
- one apple (1 serve fruit)
- a serve of fish, vegetables and rice (150g fish = 1.5 serves lean meat, 1 cup cooked vegetables = 2 serves vegetables, 1 cup rice = 2 serves grains) with a 200 ml glass of wine (2 serves 'discretionary foods')
- one serve of fruit salad (1 cup = 1 serve fruit) with 1/3 cup natural yoghurt (1/2 serve dairy).

For a **35-year-old man** over a whole day this could include:
- one cup of porridge cooked with ½ cup low fat milk and one banana (2 serves grains, 0.5 serves dairy, 1 serve fruit)
- one skim latte (1 serve dairy)
- multigrain sandwich with small tin of tuna, lettuce, tomato and cucumber (2 slices bread = 2 serves grains, 1 can tuna = 1 serve lean meat, 1 cup lettuce, ½ tomato and ½ cucumber = 2 serves vegetables) and one apple (1 serve fruit)
- three crisp breads with hummus and eggplant dip (1 serve grains, ½ serve vegetables)
- steak with cooked vegetables (200g steak = 2 serves lean meat, 1 cup cooked vegetables = 2 serves vegetables, 1/2 large sweet potato = 1.5 serves vegetables)
- one tub low fat no added sugar yoghurt (1 serve dairy)
- one slice multigrain bread with 100% natural peanut butter (1 serve grains, 1 serve nuts)
- one 'row' of a large chocolate pack (1 serve discretionary foods).

Limiting packaged and processed foods

The *Australian Guide for Healthy Eating* follows the same principles as the Mediterranean diet in that there is a focus on fresh and minimally processed foods. Unfortunately, today's supermarkets teem with highly processed, nutritionally dubious foodstuffs. At first glance, many of these can seem to be reasonable nutritional choices. Food labels proclaim they are 'wholegrain', 'low-fat', and/or 'no added sugar'. Some, if not all, of these claims may be true. However, these foods also often contain highly refined grains added as fillers. They also often add salt to make the products tastier and to preserve the food and prevent spoilage. Both fillers and salt have associations with chronic disease.

Minimising your intake of processed foods can be challenging as many packaged foods are convenient foods. The trick is (a) knowing how to choose the healthiest of the packaged foods available, and (b) swapping processed foods for unprocessed versions where possible.

Healthier packaged food choices

Some processed foods make for quite reasonable food choices. These include:

- tinned fruit, vegetables and legumes – choose no-added or reduced salt varieties
- tinned fish
- pasta and noodles
- frozen whole plain fish
- frozen vegetables.

Get in the habit of reading the label, and be wary of processed foods that are high in salt, sugar and preservatives. Be wary of reconstituted frozen fish or poultry products (such as nuggets), muesli bars, dry biscuits, breads, pasta and stir-fry sauces, packet pasta meals, instant noodles, processed meat products (such as salami, pastrami and chicken loaf) and breakfast cereals.

Shopping tips

Shopping in supermarkets can be challenging. Supermarkets are designed to encourage you to buy more, which means there is just more on offer for you to eat. The following tips will help you make healthier food choices when you are shopping.

DON'T SHOP WHEN HUNGRY

Avoid going shopping when you are hungry. Being hungry when you are shopping makes it much harder to resist the lure of unhealthy snack foods. Plan to do your shopping at times when you won't be hungry.

However, if you do get stuck and need to go shopping at a time when you are hungry, have a small snack before you go. Try eating a little dried fruit-and-nut mix or a piece of fruit.

STOP THE DAILY PICK UP

If you find you shop at the supermarket every day or two to pick up necessities, you are increasing the number of times you are being subjected to temptation.

If you have to make a quick trip to pick up a few things, use a basket rather than a trolley. This will help you to avoid overbuying.

Meal planning and shopping with a list will ensure you buy everything you need and reduce the number of times you have to visit the supermarket.

SHOP AROUND THE STORE PERIMETER

In a typical supermarket, the fresh fruit and vegetables, meat and dairy sections are located around the edges. Aim to do most of your food shopping from these areas. Try to avoid the aisles as much as possible and avoid the chip, chocolate, soft drink and biscuit aisles altogether.

HEALTHY FOODS ARE CHEAPER

We are often tempted by unhealthy foods because they are on special. Don't get tempted by the 'bargain' two-for-one, on special, or economy-size chips, chocolates and ice-cream. It's not a bargain in the long run if it means you eat more.

While fruit and vegetables can seem expensive, the price per kilogram is often much cheaper than that of the unhealthy foods. For example, a 200 gram packet of chips for $2.50 seems cheaper than a kilogram of apples at $4.99 a kilogram. But the 200 gram packet of chips actually works out to $12.50 a kilogram. The apples are less than half the price, not to mention the savings on kilojoules.

PERFORM A TROLLEY CHECK

Before you head off to pay, check your trolley (or basket) to make sure your buying habits reflect your healthy eating habits. Limit less-than-healthy foods to only two to three items. Make sure most of your groceries are fruit, vegetables, lean meat and low-fat dairy.

SHOP OUTSIDE THE SUPERMARKETS

Consider getting your food from a fruit-and-vegetable shop, a butcher shop and/or markets or farmers markets. This way you can avoid the chocolate, chip and biscuit aisles. Leave the supermarkets for buying non-food items.

USE TECHNOLOGY

Consider doing your shopping online. Both Coles and Woolworths have online shopping available. There are other options available, such as Aussie Farmers Direct who deliver fresh fruit and vegetables.

There are some apps available that may help you to choose healthier food products. An example we have found is Food Switch. Using the app, scan a product's barcode and the app will identify a 'healthier' product for you to buy. However, remember that the product suggested may still be a highly processed or 'discretionary food'.

Swapping processed foods for less processed or unprocessed options

INSTEAD OF	CHOOSE
Muesli bars	Nuts and seeds, small amount of dried fruit
Refined grains:	
White bread	Grainy, ideally sourdough breads with minimal ingredients except wholegrain flour, water and yeast
White crackers, rice crackers	Grainy crackers (such as Vitaweat or Ryvita)
Breakfast cereals (rice, wheat or corn-based)	Oat-based cereals (traditional – not instant or quick cook – oats, porridge oats or muesli)
White rice	Brown rice (ideally, long-grain versions), red or black rice, quinoa, freekeh, faro
Savoury biscuits, corn chips, potato chips, fried vegetable chips (even the 75% reduced saturated fat ones)	Air-popped popcorn, chickpea or fava bean 'nuts', wasabi peas

Reading labels

Understanding how to read nutrition information panels on food products will help you identify healthy food choices. We are focusing on reducing saturated fat in foods. However, we also consider other relevant nutrients such as sugars, sodium (salt) and fibre. You will find nutritional recommendations in the table on the following page.

Note that these recommendations are guidelines only. It can be challenging to find products that meet all the criteria. The foods closest to the recommendations given will be the best choices.

The most useful part of the food package for evaluating the nutritional value of a product is the nutrition information panel. This table is required by law to be on all packaged food products sold in Australia. To choose a healthy product, check the 'quantity per 100 g' column, which is usually (but not always) on the right-hand side of the table.

How often can I eat unhealthy foods and still have a healthy diet?

Currently the average Australian consumes one-third of their daily kilojoule intake every day from 'discretionary foods'. These are foods that should be eaten only occasionally. These are high in kilojoules, saturated fat, added sugars, added salt or alcohol. Discretionary foods (and drinks) include:

- chocolates and lollies
- sweet biscuits, cakes and slices
- savoury biscuits
- ice-cream
- potato chips and crisps
- processed meats
- sausages
- pies and pasties
- takeaway foods such as burgers, hot chips, dim sims and fried foods
- cream and butter
- sugar-sweetened beverages such as soft drinks, cordials, fruit drinks, iced tea, energy drinks and sports drinks
- alcohol.

While discretionary foods can be included (occasionally and in small quantities) within an overall healthy diet, many of us eat far too much of these foods. The foods listed above should not be eaten on a daily basis. Eat these foods no more than once or twice a week if you are within the healthy weight range. If you are trying to lose or manage your weight, limit these foods to once to twice a month. Artificially sweetened beverages should be kept to a minimum. Water is the healthiest drink choice.

When and how often to eat

We commonly hear that we should eat three meals plus snacks over the day. In the modern environment – where meal and snack options are often high kilojoule foods and are served in excessive portion sizes – this frequency of eating can simply lead to more opportunities to overeat. There is no biological need to eat every three to four hours, so having three meals a day will ensure opportunity to have a healthy, balanced and nutritionally adequate diet. Having snacks is often a matter of personal preference. People who choose to snack if they are hungry should compensate by having smaller meals.

The timing of when you eat your meals, however, can play an important role. Diet-induced thermogenesis is the amount of energy the body produces after a meal. Diet-induced thermogenesis is 45–50% lower in the evening compared to the morning. Eating later in the evening is associated with a higher total kilojoule intake. This may be because people who eat after their dinner meal have just had another occasion to consume extra kilojoules.

Overall there is no one size fits all approach to eating over the day. However, having regular meals, while not overeating at dinner or during the evening, appears to be the best for preventing disease.

Nutritional value on food labels - listed in order of importance

NUTRIENTS	AIM FOR	NOTES
Saturated fat – per 100 g	• Nuts – 10 g/100 g or less • Cheese – 10 g/100 g or less • Oils – 20 g/100 g or less • Margarines – 15 g/100 g or less • All other products – 2 g/100 g or less	At these low levels of saturated fat normal consumption of the product will be unlikely to result in a total saturated fat intake above the recommendation. If the product contains more than the suggested limit of saturated fat per 100 g for that product, it should be consumed rarely.
Sugar – per 100 g	• Fruit-based products (fruit is listed in the first three ingredients) – 25 g/100 g or less • All other products – 15 g/100 g or less.	Sugar content can be confusing on the nutrition information panel, as it will include both natural sugars from foods, like dairy and fruit-based foods, and added sugars. Remember that ingredients are listed in the order of most to least, by weight. So it is best to avoid products that list sugar (or alternative names for sugar) in the first three ingredients. This ensures the product will be low in added sugars. The requirement for nutrition labels does not include listing fructose, so food products cannot be assessed based on fructose levels. However, the recommended levels for sugars will ensure all products meeting these criteria will also contain low levels of fructose. If the product contains more than the suggested limit of sugar per 100 g for that product it should be consumed rarely.
Fibre – per 100 g	• 8 g/100 g or more	Note that fibre is the only nutrient where **more** is better. This ensures the product will be high in fibre and may also contain soluble fibre, and normal consumption of the product will promote achieving the total fibre and soluble fibre recommendation. It can be very difficult to find foods that meet that criterion so choose the highest fibre option.
Sodium – per 100 g	120 mg/100 g or less (It can be very difficult to find foods that meet this criterion, so a higher limit of 400 mg/100 g or less can be used.)	A high sodium intake is one contributing factor to high blood pressure, however a low added salt diet will benefit you even if you don't have high blood pressure. If the product contains more than the suggested limit of sodium per 100 g for that product, it should be consumed rarely.

Intermittent fasting

In addition, recent studies have shown that intermittent fasting can improve markers of disease such as insulin resistance and inflammation. These fasts usually mean not eating in a 16-hour period between meals – for example, not eating anything between dinner one night and lunch the following day. It may actually be beneficial for humans to have occasional short periods without food. However, there have been no studies showing that intermittent fasting can reduce disease or increase lifespan. It is also not recommended for everyone. Some people find fasting more difficult than others. They may feel faint or unwell. These people should not force themselves to fast.

Portion sizes

With plate sizes and restaurant and café meals ever-increasing in size, it's not surprising that many of us eat too much. Our portion sizes are overlarge. We need to re-learn what an appropriate portion size looks like.

GET THE RIGHT SIZE PLATE

Most dinner plates and bowls are oversized. This makes portion control a challenging concept. Having the right size plate makes it easier to avoid overfilling your plate and your stomach.

Aim to use a dinner plate or bowl that is less than 25 centimetres wide (see plate overleaf). Take the measurement from the outer rim.

Have a balanced meal

To have a balanced meal, your plate should contain three elements:
- a lower GI carbohydrate – such as pasta, rice, bread, sweet potato, corn, lentils and legumes
- some lean protein – such as trimmed meat, skinless chicken, fish, seafood, tofu, egg
- cooked vegetables or salad – such as carrot, broccoli, peas, capsicum, cucumber, beans, beetroot, cabbage, bok choy, eggplant.

The table and picture on the following page show the recommended portion sizes for these elements. Use these portions as a guide when you are serving meals at home. When you are out, try to order so that you are following this guide as closely as you can. This may mean leaving some food on your plate, sharing a plate with someone else or ordering an extra serving of vegetables or salad.

How to eat

How we eat can be as important as what we choose to eat. Many eating habits can be unhealthy and lead to over-consumption. Overeating healthy foods can still lead to weight gain and chronic disease.

SIT DOWN AND SLOW DOWN

Many of us eat on the run, which makes it easy to not appreciate our foods and miss satiety (feelings of fullness and satisfaction) signals.

Good habits to develop include:
- sit down – don't eat while standing in front of the fridge or at the kitchen bench
- portion your foods out – don't eat straight from the box, packets or tub
- avoid taste-testing your food – it's easy to eat a meal amount while you are cooking
- quench your thirst with water, not alcohol or soft drinks
- be mindful with your alcoholic drinks – pour yourself one standard drink and then re-seal the bottle.

A balanced meal

Choose one serving from each of the following categories.

LOW GI CARBOHYDRATES

Pasta or noodles	1 cup cooked or 50 g dry
Rice – basmati/Mahatma/Doongara	2/3 cup cooked or 40 g dry
Sweet potato or Carisma potato	200 g (leave skin on where possible)
Corn	1 cob or ½ cup corn kernels
Grain bread or wholemeal flat bread	1–2 slices, or 1 small chapatti/pita/roti
Legumes or lentils	150g cooked or canned

LEAN PROTEIN

Lean meat – beef, lamb, pork	150 g raw or 120 g cooked
Skinless chicken or turkey	150 g raw or 120 g cooked
Fish and seafood	170 g raw or 150 g cooked
Tofu	150 g
Egg	2 whole
Legumes or lentils	150g cooked or canned

VEGETABLES

Salad	2–3 cups
Stir-fried or raw vegetables	2–3 cups
Cooked vegetables	1.5–2 cups

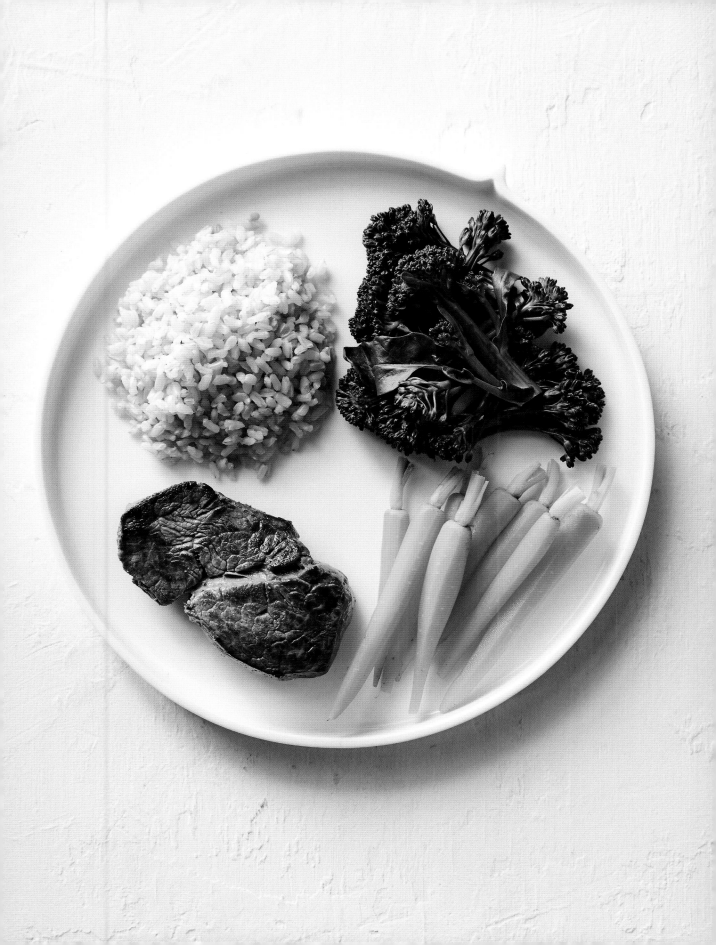

It is easy to fall into bad eating habits if you are not paying attention to your food and the way that you are eating it. Eating slowly and mindfully will help you to eat less yet enjoy your food more. Start by eating your food at a table, and remove distractions. Don't eat in front of the TV, or eat while you are reading. Take the time to slow down and actually taste your food. Pay attention to flavours, textures, temperature and allow yourself to note how much you enjoy these elements.

Some things you can do to slow down your eating include:

- **serve smaller portions, use smaller plates** – remove the temptation to eat everything left on your plate
- **eat with other people**
- **chat to the other people at the table** – you can't eat and talk at the same time
- **use a smaller fork or spoon** – don't overload your fork or spoon
- **eat with chopsticks** – these will slow the speed of food to your mouth
- **cut your food into smaller bites**
- **chew and swallow your food completely before selecting another bite**
- **put the fork or spoon down after each bite** – this will slow down the automatic fork-to-mouth motion
- **put handheld food (like a sandwich) down between each bite**
- **chew for longer** – chew every bite a minimum of 10 times
- **sip water in between bites** – this will slow you down, and the water will help fill you up
- **take a break** – stop once or twice during your meal for at least 1–2 minutes. Use the break to assess how you are feeling. Are you still hungry, satisfied or full?

Checking your hunger using a 'hunger and fullness scale' can be a great way to assess your hunger level.

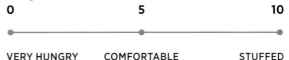

0	5	10
VERY HUNGRY	COMFORTABLE	STUFFED

Before each meal or snack you should be aiming to be a 2–3 on the scale. After each meal or snack, you should feel about a 7 on the scale. Rating your hunger half-way through a meal will help you slow down and prevent overeating.

Feeling 'very hungry' or a 0 on the scale may lead to overeating.

Feeling 'stuffed' or a 10 on the scale often means you have overeaten.

Healthy eating for the family

Eating socially is an important part of a healthy food experience. Healthy eating is important for the whole family and having all family members involved in eating healthy foods is essential to promoting a healthy food environment. It can be hard to get the whole family together with so many competing tasks and places to be, however try to make time where possible for the family to share a meal together at least a few meals each week. Don't feel this has to be dinners, as shared breakfasts and lunches (or snacks) can be just as good an opportunity for the family to share healthy foods together.

MODEL HEALTHY FOOD RELATIONSHIPS AND BEHAVIOURS

Kids learn from their parents, so who better to show them how important a healthy lifestyle is by leading by example. It also works the other way; if parents don't eat their vegetables, how can kids be expected to get excited about (or just tolerate) eating theirs?

Kids (of all ages) can be fussy eaters. This can be tricky to manage, but it shouldn't be an excuse for kids to get away with eating unhealthy foods, because that's all they will eat. However, some parents can end up offering mainly unhealthy foods so that their kids will at least eat something. Kids soon learn that if they refuse healthy foods they may get their preferred unhealthy foods.

Refusing food can simply be a way that a kid can establish some autonomy. Giving kids a choice of two healthy options ('would you prefer the carrot sticks or the apple for a snack today?') can both teach kids what healthy options are, and give them a feeling of choice. Helping choose the salad ingredients for dinner or the fruit when you go shopping can also be ways to give kids choices in building their own healthy eating habits.

If kids refuse both foods, don't immediately offer them an unhealthier alternative. If possible leave the healthy option available for a later time ('Ok, so you don't want it now. The apple is here on the bench if you feel hungry later'). Kids will eat when they are hungry so letting them know that the healthy option will still be the option later may prompt them to have it now.

Eating when you are hungry is an important skill to learn. Many adults feel they must finish everything on their plate, even if they feel satisfied or full, due to the habits they learnt as children.

Avoid passing on those unhealthy eating habits to your kids. If kids don't want to finish their meal, it could be saved for later if they do become hungry. If they continually don't finish their meals and choose not to eat them later, you may be serving them too much food.

Avoid the trap of using dessert as a reward. While high sugar or high-fat desserts should be an occasional treat, forcing kids to finish a meal so they can have dessert is simply encouraging them to overeat and normalising feelings of overfullness. If the whole family is having dessert, allow kids to eat until they feel full, but give them a smaller portion of dessert. Overeating dessert is just as harmful as overeating healthy foods. Don't allow them to eat little of their healthy dinner and then eat multiple serves of dessert!

Ways to add healthy foods

Sometimes finding ways to add healthy foods to your diet can be challenging. Here are some suggestions to help you make healthy choices and healthier meals.

Variety is the spice of life. Use a mix of seeds, including sesame seeds, poppy seeds, linseeds/flaxseeds, chia seeds, sunflower seeds and pepitas. Remember that there are many types of nuts, including almonds, walnuts, cashews, peanuts, macadamias, pecans, pine nuts, pistachios, hazelnuts. You can also use spice mixes such as dukkah, zaatar, ras el hanout or garam marsala that contain seeds, nuts and/or spices.

Don't forget that a lot of spices come from seeds, including coriander, cumin, celery seed, onion seed, allspice, nutmeg, star anise, caraway, fennel, cardamom, dill, fenugreek, mustard, nigella (black cumin) or wattleseed.

Add a sprinkle of chopped or whole seeds and/or nuts:
- on porridge or breakfast cereals
- on yoghurt
- in salads
- on baked vegetables
- on open sandwiches (particularly over mashed avocado, chopped tomatoes, hummus, tinned tuna or chopped boiled eggs).

You can also use 100%, no-added-sugar nut butters on toast, or dip fruit slices (apple and pear work especially well) or vegetables (capsicum, celery) in nut butter for a snack.

Herbs can add lots of flavour, as well as antioxidants. Don't be shy with using flavourful fresh or dried culinary herbs in cooking, such as parsley, dill, basil, Thai basil, lemongrass, coriander leaf, oregano, mint, lemon balm, chives, rosemary, tarragon, sage, thyme.

You can also drink herbal teas like chamomile, mint, rosehip or licorice as a way to add extra herbs to your day. Add them to hot or iced water to add flavour – just avoid adding sugar.

Some ways that you can get extra herbs into your diet include:
- using the whole leaf of herbs like mint, basil, coriander or parsley in salads
- adding finely chopped herbs to a vinaigrette-style dressing
- adding fresh herbs to green smoothies
- mixing chopped mint, basil or oregano with cottage or cream cheese to use as a topping for dry biscuits or an open sandwich
- adding chopped herbs to omelettes or frittatas
- using fresh or dried herbs on baked vegetables
- using sweet herbs like lavender (in small quantities) in breakfast cereals.

Many people don't like lentils and legumes, but there are lots of ways to prepare lentils or legumes to make them tasty. If you do not currently eat legumes, add them in small amounts to your meals so they don't overwhelm your taste buds.

If you don't tolerate legumes well or experience gut discomfort after eating them, you may find eating small quantities regularly will be more tolerable. Try eating a few tablespoons of hummus served with vegetable sticks, or some beans in a salad.

Try a variety of legumes in your meals, such as chickpeas, kidney beans, four-bean mix, cannellini beans, red, brown or puy lentils, split peas, borlotti beans, black-eyed beans, mung beans, soy beans, broad beans or flageolet beans.

Lentils and legumes can be bland on their own, so they often work best in dishes with strong flavours, like Indian and Mexican dishes.

Some ways that you can get extra beans into your diet include:
- **using tinned** (try to find ones with no added salt) or sprouted legumes (like mung beans or chickpeas) in salads
- **using fresh beans like broad beans** – especially if you are just starting to add beans to your diet – some people find the taste of fresh beans easier to handle at first; later you can start trying some of the heavier-style legumes
- **adding legumes to soups**
- **using red lentils in stews and sauces** – red lentils cook down and add thickness to a sauce; try substituting some of the meat in your recipe with lentils
- **using dahl** – highly spiced dishes like dahl can be a great way to make bland food much tastier
- **eating felafels and hummus** – a great way to eat chickpeas (particularly if you don't like the texture of whole beans).

Making healthier meals

Choosing healthy ingredients is one piece of the healthy-eating puzzle. How you cook those ingredients – what you do with them – is another piece. Adopting healthy ways to prepare your meals can make a difference to your overall diet.

Some healthier cooking methods that you can use include:

- **cooking with foil parcels** – these are great for vegetables (like potato, beetroot, pumpkin and turnip), fish, roast meats and chicken. Herbs like rosemary and parsley can be added to the parcels to add flavour.
- **cooking stews and casseroles** – you can cook a stew or casseroles by browning lean red meat or chicken and vegetables in 2 tablespoons of oil in a pan, adding a bit of water if the mixture gets too dry. Sprinkle a tablespoon of flour over the meat, then add salt-reduced stock or a can of tomatoes (adding a little extra water). Simmer for 1–2 hours. Serve the stew immediately – or if possible, cool it in the fridge and skim the fat off the top before reheating to serve.
- **steaming** – this allows you to cook skinless chicken, fish or vegetables. For a simple one-pot meal, place chicken or fish in the steamer and cook for 15–20 minutes. Add vegetables and cook for an extra 5 minutes.
- **oven-baking** – lay some lean meat, skinless chicken or fish on baking paper in an oven dish and drizzle over some extra virgin olive oil. Bake in the oven.
- **barbecuing or grilling** – you can grill lean meat, skinless chicken, fish or vegetables on the BBQ, or on a grill pan on your stovetop. Use a little oil on the meat/vegetables so they don't stick.
- **stir-frying** – cook finely sliced chicken, pork or beef in a little peanut or sunflower oil on a high heat. Add lots of finely sliced vegetables (such as cabbage, Asian vegetables, snow peas, capsicum, broccoli or carrot). Stir through some bean shoots just before serving for a bit of extra crunch.
- **poaching** – this is a great way to cook chicken or eggs. Place some water (5–10 cms depth) in a pan over a medium-low heat. When little bubbles appear on the bottom of the pan, add the chicken or eggs. Cook for 2–3 minutes for eggs, 15–20 minutes for a skinless chicken breast.
- **microwaving** – to cook a delicious meal, place some lean meat, skinless chicken, fish or vegetables in a microwave-safe container or bowl, adding a little water and herbs for extra flavour. Microwave on medium-high until cooked.

PART 3

MENU PLANS

AND RECIPES

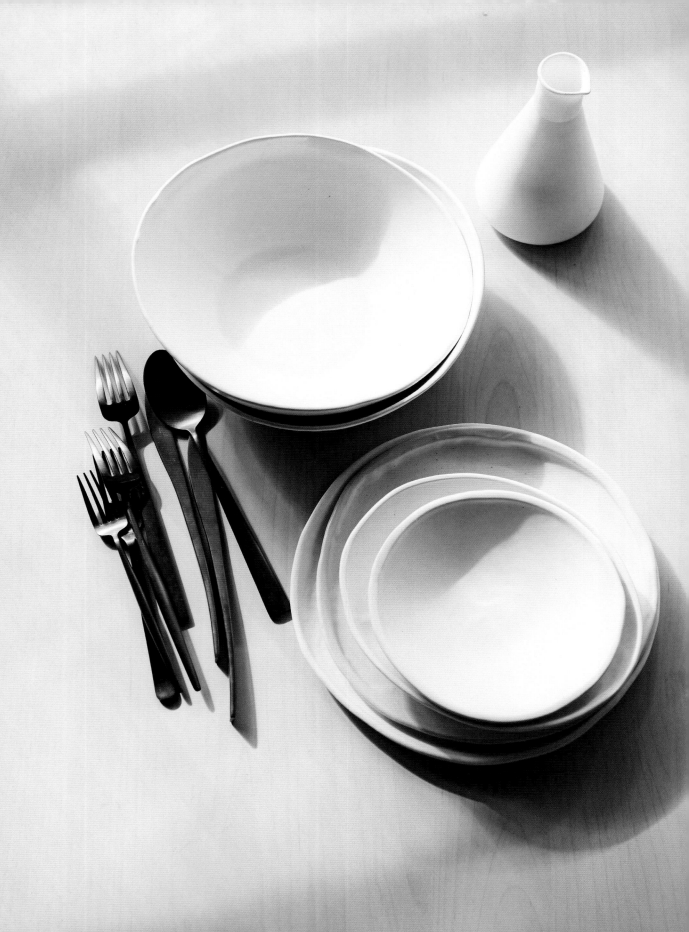

How to use the menu plans

The following menu plans have been designed to help you construct a dietary plan using the recipes in this book.

While this is not a weight loss book, maintaining a healthy weight or losing weight if you are overweight is an important part of disease prevention. Choosing the correct menu plan will assist with this.

Two menu plans have been developed, one of 6500kJ per day and one of 8500kJ per day. All menu plans are based on one serving size of the recipe mentioned unless otherwise stated.

Both men and women who want to lose weight should use the menu plan for 6500kJ per day. If you find you are not losing weight you may need to reduce your energy intake further by reducing the snack items within the menu plan. If you are losing weight more quickly than desired you may choose to increase the portion sizes a little, or add in an extra snack or two (follow the snack suggestions listed in the meal plans).

Both men and women who wish to maintain their existing weight should use the menu plan for 8500kJ per day. If you are gaining weight on this plan you may need to reduce the snack items within the menu plan. If you are losing weight you may choose to increase the portion sizes a little, or add in an extra snack or two (follow the snack suggestions listed in the meal plans).

How to use the recipes

The recipes are designed to assist you with making meals that meet the nutritional targets outlined in the previous chapters. Each recipe contains a nutritional analysis to help you understand more about your food intake and make choices on the best meals for your individual requirements.

The recipes specify low saturated fat, low added sugar and low salt ingredients. To ensure the recipes are suitable it is required that you use the correct ingredients.

The recipes all include nutritional information per serve including energy (kilojoules), saturated fat, protein, carbohydrate, fibre and sodium.

Those with specific dietary requirements may use this information to choose the best recipe options within the healthy recipes provided in this book.

Energy – Consider choosing higher or lower energy recipes depending on your energy and weight management needs.

Saturated fat – Linked with risk of heart disease and insulin resistance. If you are at high risk of, or have heart disease or diabetes, choose recipes under 4g saturated fat per serve.

Protein – Most recipes include lean protein sources. Balance your protein sources; include red meat 2-3 times a week, poultry 1-2 times a week and fish 2-3 times a week, and at least one meat free meal per week. Some people may benefit from a higher protein diet for weight management. Choose recipes with a higher protein and lower carbohydrate amount to aid weight management.

Carbohydrate – Most carbohydrate foods included in the recipes are from wholegrain, high fibre and low GI sources. All recipes are low in added sugars. However some people may benefit from a lower carbohydrate intake for weight management. Choose lower carbohydrate recipes to aid weight management. People who are very physically active may require more carbohydrate and should choose higher carbohydrate recipes.

Fibre – Most recipes are high in fibre. A high fibre diet can aid weight management and reduce the risk of bowel cancer. Choose recipes more than 5g fibre per serve.

Sodium – Most recipes are low in sodium. Sodium is linked with blood pressure and risk of heart disease. If you are at high risk of heart disease or have high blood pressure, choose recipes under 600mg sodium per serve.

6,500 kJ plan - Week 1

	DAY 1	DAY 2	DAY 3
BREAKFAST	• 1 serve oat, barley and buckwheat bircher muesli (see p 126) Snacks: apple	• 2 slices wholegrain sourdough toast with ¼ avocado, • 1 medium tomato and a sprinkle of dukkah (see p 293) Snacks: tub of healthy choice yoghurt**	• 30 g traditional oats with ½ cup skim milk, 1 tablespoon dried fruit and 1 teaspoon honey Snacks: 200 g reduced-fat Greek-style yoghurt, 5 strawberries
LUNCH	• Chopped salad with smoked rainbow trout (see p 171) Snacks: peach, tub of healthy choice yoghurt**	• Carrot, zucchini and chickpea slice (see p 149) Snacks: orange, 30 g mixed raw, unsalted nuts	• Scallop and noodle lettuce cups (see p 158) Snacks: small carrot, Lebanese cucumber, Pumpkin and red lentil dip (see p 263)
DINNER	• Beef and vegetable curry (see p 207)	• Okonomiyaki with pork leg steaks (see p 223)	• Rocket, potato and chickpea soup (p 193)

* ie, no added salt or sugar – check the ingredients list

** Healthy yoghurt options include low fat, natural or Greek yoghurt, or flavoured low fat yoghurt with no added sugar (Tamar Valley No Added Sugar, Nestle Soleil and Yoplait Forme)

*** Healthy multigrain biscuit options include Vita-Weat or Ryvita

6,500 kJ plan - Week 1

DAY 4	DAY 5	DAY 6	DAY 7
• 2 slices wholegrain sourdough toast with 2 tablespoons 100% peanut butter* and ½ banana	• 1 serve oat, barley and buckwheat bircher muesli (see p 126) Snacks: apple, 20 almonds, tub of healthy choice yoghurt**	• Roasted mushrooms with spinach and poached eggs (see p 128) Snacks: tub of healthy choice yoghurt**	• Breakfast banana split (see p 122) Snacks: Pumpkin and red lentil dip (see p 263), 1 serve healthy multigrain biscuits***
• Lamb souvlaki wrap with garlic sauce (see p 142) Snacks: apple	• Broccolini, broccoli and tofu salad (see p 168) Snacks: Pumpkin and red lentil dip (see p 263), 1 serve healthy multigrain biscuits***	• Hot and sour seafood soup (see p 189) Snacks: apple	• Cauliflower and cannellini bean pizza crust with smoked salmon (see p 141) Snacks: orange
• Black bean and jalapeño burgers with avocado tomato salsa (see p 215) • Coconut and lime chia pudding (see p 278)	• Chargrilled chicken with charred peach salsa (see p 237)	• Dukkah-crusted butterflied sardines with freekeh and cauliflower pilaf (see p 253) • Berry tiramisu (see p 274)	• Italian-herb stuffed roast beef and cavolo nero with anchovy crumbs (see p 238)

6,500 kJ plan - Week 2

	DAY 1	DAY 2	DAY 3
BREAKFAST	• 2 slices wholegrain sourdough toast with 2 tablespoons 100% peanut butter* and 1 medium tomato Snacks: 2 kiwifruit, tub of healthy choice yoghurt**	• ½ serve oat, barley and buckwheat bircher muesli (see p 126) with ½ cup skim milk and ½ banana Snacks: apple	• 2 slices wholegrain sourdough toast with 2 tablespoons 100% peanut butter* and ½ banana
LUNCH	• Roasted cauliflower and black lentil salad (see p 176) Snacks: 20 g mixed raw, unsalted nuts	• Prawn and mushroom pot stickers (see p 153) Snacks: peach, tub of healthy choice yoghurt**	• Pan-seared squid with tarragon dressing (see p 175) Snacks: Spiced baked apple chips (see p 271)
DINNER	• Tuna, lemon and herb 'meatballs' (see p 227)	• Kangaroo, lentil and eggplant moussaka (see p 220)	• Chicken, lemon and dill soup (see p 185) • No-churn avocado, lime and cardamom ice cream (see p 285)

* ie, no added salt or sugar – check the ingredients list

** Healthy yoghurt options include low fat, natural or Greek yoghurt, or flavoured low fat yoghurt with no added sugar (Tamar Valley No Added Sugar, Nestle Soleil and Yoplait Forme)

*** Healthy multigrain biscuit options include Vita-Weat or Ryvita

6,500 kJ plan - Week 2

DAY 4	DAY 5	DAY 6	DAY 7
• 2 slices wholegrain sourdough toast with 125 g low-fat cottage cheese, 1 medium tomato and 1 tablespoon pesto Snacks: apple	• ½ serve oat, barley and buckwheat bircher muesli (see p 126) with ½ cup skim milk and 5 strawberries Snacks: 1 cup grapes	• 1 serve oat, barley and buckwheat bircher muesli (see p 126) Snacks: 1 cup fruit salad, 100 g reduced-fat Greek-style yoghurt	• Breakfast rice with poached eggs, kimchi and choy sum (see p131)
• Thai turkey omelette wrap (see p 154) Snacks: Black bean dip (see p 262), small carrot, Lebanese cucumber	• Chunky beetroot, farro and vegetable soup (see p 186) Snacks: tub of healthy choice yoghurt**	• Spicy fish tacos (see p 150) Snacks: Cauliflower 'popcorn' (see p 260)	• Tarragon chicken with celeriac-mustard mash (see p 231) Snacks: Spiced baked apple chips (see p 271)
• Braised lentils and silverbeet with teff and poached eggs (see p 216)	• Roast beef with cauliflower 'steaks' and salsa verde (see p 200)	• Pork steaks with pear and cider sauce and celeriac-borlotti bean mash (see p 241) • Maple-baked pears with whipped ricotta (see p 282)	• Grilled blue-eye trevalla with roasted capsicums, tomatoes and butter beans (see p 257)

6,500 kJ plan - Week 3

	DAY 1	DAY 2	DAY 3
BREAKFAST	• 2 slices wholegrain sourdough toast with 125 g low-fat cottage cheese, 1 medium tomato and 1 tablespoon pesto Snacks: ½ mango, 150 g reduced-fat Greek-style yoghurt	• ½ serve oat, barley and buckwheat bircher muesli (see p 126) with ½ cup skim milk and ½ banana Snacks: Baba ganoush (see p 262), 1 serve healthy multigrain biscuits***	• 2 slices wholegrain sourdough toast with ¼ avocado, 1 medium tomato and a sprinkle of dukkah (see p 293) Snacks: 200 g reduced-fat Greek-style yoghurt, 5 strawberries
LUNCH	• Ocean trout ramen (see p 194)	• Baked ricotta with roasted cherry tomatoes (see p 148) Snacks: apple, 30 g mixed raw, unsalted nuts	• Tuna, tomato, lentil and chickpea salad (see p 179) Snacks: Baba ganoush (see p 262), 1 serve healthy multigrain biscuits***
DINNER	• Lamb cutlets with fattoush and baba ganoush (see p 208)	• Smokey braised pork and black beans (see p 224)	• Turkey and zucchini kofte with iceberg salad (see p 228)

* ie, no added salt or sugar – check the ingredients list

** Healthy yoghurt options include low fat, natural or Greek yoghurt, or flavoured low fat yoghurt with no added sugar (Tamar Valley No Added Sugar, Nestle Soleil and Yoplait Forme)

*** Healthy multigrain biscuit options include Vita-Weat or Ryvita

6,500 kJ plan - Week 3

DAY 4	DAY 5	DAY 6	DAY 7
• 2 slices wholegrain sourdough toast with 2 tablespoons 100% peanut butter* and 1 medium tomato Snacks: apple	• ½ serve oat, barley and buckwheat bircher muesli (see p 126) with ½ cup skim milk and 5 strawberries Snacks: pear, tub of healthy choice yoghurt**	• Baked pear and blueberry porridge (see p 127)	• Wholegrain sourdough with green smash and shredded chicken (see p 135) Snacks: 2 apricots
• Gado gado (see p 172) Snacks: Chocolate and pistachio madeleines (see p 267)	• Super greens soup (see p 197) Snacks: 20 g 70% cocoa dark chocolate, 30 g mixed raw, unsalted nuts	• Mexican chicken wrap (see p 146)	• Freekeh salad with chargrilled prawns (see p 145) Snacks: 5 strawberries, tub of healthy choice yoghurt**
• Caramelised leek, lentil, mushroom and thyme tarts (see p 254)	• Spicy Italian mussels with tomato and pearl couscous (see p 250)	• Baked rainbow trout with roasted vegetables and caper-parsley sauce (see p 234) • Milk and rosewater jelly with tropical fruit (see p 281)	• Slow-cooked lamb with green rice (see p 246)

6,500 kJ plan - Week 4

	DAY 1	DAY 2	DAY 3
BREAKFAST	• 30 g traditional oats with ½ cup low fat milk, 1 tablespoon dried fruit and 1 teaspoon honey Snacks: **30 g mixed raw, unsalted nuts**	• 2 slices wholegrain sourdough toast with 2 tablespoons 100% peanut butter* and 1 medium tomato Snacks: **apple**	• ½ serve oat, barley and buckwheat bircher muesli (see p 126) with ½ cup skim milk and ½ banana Snacks: **Canellini bean, pea and parsley dip (see p 263), 1 serve healthy multigrain biscuits***
LUNCH	• Asian slaw with poached turkey (see p 164) Snacks: **mango, tub of healthy choice yoghurt****	• Broccoli and pea soup with scallops (see p 182) Snacks: **Eggplant and zucchini 'fries' (see p 264)**	• Beef and bean quesadillas (see p 138) Snacks: **1 cup chopped pineapple, tub of healthy choice yoghurt****
DINNER	• Salmon with parsnip fries and cannellini bean and pea puree (see p 249)	• Mushroom bolognese (see p 211)	• Harissa fish with freekeh and cauliflower pilaf (see p 212)

* ie, no added salt or sugar – check the ingredients list

** Healthy yoghurt options include low fat, natural or Greek yoghurt, or flavoured low fat yoghurt with no added sugar (Tamar Valley No Added Sugar, Nestle Soleil and Yoplait Forme)

*** Healthy multigrain biscuit options include Vita-Weat or Ryvita

6,500 kJ plan - Week 4

DAY 4	DAY 5	DAY 6	DAY 7
• 2 slices wholegrain sourdough toast with ¼ avocado, 1 medium tomato and a sprinkle of dukkah (see p 293) Snacks: Fruity yoghurt popsicles (see p 268)	• 2 slices wholegrain sourdough toast with 2 tablespoons 100% peanut butter* and ½ banana Snacks: orange	• Wholemeal buckwheat pancakes with rhubarb, strawberries and whipped ricotta (see p 125)	• Smoky baked beans and chickpeas (see p 132) Snacks: 30 g mixed raw, unsalted nuts
• Moroccan pumpkin and lentil soup with dukkah-dusted rainbow trout (see p 190) Snacks: apple, 125g low-fat cottage cheese, 1 serve healthy multigrain biscuits***	• Black-eyed bean salad with flaked chia flathead (see p 167) Snacks: Canellini bean, pea and parsley dip (see p 263), 1 serve healthy multigrain biscuits***	• Spinach and chickpea pakoras with tomato sambal (see p 161) Snacks: 125 g low-fat cottage cheese, 1 serve healthy multigrain biscuits***	• Salmon ceviche with witlof salad (see p 157) Snacks: 1 cup fruit salad, 200 g reduced-fat Greek-style yoghurt
• Bibimbap (see p 219)	• Maple and soy-glazed pork with vegetable stir-fry (see p 203)	• Provencal fish stew with red capsicum rouille (see p 242) • Baked custard with peaches (see p 277)	• Braised lamb shanks with eggplant and zucchini (see p 245)

6,500 kJ meal plan disclaimer

This dietary intake, if using standard dairy products, is inadequate in calcium for adult men and women of all ages. It is recommended people following this meal plan take a calcium supplement (a dose containing at least 500 mg calcium if you are aged under 65 years, and containing at least 800 mg calcium if you are aged over 65 years).

Menstruating women following this meal plan will have an inadequate intake of iron. It is recommended menstruating women following this meal plan take an iron supplement containing 5 mg iron per day and have their iron levels monitored by their GP if following this plan for longer than 3 months.

Adult men following this meal plan will have an inadequate intake of zinc. It is recommended men following this meal plan take a zinc supplement containing 5 mg zinc per day.

This dietary intake is not suitable for women who are pregnant or who are trying to fall pregnant.

8,500 kJ plan - Week 1

	DAY 1	DAY 2	DAY 3
BREAKFAST	• 1 serve oat, barley and buckwheat bircher muesli (see p 126) • 250 ml skim milk**** or 120 g low-fat ricotta or cottage cheese Snacks: **40 g reduced-fat cheese, 1 serve healthy multigrain biscuits***	• 2 slices wholegrain sourdough toast with ¼ avocado, 1 medium tomato and a sprinkle of dukkah (see p 293) • 250 ml skim milk**** or 120 g low-fat ricotta or cottage cheese Snacks: **orange, tub of healthy choice yoghurt**	• 30 g traditional oats with ½ cup skim milk, 1 tablespoon dried fruit and 2 teaspoons honey • 250 ml skim milk**** or 120 g low-fat ricotta or cottage cheese Snacks: **Pumpkin and red lentil dip (see p 263), small carrot, Lebanese cucumber**
LUNCH	• Chopped salad with smoked rainbow trout (see p 171) Snacks: **apple, 2 peaches, tub of healthy choice yoghurt**	• Carrot, zucchini and chickpea slice (see p 149) Snacks: **50 g mixed raw, unsalted nuts**	• Scallop and noodle lettuce cups (see p 158) Snacks: **200 g reduced-fat Greek-style yoghurt, 5 strawberries**
DINNER	• Beef and vegetable curry (see p 207)	• Okonomiyaki with pork leg steaks (see p 223)	• Rocket, potato and chickpea soup (p 193)

* ie, no added salt or sugar – check the ingredients list

** Healthy yoghurt options include low fat, natural or Greek yoghurt, or flavoured low fat yoghurt with no added sugar (Tamar Valley No Added Sugar, Nestle Soleil and Yoplait Forme)

*** Healthy multigrain biscuit options include Vita-Weat or Ryvita

**** or medium size coffee made on milk (e.g. skinny cafe latte)

8,500 kJ plan - Week 1

DAY 4	DAY 5	DAY 6	DAY 7
• 2 slices wholegrain sourdough toast with 3 tablespoons 100% peanut butter* and 1 banana • 250 ml skim milk**** or 120 g low-fat ricotta or cottage cheese Snacks: apple, 1 cup grapes, tub of healthy choice yoghurt**	• 1 serve oat, barley and buckwheat bircher muesli (see p 126) • 250 ml skim milk**** or 120 g low-fat ricotta or cottage cheese Snacks: Pumpkin and red lentil dip (see p 263), 1 serve healthy multigrain biscuits***	• Roasted mushrooms with spinach and poached eggs (see p 128) with 1 slice wholegrain sourdough bread • 250 ml skim milk**** or 120 g low-fat ricotta or cottage cheese Snacks: apple, tub of healthy choice yoghurt**	• Breakfast banana split (see p 122) • 250 ml skim milk**** or 120 g low-fat ricotta or cottage cheese Snacks: Pumpkin and red lentil dip (see p 263), 1 serve healthy multigrain biscuits***
• Lamb souvlaki wrap with garlic sauce (see p 142) Snacks: Pumpkin and red lentil dip (see p 263), small carrot, Lebanese cucumber	• Broccolini, broccoli and tofu salad (see p 168) Snacks: apple, 40 almonds, tub of healthy choice yoghurt**	• Hot and sour seafood soup (see p 189) Snacks: ½ avocado, 1 teaspoon dukkah (see p 293), 1 serve healthy multigrain biscuits***	• Cauliflower and cannellini bean pizza crust with smoked salmon (see p 141) Snacks: orange, 200 g reduced-fat Greek-style yoghurt, 2 teaspoons honey, 30 g mixed raw, unsalted nuts
• Black bean and jalapeño burgers with avocado tomato salsa (see p 215) • Coconut and lime chia pudding (see p 278)	• Chargrilled chicken with charred peach salsa (see p 237)	• Dukkah-crusted butterflied sardines with freekeh and cauliflower pilaf (see p 253) • Berry tiramisu (see p 274)	• Italian-herb stuffed roast beef and cavolo nero with anchovy crumbs (see p 238)

8,500 kJ plan - Week 2

	DAY 1	DAY 2	DAY 3
BREAKFAST	• 2 slices wholegrain sourdough toast with 2 tablespoons 100% peanut butter* and 1 medium tomato • 250 ml skim milk**** Snacks: 1 serve healthy multigrain biscuits***, 125 g low-fat cottage cheese	• 1 serve oat, barley and buckwheat bircher muesli (see p 126) with ¾ cup skim milk and 1 banana • 250 ml skim milk**** or 120 g low-fat ricotta or cottage cheese Snacks: 1 tablespoon 100% peanut butter*, 1 serve healthy multigrain biscuits***	• 2 slices wholegrain sourdough toast with 2 tablespoons 100% peanut butter* and 1 banana • 250 ml skim milk**** or 120 g low-fat ricotta or cottage cheese Snacks: Spiced baked apple chips (see p 271)
LUNCH	• Roasted cauliflower and black lentil salad (see p 176), • ½ avocado Snacks: 2 kiwifruit, 30 g mixed raw, unsalted nuts, tub of healthy choice yoghurt**	• Prawn and mushroom pot stickers (see p 153) Snacks: apple, 2 peaches, tub of healthy choice yoghurt**	• Pan-seared squid with tarragon dressing (see p 57), 1 slice wholegrain sourdough bread Snacks: 100 g reduced-fat Greek-style yoghurt
DINNER	• Tuna, lemon and herb 'meatballs' (see p 109)	• Kangaroo, lentil and eggplant moussaka (see p 220)	• Chicken, lemon and dill soup (see p 185) • No-churn avocado, lime and cardamom ice cream (see p 285)

* ie, no added salt or sugar – check the ingredients list

** Healthy yoghurt options include low fat, natural or Greek yoghurt, or flavoured low fat yoghurt with no added sugar (Tamar Valley No Added Sugar, Nestle Soleil and Yoplait Forme)

*** Healthy multigrain biscuit options include Vita-Weat or Ryvita

**** or medium size coffee made on milk (e.g. skinny cafe latte)

8,500 kJ plan - Week 2

DAY 4	DAY 5	DAY 6	DAY 7
• 2 slices wholegrain sourdough toast with 125 g low-fat cottage cheese, 1 medium tomato and 1 tablespoon pesto • 250 ml skim milk**** or 120 g low-fat ricotta or cottage cheese Snacks: Black bean dip (see p 262), small carrot, Lebanese cucumber	• 1 serve oat, barley and buckwheat bircher muesli (see p 126) with ¾ cup skim milk and 6 strawberries • 250 ml skim milk**** or 120 g low-fat ricotta or cottage cheese Snacks: 1 cup grapes, tub of healthy choice yoghurt**	• 1 serve oat, barley and buckwheat bircher muesli (see p 126) • 250 ml skim milk**** or 120 g low-fat ricotta or cottage cheese Snacks: Cauliflower 'popcorn' (see p 260)	• Breakfast rice with poached eggs, kimchi and choy sum (see p 131) • 250 ml skim milk**** or 120 g low-fat ricotta or cottage cheese Snacks: Spiced baked apple chips (see p 271), tub of healthy choice yoghurt**
• Thai turkey omelette wrap (see p 154) Snacks: apple, 80 g can tuna in sunflower oil, drained	• Chunky beetroot, farro and vegetable soup (see p 186), 1 slice wholegrain sourdough bread Snacks: 20 g reduced-fat cheese, ¼ avocado, 1 serve healthy multigrain biscuits***	• Spicy fish tacos (see p 150) Snacks: banana, 1 cup fruit salad, 100 g reduced-fat Greek-style yoghurt	• Tarragon chicken with celeriac-mustard mash (see p 231) Snacks: Cauliflower 'popcorn' (see p 260)
• Braised lentils and silverbeet with teff and poached eggs (see p 216)	• Roast beef with cauliflower 'steaks' and salsa verde (see p 200)	• Pork steaks with pear and cider sauce and celeriac-borlotti bean mash (see p 241) • Maple-baked pears with whipped ricotta (see p 282)	• Grilled blue-eye trevalla with roasted capsicums, tomatoes and butter beans (see p 257)

8,500 kJ plan - Week 3

	DAY 1	DAY 2	DAY 3
BREAKFAST	• 3 slices wholegrain sourdough toast with 200 g low-fat cottage cheese, 1 large tomato and 2 tablespoons pesto • 250 ml skim milk**** or 120 g low-fat ricotta or cottage cheese Snacks: apple, 20 almonds	• 3 slices wholegrain sourdough toast with 1 boiled egg, ½ avocado, 1 medium tomato and 2 teaspoons dukkah (see p 293) • 250 ml skim milk**** or 120 g low-fat ricotta or cottage cheese Snacks: apple, 50 g mixed raw, unsalted nuts	• 1 serve oat, barley and buckwheat bircher muesli (see p 126) with ¾ cup skim milk, 1 banana • 250 ml skim milk**** or 120 g low-fat ricotta or cottage cheese Snacks: Baba ganoush (see p 262), 1 serve healthy multigrain biscuits***
LUNCH	• Ocean trout ramen (see p 194) Snacks: mango, 150 g reduced-fat Greek-style yoghurt	• Baked ricotta with roasted cherry tomatoes (see p 148) Snacks: banana, Baba ganoush (see p 262), 1 serve healthy multigrain biscuits***	• Tuna, tomato, lentil and chickpea salad (see p 179) Snacks: 200 g reduced-fat Greek-style yoghurt, 5 strawberries, 50 g mixed raw, unsalted nuts
DINNER	• Lamb cutlets with fattoush and baba ganoush (see p 208)	• Smokey braised pork and black beans (see p 224)	• Turkey and zucchini kofte with iceberg salad (see p 228)

* ie, no added salt or sugar – check the ingredients list

** Healthy yoghurt options include low fat, natural or Greek yoghurt, or flavoured low fat yoghurt with no added sugar (Tamar Valley No Added Sugar, Nestle Soleil and Yoplait Forme)

*** Healthy multigrain biscuit options include Vita-Weat or Ryvita

**** or medium size coffee made on milk (e.g. skinny cafe latte)

8,500 kJ plan - Week 3

DAY 4	DAY 5	DAY 6	DAY 7
• 1 serve oat, barley and buckwheat bircher muesli (see p 126) with ½ cup skim milk and 5 strawberries • 250 ml skim milk**** or 120 g low-fat ricotta or cottage cheese Snacks: pear, 40 g reduced-fat cheese, 1 serve healthy multigrain biscuits***	• 1 serve oat, barley and buckwheat bircher muesli (see p 126) with ¾ cup skim milk and 6 strawberries • 250 ml skim milk**** or 120 g low-fat ricotta or cottage cheese Snacks: 1 cup grapes, tub of healthy choice yoghurt**	• Baked pear and blueberry porridge (see p 127) • 250 ml skim milk**** or 120 g low-fat ricotta or cottage cheese	• Wholegrain sourdough with green smash and shredded chicken (see p 135) with additional slice wholegrain sourdough • 250 ml skim milk**** or 120 g low-fat ricotta or cottage cheese Snacks: 2 apricots, 50 g mixed raw, unsalted nuts, 30 g dried fruit
• Gado gado (see p 172) Snacks: Chocolate and pistachio madeleines (see p 267)	• Super greens soup (see p 197) with 1 slice wholegrain sourdough bread Snacks: 20 g 70% cocoa dark chocolate, 30 g mixed raw, unsalted nuts, tub of healthy choice yoghurt**	• Mexican chicken wrap (see p 146) with ¼ avocado Snacks: 40 g reduced-fat cheese, 1 serve healthy multigrain biscuits***	• Freekeh salad with chargrilled prawns (see p 145) Snacks: 5 strawberries, tub of healthy choice yoghurt**
• Caramelised leek, lentil, mushroom and thyme tarts (see p 254)	• Spicy Italian mussels with tomato and pearl couscous (see p 250)	• Baked rainbow trout with roasted vegetables and caper-parsley sauce (see p 234) • Milk and rosewater jelly with tropical fruit (see p 281)	• Slow-cooked lamb with green rice (see p 246)

8,500 kJ plan - Week 4

	DAY 1	DAY 2	DAY 3
BREAKFAST	• 60 g traditional oats with 1 cup skim milk, 2 tablespoons dried fruit and 2 teaspoons honey • 250 ml skim milk**** or 120 g low-fat ricotta or cottage cheese Snacks: 50 g mixed raw, unsalted nuts	• 3 slices wholegrain sourdough toast with 3 tablespoons 100% peanut butter* and 1 medium tomato • 250 ml skim milk**** or 120 g low-fat ricotta or cottage cheese Snacks: apple, orange	• 1 serve oat, barley and buckwheat bircher muesli (see p 126) with 1 cup skim milk and 1 banana • 250 ml skim milk**** or 120 g low-fat ricotta or cottage cheese Snacks: Canellini bean, pea and parsley dip (see p 263), 1 serve healthy multigrain biscuits***
LUNCH	• Ocean trout ramen (see p 194) Snacks: mango, 150 g reduced-fat Greek-style yoghurt	• Broccoli and pea soup with scallops (see p 182) Snacks: Eggplant and zucchini 'fries' (see p 264)	• Beef and bean quesadillas (see p 138) Snacks: 1 cup pineapple, tub of healthy choice yoghurt**
DINNER	• Salmon with parsnip fries and cannellini bean and pea puree (see p 249)	• Mushroom bolognese (see p 211)	• Bibimbap (see p 219)

* ie, no added salt or sugar – check the ingredients list

** Healthy yoghurt options include low fat, natural or Greek yoghurt, or flavoured low fat yoghurt with no added sugar (Tamar Valley No Added Sugar, Nestle Soleil and Yoplait Forme)

*** Healthy multigrain biscuit options include Vita-Weat or Ryvita

**** or medium size coffee made on milk (e.g. skinny cafe latte)

8,500 kJ plan - Week 4

DAY 4	DAY 5	DAY 6	DAY 7
• 2 slices wholegrain sourdough toast with ½ avocado, 1 medium tomato and a sprinkle of dukkah (see p 175) • 250 ml skim milk**** or 120 g low-fat ricotta or cottage cheese Snacks: 1½ serves healthy multigrain biscuits***, 150 g low-fat cottage cheese, apple	• 3 slices wholegrain sourdough toast with 3 tablespoons 100% peanut butter* and ½ banana • 250 ml skim milk**** or 120 g low-fat ricotta or cottage cheese Snacks: orange, 30 g mixed raw, unsalted nuts	• Wholemeal buckwheat pancakes with rhubarb, strawberries and whipped ricotta (see p 125) • 250 ml skim milk**** or 120 g low-fat ricotta or cottage cheese Snacks: 50 g mixed raw, unsalted nuts	• Smoky baked beans and chickpeas (see p 132) • 250 ml skim milk**** or 120 g low-fat ricotta or cottage cheese Snacks: 1 serve healthy multigrain biscuits***, 2 teaspoons pesto, medium tomato
• Moroccan pumpkin and lentil soup with dukkah-dusted rainbow trout (see p 190) Snacks: Fruity yoghurt popsicles (see p 268)	• Black-eyed bean salad with flaked chia flathead (see p 167) Snacks: Canellini bean, pea and parsley dip (see p 263), 1 serve healthy multigrain biscuits***	• Spinach and chickpea pakoras with tomato sambal (see p 161) Snacks: 125 g low-fat cottage cheese, 1 serve healthy multigrain biscuits***	• Salmon ceviche with witlof salad (see p 157) Snacks: apple, 1 cup fruit salad, 200 g reduced-fat Greek-style yoghurt
• Maple and soy-glazed pork with vegetable stir-fry (see p 203)	• Spicy Italian mussels with tomato and pearl couscous (see p 250)	• Provincial fish stew with red capsicum rouille (see p 242) • Baked custard with peaches (see p 277)	• Slow-cooked lamb with green rice (see p 246)

8,500 kJ meal plan disclaimer

This dietary intake, if using standard dairy products, is inadequate in calcium for adult men over 75 years of age and adult women over 65 years of age. It is recommended people of these ages following this meal plan take a calcium supplement dose containing at least 400 mg calcium.

Menstruating women following this meal plan will have a slightly inadequate intake of iron. It is recommended menstruating women following this meal plan have their iron levels monitored by their GP if following this plan for longer than 3 months.

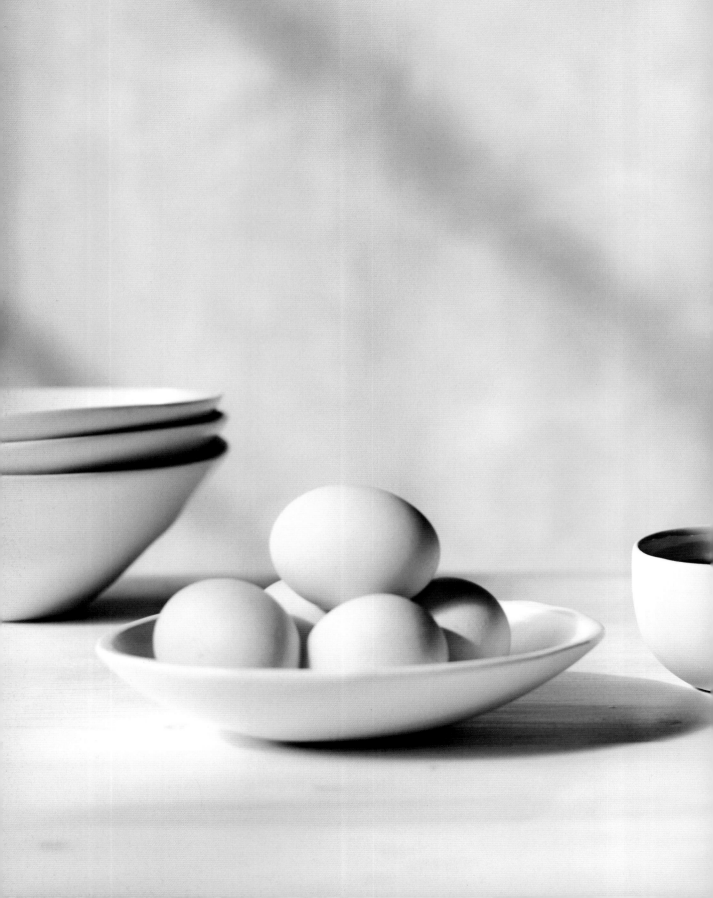

BREAKFASTS

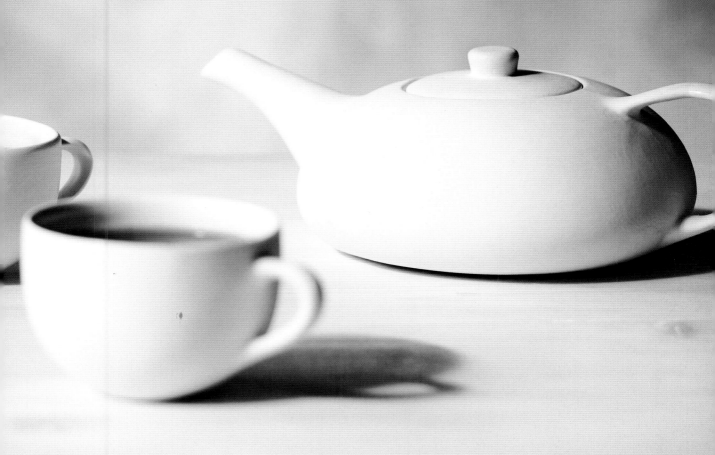

Breakfast banana split

This yummy breakfast really sets you up for the day. The bananas and muesli give you energy while the refreshing watermelon and yoghurt add a lightness to the dish that is topped off with the decadent sweetness of the passionfruit.

SERVES 4

PREP TIME 15 MINUTES, PLUS 2 HOURS OR OVERNIGHT SOAKING

COOKING TIME NIL

4 small bananas, peeled

⅔ cup (190 g) reduced-fat natural Greek-style yoghurt

½ quantity homemade oat, barley and buckwheat bircher muesli (see page 126), omitting the berries, nuts and seeds (the nashi pear should still be stirred in)

1 cup (160 g) diced watermelon

2 passionfruit

2 tablespoons roughly chopped unsalted macadamias

2 tablespoons sunflower seeds

1. Cut each of the bananas in half lengthways, and divide among 4 shallow serving bowls. Top each split banana with one-quarter of the yoghurt, bircher muesli and watermelon.

2. Cut both passionfruit in half, and scoop the pulp from each half to drizzle over the top of each dish.

3. Sprinkle with the nuts and seeds, then serve.

NUTRITIONAL ANALYSIS	ENERGY (KJ)	1552	CARBOHYDRATE (G)	52	SODIUM (MG)	51
TO SERVE 4 (PER SERVE)	PROTEIN (G)	9	SATURATED FAT (G)	3.8	FIBRE (G)	8

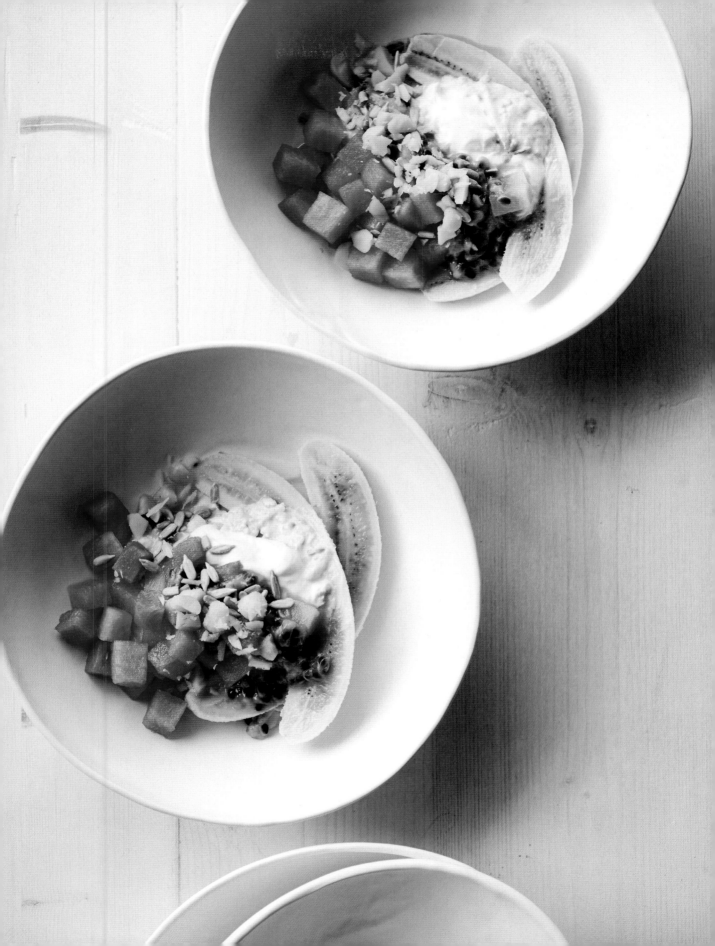

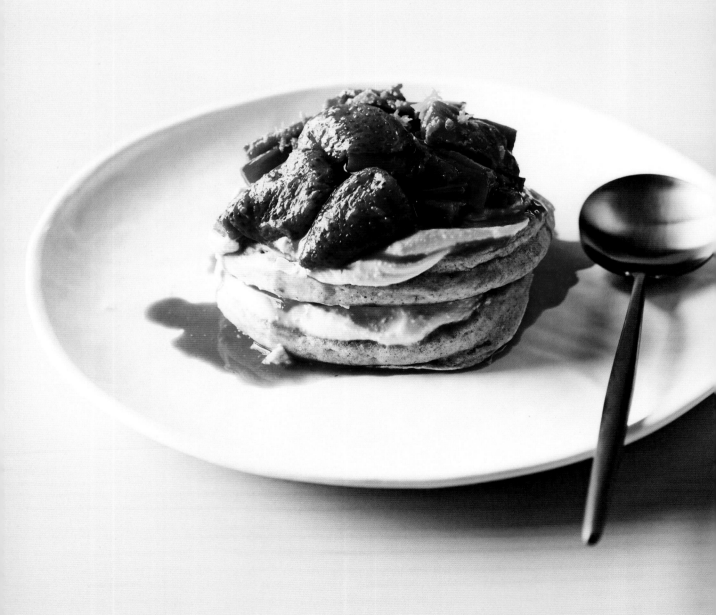

Wholemeal buckwheat pancakes with rhubarb, strawberries and whipped ricotta

These light, fluffy pancakes have an earthy flavour, which is complemented by the sweet and tangy fruit and creamy ricotta. If the rhubarb and strawberries are not at their peak or if they are slightly tart, add a teaspoon or two of maple syrup or honey to sweeten when you serve.

SERVES 4
PREP TIME 20 MINUTES
COOKING TIME 30 MINUTES

500 g strawberries, hulled, and halved if large
300 g trimmed rhubarb stalks, cut into 4 cm lengths
finely grated zest of 1 orange
juice of 2 oranges, including pulp
1½ cups (300 g) fresh, firm low-fat ricotta

WHOLEMEAL BUCKWHEAT PANCAKES
⅔ cup (160 ml) buttermilk
2 large eggs
½ cup (80 g) wholemeal plain flour
½ cup (75 g) buckwheat flour
1 teaspoon baking powder
¼ teaspoon bicarbonate of soda
light olive oil spray, for cooking

1. Place the strawberries and rhubarb in a large, heavy-based saucepan. Add half of the orange zest, reserving the remainder for serving, along with the orange juice and pulp. Bring to the boil over medium heat, then reduce the heat to low and simmer, stirring occasionally, for 5–6 minutes or until the fruit is tender. Remove from the heat and, using a sieve, strain over a bowl, pushing down on the solid fruit to strain all the liquid.

2. Set the solid fruit aside to cool, and return the liquid to the pan. Boil over high heat for 4–5 minutes or until thickened and syrupy. Transfer to a small heatproof bowl and set aside to cool.

3. Whip the ricotta and ¼ cup (60 ml) of the cooled syrup in a food processor or blender until smooth. Add a little more syrup to adjust the consistency if required. It should be smooth, but not runny.

4. Preheat the oven to 100°C (80°C fan-forced). Line a baking tray with baking paper.

5. For the pancakes, whisk the buttermilk and eggs in a large bowl until combined. Sift the flours, baking powder and bicarbonate of soda over the buttermilk mixture, tipping the husks from the sieve into the bowl. Whisk until well combined.

6. Heat a large non-stick frying pan over low–medium heat. Spray the pan lightly with oil then, working in batches, measure just less than ¼ cup (60 ml) of the batter into the pan for each pancake. Gently tilt the pan to spread out the batter to a thickness of about 1 cm. Cook for 2 minutes or until the pancakes begin to set around the edge and bubbles start to appear on the surface. Flip them over and cook on the other side for another 1–2 minutes until puffed, lightly browned and cooked through. Transfer to the prepared tray, cover loosely with foil and keep warm in the oven. Repeat with the remaining batter to make a total of 8 pancakes.

7. Serve 2 pancakes per person, topped with one-quarter of the whipped ricotta, drained fruit, remaining syrup and zest. You could also dollop some of the ricotta between the pancakes, if you like.

Transfer to a small bowl, then cover with plastic film and refrigerate until required. Reserve the remaining syrup for serving.

NUTRITIONAL ANALYSIS	ENERGY (KJ)	1401	CARBOHYDRATE (G)	38	SODIUM (MG)	791
TO SERVE 4 (PER SERVE)	PROTEIN (G)	20	SATURATED FAT (G)	4.5	FIBRE (G)	7

Oat, barley and buckwheat bircher muesli

The raw buckwheat adds an interesting flavour – earthy, and slightly nutty – and gives this breakfast favourite a lovely crunch. The use of rolled barley is also a bit different, but you can make up the quantity with rolled oats if you'd prefer. Similarly, the nashi pear can be replaced with grated apple or pear, or even fresh figs.

SERVES 4
PREP TIME 15 MINUTES, PLUS 2 HOURS OR OVERNIGHT SOAKING
COOKING TIME NIL

¾ cup (65 g) rolled oats
¼ cup (45 g) raw unhulled buckwheat, rinsed
¼ cup (30 g) rolled barley
juice of 2 oranges, including pulp
1 nashi pear, unpeeled and grated
1 cup (280 g) reduced-fat natural Greek-style yoghurt
125 g raspberries
125 g blueberries
1 tablespoon natural flaked almonds, toasted
1 tablespoon sunflower seeds
1 tablespoon sesame seeds, toasted
1 tablespoon honey (optional)

1. Combine the oats, buckwheat, barley and orange juice in a bowl. Add about ⅓ cup (80 ml) water, or just enough to ensure the mixture is almost covered in liquid. Cover and refrigerate for a minimum of 2 hours, or overnight.

2. Just before serving, stir in the nashi and yoghurt. Divide the muesli among 4 bowls and scatter evenly with the berries, almonds and seeds. Drizzle with the honey (if using).

NUTRITIONAL ANALYSIS	ENERGY (KJ)	1392	CARBOHYDRATE (G)	51	SODIUM (MG)	45
TO SERVE 4 (PER SERVE)	PROTEIN (G)	9	SATURATED FAT (G)	2.8	FIBRE (G)	8

Baked pear and blueberry porridge

The blueberries provide a lovely 'pop' of sweetness when you bite into them.
A drizzle of honey or maple syrup would also work well as a sweet topping.

SERVES 4

PREP TIME 10 MINUTES, PLUS 10 MINUTES STANDING

COOKING TIME 40 MINUTES

2 ripe pears, cored and thinly sliced
½ teaspoon mixed spice
1½ cups (135 g) rolled oats
3 cups (750 ml) skim milk
125 g blueberries
2 tablespoons roughly chopped walnuts
2 tablespoons sunflower seeds
1 tablespoon linseeds
⅔ cup (190 g) reduced-fat natural Greek-style yoghurt

1. Preheat the oven to 180°C (160°C fan-forced).

2. Spread the pear slices over the base of a 1 litre-capacity baking dish, and sprinkle with the mixed spice. Combine the oats and milk in a large bowl. Pour gently and evenly over the pears.

3. Bake for 20 minutes, then carefully and lightly stir the oat mixture over the top of the pear. Sprinkle with the blueberries, walnuts and seeds, and return to the oven to bake for a further 15–20 minutes or until the oats are tender and the mixture has slightly thickened.

4. Set aside for 5–10 minutes to cool. Divide among 4 bowls and serve warm, topped with the yoghurt.

NUTRITIONAL ANALYSIS	ENERGY (KJ)	1617	CARBOHYDRATE (G)	51	SODIUM (MG)	118
TO SERVE 4 (PER SERVE)	PROTEIN (G)	15	SATURATED FAT (G)	2.8	FIBRE (G)	5

Roasted mushrooms with spinach and poached eggs

This is a really satisfying vegetarian breakfast dish. The sauce is packed with flavour and adds texture, so it's worth spreading it on the toast as well as serving it on the side.

SERVES 4
PREP TIME 15 MINUTES
COOKING TIME 20 MINUTES

4 large portobello (flat field) mushrooms, stems trimmed
2 cloves garlic, very thinly sliced
1 teaspoon thyme leaves
2 teaspoons olive oil
240 g baby spinach leaves
4 large eggs
4 slices wholegrain bread
1 handful flat-leaf parsley, roughly chopped (optional)

YOGHURT SAUCE
½ cup (140 g) reduced-fat natural Greek-style yoghurt
1 small handful flat-leaf parsley, roughly chopped
3 teaspoons hulled tahini
½ small clove garlic, crushed (optional)

1. Preheat the oven to 200°C (180°C fan-forced).

2. Place the mushrooms, upside down, in a large baking dish. Sprinkle evenly with the garlic and thyme, drizzle with the oil and season with freshly ground black pepper. Roast for 15–20 minutes or until tender.

3. Meanwhile, for the yoghurt sauce, combine the yoghurt, parsley, tahini and garlic (if using) in a small bowl. Cover with plastic film and refrigerate until required.

4. Heat a large, heavy-based non-stick frying pan over medium heat. Add the spinach and cook, turning occasionally, for 2–3 minutes or until just wilted. Transfer to a plate and set aside.

5. To poach the eggs, fill a deep, heavy-based frying pan or wide saucepan with water until about 7.5 cm deep, and bring to the boil. Carefully break each egg into a separate saucer or small ramekin. Stir the water to form a whirlpool, and quickly slide the eggs into the whirlpool (you can cook them one at a time if you prefer). Reduce the heat so the water is just simmering, and poach the eggs for 3–4 minutes or until the whites are set. Lift out the eggs with a slotted spoon and briefly drain on paper towel. (Alternatively, use an egg poacher if you have one.)

6. Toast the bread and spread a little yoghurt sauce over each slice. Divide among 4 plates and top each piece with a roasted mushroom, one-quarter of the spinach and a poached egg. Sprinkle with parsley (if using), and serve with the remaining yoghurt sauce.

NUTRITIONAL ANALYSIS	ENERGY (KJ)	1211	CARBOHYDRATE (G)	21	SODIUM (G)	241
TO SERVE 4 (PER SERVE)	PROTEIN (G)	17	SATURATED FAT (G)	4.1	FIBRE (G)	6

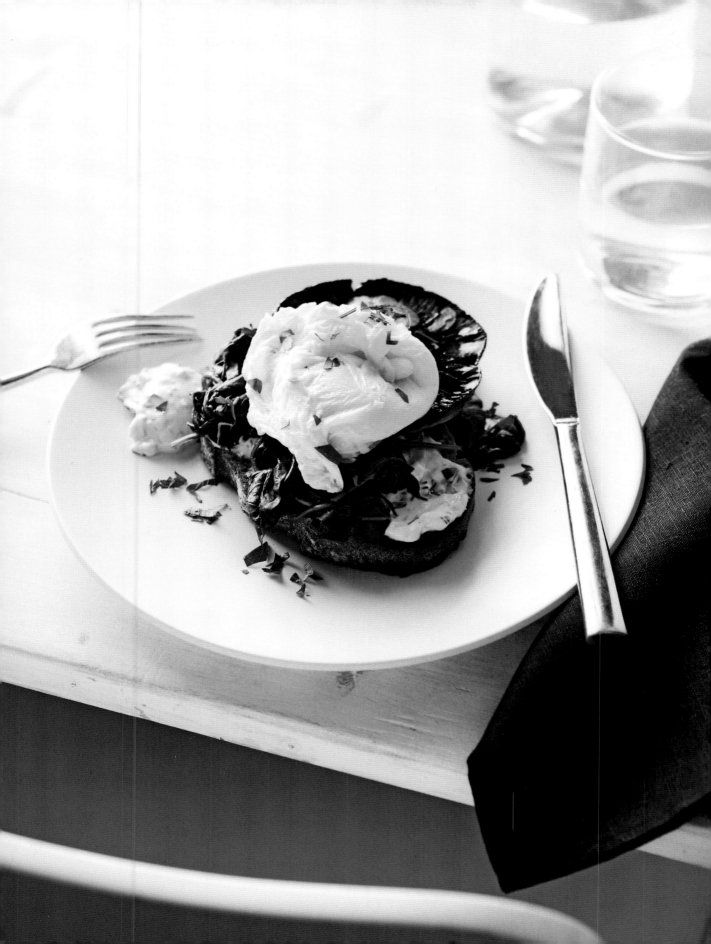

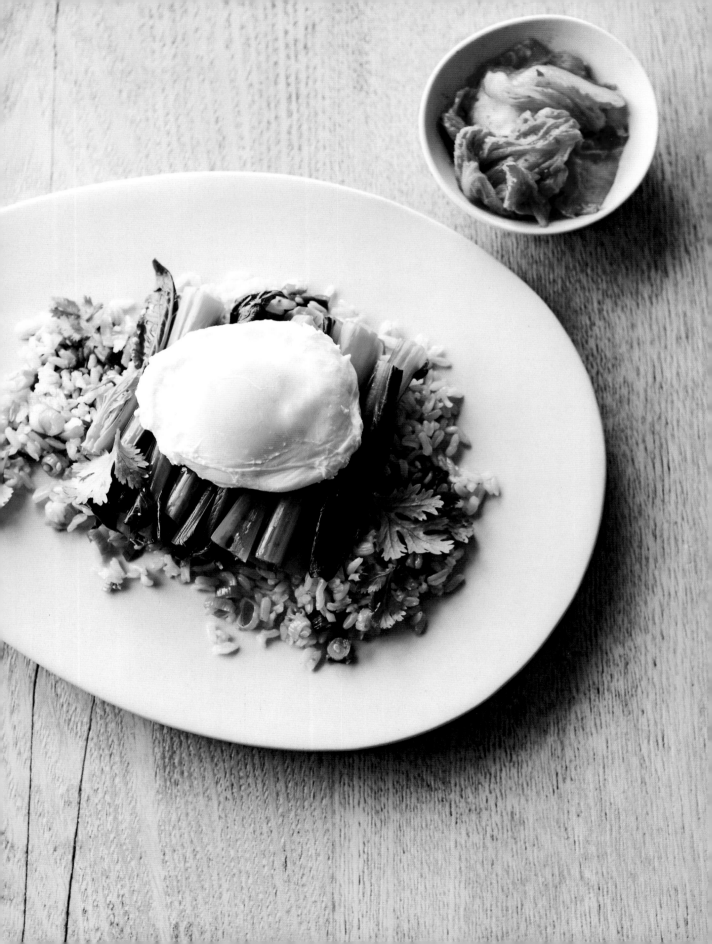

Breakfast rice with poached eggs, kimchi and choy sum

Kimchi is a spicy and sour Korean pickle, usually made with cabbage and
ground chillies, which gives a distinctive tang to this dish. You can pick up kimchi
from some large supermarkets and Korean grocery stores.

SERVES 4

PREP TIME 15 MINUTES

COOKING TIME 40 MINUTES

1 cup (200 g) long-grain brown basmati rice

2 teaspoons peanut oil

4 spring onions, trimmed and finely chopped

1 tablespoon sesame seeds

1 teaspoon finely grated ginger

1 clove garlic, very thinly sliced

400 g choy sum, trimmed and
    cut into 10 cm lengths

4 large free-range eggs

1 teaspoon sesame oil

2 teaspoons reduced-salt soy sauce

1 handful coriander leaves

⅔ cup (170 g) kimchi

1. Place the rice in a large heavy-based saucepan of
   boiling water and simmer for 25–30 minutes or
   until tender. Drain well.

2. Heat the peanut oil in a large non-stick frying pan
   or wok over medium heat. Add the spring onions,
   sesame seeds, ginger and garlic, and cook, stirring,
   for 1 minute or until fragrant. Add the cooked rice
   and continue to cook, stirring gently, for 3 minutes
   or until heated through.

3. Meanwhile, steam the choy sum in a steamer
   basket over a large saucepan of simmering water
   for 2 minutes or until tender but still crisp.

4. To poach the eggs, fill a deep, heavy-based frying
   pan or wide saucepan with water until about
   7.5 cm deep, and bring to the boil. Carefully break
   each egg into a separate saucer or small ramekin.
   Stir the water to form a whirlpool, and quickly
   slide the eggs into the whirlpool (you can cook
   them one at a time if you prefer). Reduce the heat
   so the water is just simmering, and poach the eggs
   for 3–4 minutes or until the whites are set. Lift out
   the eggs with a slotted spoon and briefly drain
   on paper towel. (Alternatively, use an egg poacher
   if you have one.)

5. Divide the fried rice evenly among 4 plates. Top
   each plate with one-quarter of the choy sum and
   a poached egg. Sprinkle with the sesame oil and
   soy sauce, scatter the coriander over the top,
   and serve with kimchi on the side.

NUTRITIONAL ANALYSIS	ENERGY (KJ)	1168	CARBOHYDRATE (G)	16	SODIUM (MG)	363
TO SERVE 4 (PER SERVE)	PROTEIN (G)	12	SATURATED FAT (G)	3.9	FIBRE (G)	4

Smoky baked beans and chickpeas

This bean mixture has a wonderfully mellow smoky flavour. The soft-boiled eggs go deliciously well, but scrambled or poached eggs would be equally good.

SERVES 4
PREP TIME 15 MINUTES
COOKING TIME 30 MINUTES

2 teaspoons olive oil
1 leek, washed and thinly sliced
1 tablespoon low-salt tomato paste
2 teaspoons smoked paprika
1 clove garlic, very thinly sliced
1 × 400 g tin low-salt chopped tomatoes
1 × 400 g tin low-salt borlotti beans, drained and rinsed
1 × 400 g tin low-salt chickpeas, drained and rinsed
2 teaspoons white vinegar
4 large eggs, at room temperature
4 thin slices sourdough bread
1 handful flat-leaf parsley leaves (optional)

1. Heat the oil in a large, heavy-based, non-stick frying pan over low–medium heat. Add the leek and cook, stirring occasionally, for 8–10 minutes or until tender. Add a little splash of water if the leek starts to stick. Add the tomato paste, smoked paprika and garlic. Increase the heat to medium and cook, stirring, for 1 minute or until fragrant. Stir in the tomatoes, beans, chickpeas and ½ cup (125 ml) water. Bring to the boil, then reduce the heat to low and simmer for 10–15 minutes or until thickened.

2. Meanwhile, add the vinegar to a small saucepan of boiling water. Using a spoon, carefully lower the eggs, one at a time, into the saucepan, and boil for 6 minutes. Drain and cool the eggs under cold running water. Peel and set aside.

3. Toast the bread and divide among 4 plates. Top each with an egg, then gently cut the eggs in half; the yolks should be a little runny. Divide the bean mixture evenly among the plates, scatter with parsley (if using) and serve.

NUTRITIONAL ANALYSIS	ENERGY (KJ)	1441	CARBOHYDRATE (G)	38	SODIUM (G)	992
TO SERVE 4 (PER SERVE)	PROTEIN (G)	19	SATURATED FAT (G)	2.6	FIBRE (G)	4

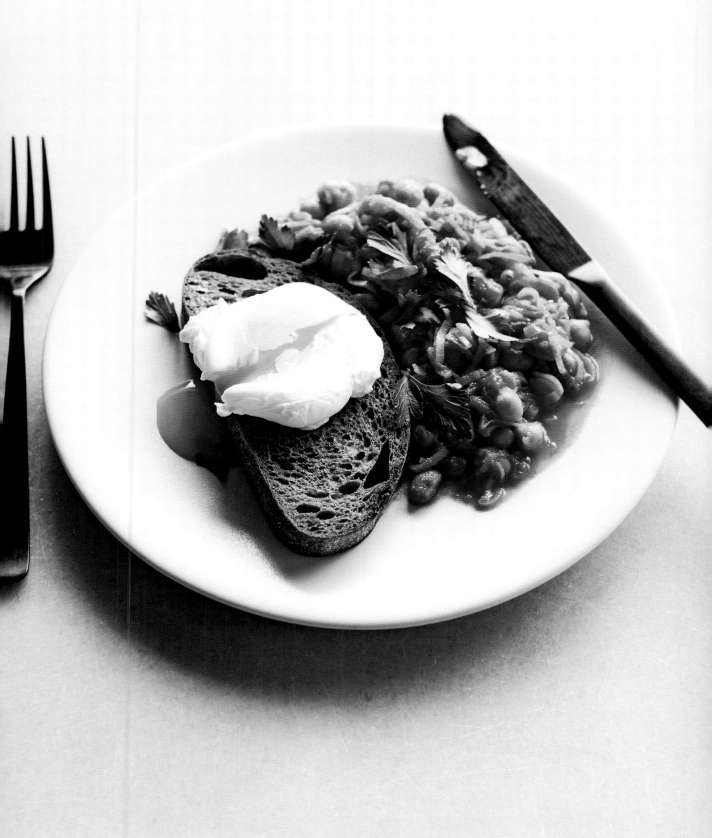

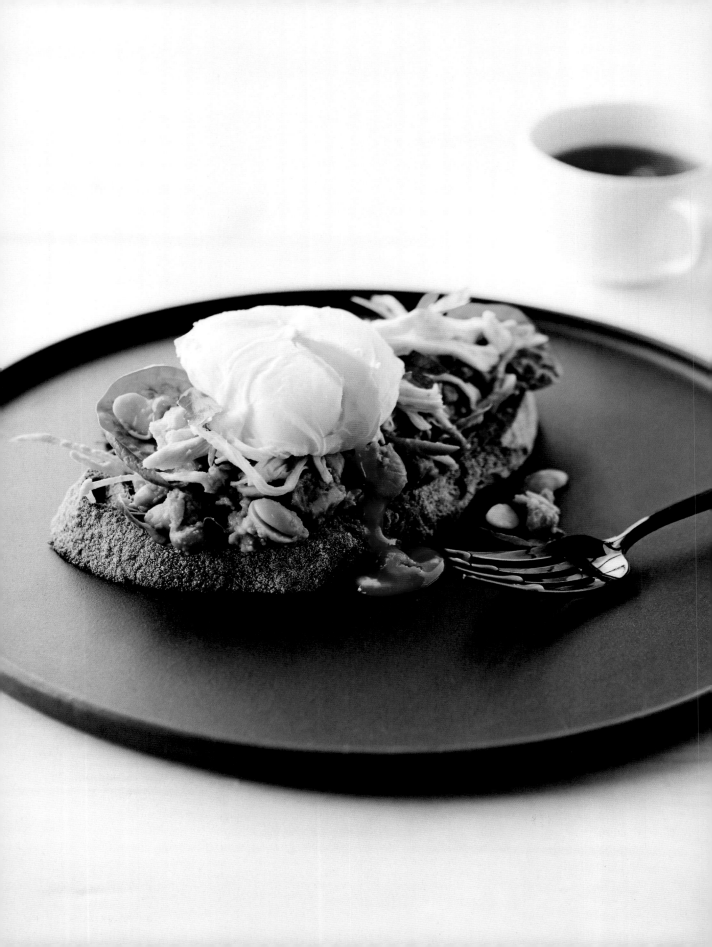

Wholegrain sourdough with green smash and shredded chicken

The crispness of the snow peas gives a pleasing bite to this wonderfully simple dish.
The peas and edamame add a nutritious twist to the smashed avocado,
and the runny yolk of the poached egg creates the perfect dressing.

SERVES 4
PREP TIME 20 MINUTES
COOKING TIME 25 MINUTES

1 × 180 g chicken breast fillet
1 onion, thinly sliced
2 cloves garlic, thinly sliced
1 cup (150 g) frozen shelled edamame (soybeans)
1 cup (120 g) frozen peas
1 large avocado, stone removed, peeled
   and roughly chopped
100 g snow peas (mangetout), thinly sliced lengthways
40 g baby spinach
3 teaspoons lemon juice
4 large eggs, at room temperature
4 thick slices wholegrain sourdough bread
1 handful flat-leaf parsley leaves (optional)

1. Score the thickest part of the chicken breast 3 times to a depth of about 1 cm. Place the chicken, onion and garlic in a heavy-based saucepan, and add just enough water to cover the chicken. Bring to the boil over medium heat, then reduce the heat to low and simmer for 6–8 minutes or until the chicken is just cooked through. Transfer the chicken to a plate and leave to rest, covered with foil.

2. Discard the onion and garlic, then add the edamame to the water. Return to the boil, then reduce the heat and simmer for 4 minutes. Add the peas and simmer for a further 2 minutes or until the edamame and peas are just tender. Drain, discarding the liquid. Transfer the edamame and peas mixture to a large bowl and set aside to cool slightly.

3. Roughly mash the edamame mixture with a masher. Add the avocado and roughly mash again, this time with a fork (try to retain some lumps for texture in the avocado). Fold in the snow peas, baby spinach and lemon juice, and season with freshly ground black pepper.

4. To poach the eggs, fill a deep, heavy-based frying pan or wide saucepan with water until about 7.5 cm deep, and bring to the boil. Carefully break each egg into a saucer or small ramekin. Stir the water to form a whirlpool, and quickly slide the eggs into the whirlpool (you can cook them one at a time if you prefer). Reduce the heat so the water is just simmering, and poach the eggs for 3–4 minutes or until the whites are set. Lift out the eggs with a slotted spoon and briefly drain on paper towel. (Alternatively, use an egg poacher if you have one.)

5. Using two forks, shred the chicken. Toast the bread and divide among 4 plates. Spread each slice with one-quarter of the green smash. Top with one-quarter of the shredded chicken and a poached egg, then scatter with parsley (if using) and serve.

NUTRITIONAL ANALYSIS	ENERGY (KJ)	1647	CARBOHYDRATE (G)	21	SODIUM (MG)	191
TO SERVE 4 (PER SERVE)	PROTEIN (G)	27	SATURATED FAT (G)	5.3	FIBRE (G)	7

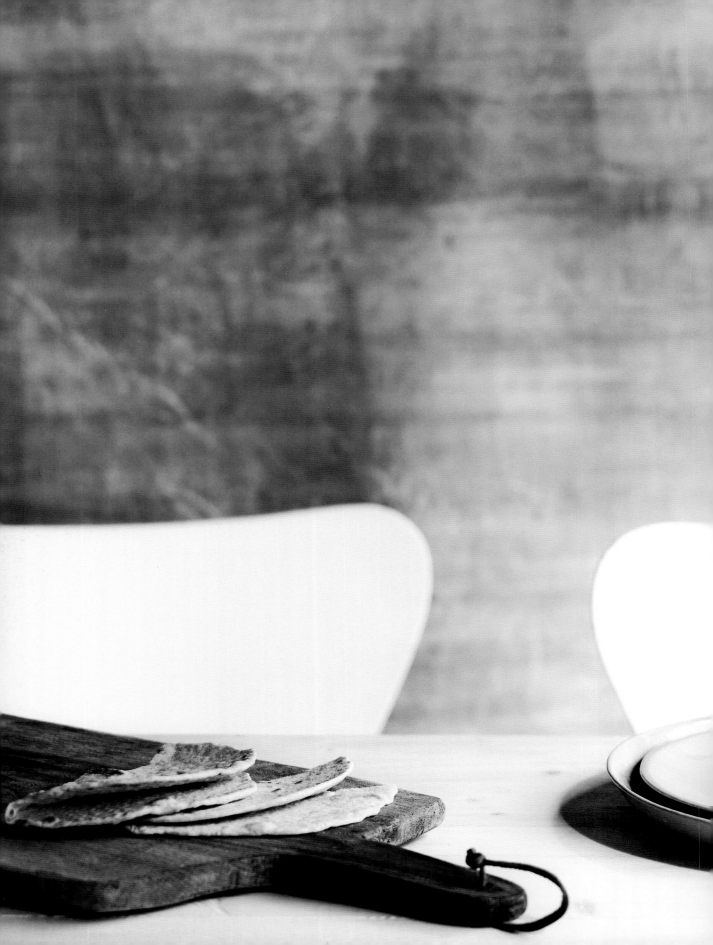

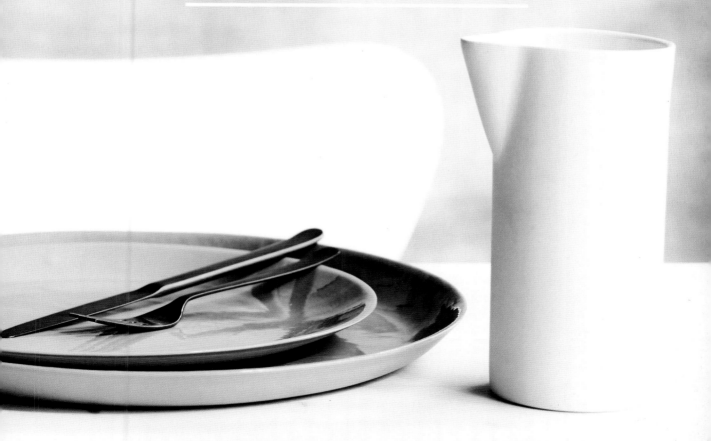

LUNCHES AND

LIGHT MEALS

Beef and bean quesadillas

These quesadillas burst at the seams with both filling and flavour.
If you don't like too much spice, you can leave out the chipotle chilli ingredients.

SERVES 4
PREP TIME 20 MINUTES
COOKING TIME 20 MINUTES

½ red onion, thinly sliced
2 tablespoons red wine vinegar
1 × 400 g tin black beans or low-salt kidney beans,
    drained and rinsed
2 large tomatoes, diced
2 spring onions, chopped
1 handful coriander, including stalks, chopped
1 teaspoon ground cumin
¼ teaspoon chipotle chilli powder or 1 teaspoon tinned
    chipotle peppers, chopped in adobo sauce (optional)
4 wholegrain wraps
4 thin slices (150 g) lean roast beef
¾ cup (150 g) low-fat fresh ricotta
1 small baby cos lettuce, quartered lengthways
1 zucchini (courgette), quartered lengthways
    and thinly sliced
1 avocado, stone removed, peeled and quartered (optional)
1 tablespoon homemade classic salad dressing
    (see page 289)

1. Place the onion and red wine vinegar in a small
   bowl, and mix well. Set aside.

2. Place the black beans or kidney beans in a bowl and
   roughly mash with a fork. Add the tomatoes and
   roughly mash until combined. Mix in the spring
   onions, coriander, cumin and chipotle chilli powder.

3. Spoon one-quarter of the bean mixture onto
   each wrap, spreading it over half of the wrap in
   a semicircle. Share the beef and ricotta between
   the wraps, spreading them evenly across the bean
   mixture semicircles. Drain the onion from the
   vinegar, discarding the vinegar, and sprinkle over
   the wrap fillings. Fold over each wrap to cover
   its filling.

4. Heat a sandwich press and toast the filled wraps,
   in batches if necessary, for 4–5 minutes or until
   lightly browned and heated through. (Alternatively,
   heat a large, heavy-based, non-stick frying pan
   over low–medium heat. Cook the quesadillas, one
   at a time, for 4–5 minutes on each side, pressing
   down lightly with a spatula and making sure they
   remain flat. They should be golden and crisp
   around the edges, and heated through.)

5. Cut the quesadillas into wedges. Serve with a side
   of lettuce and avocado (if using), scattered with
   the zucchini and drizzled with the dressing.

NUTRITIONAL ANALYSIS	ENERGY (KJ)	1990	CARBOHYDRATE (G)	35	SODIUM (MG)	876
TO SERVE 4 (PER SERVE)	PROTEIN (G)	24	SATURATED FAT (G)	7.1	FIBRE (G)	10

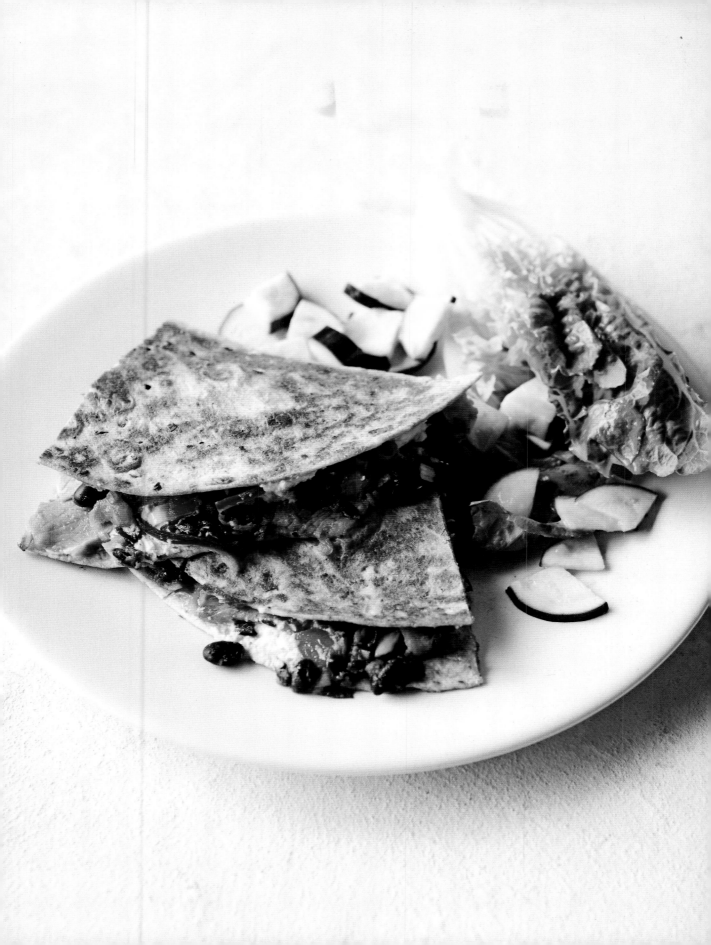

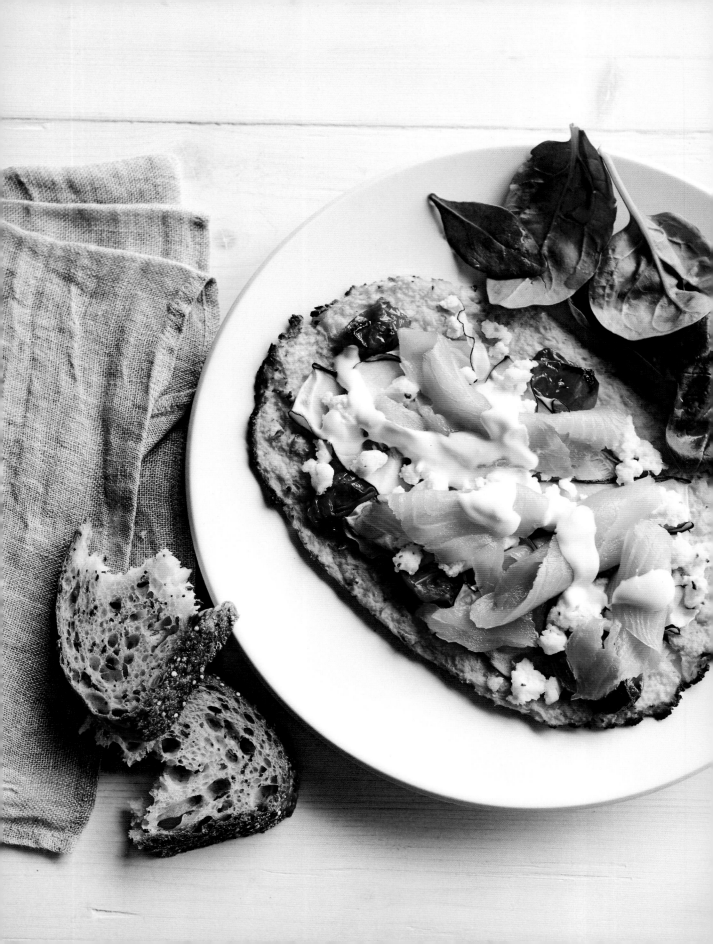

Cauliflower and cannellini bean pizza crust with smoked salmon topping

This gluten-free pizza-base alternative is worth the effort; the cauliflower crisps up to give a wonderful snap as you bite into it. If you're unable to fit three baking trays in your oven at the same time, roast the tomatoes before cooking the pizza bases.

SERVES 4
PREP TIME 30 MINUTES, PLUS COOLING
COOKING TIME 35 MINUTES

10 cups (1 kg) cauliflower florets
1 × 400 g tin low-salt cannellini beans, drained and rinsed
3 large eggs, lightly whisked
3 spring onions, finely chopped
olive oil spray, for cooking
250 g cherry tomatoes, halved
1 zucchini (courgette), peeled into thin ribbons
¾ cup (150 g) reduced-fat fresh firm ricotta cheese
200 g salt-reduced sliced smoked salmon, torn
¼ cup (70 g) reduced-fat natural Greek-style yoghurt
1 handful baby spinach, rocket or mixed salad leaves
4 small slices wholemeal sourdough bread
lemon wedges, to serve (optional)

1. Preheat the oven to 220°C (200°C fan-forced). Line 3 baking trays with baking paper.

2. Working in batches, use a food processor to process the cauliflower until it resembles couscous. Transfer the processed cauliflower to a large microwave-safe dish, cover with a microwave-safe lid and microwave on the high setting for 4 minutes. Stir, then microwave on high for a further 2–4 minutes, until just tender. Drain in a sieve lined with muslin or a clean tea towel, and set aside to cool. When cool, squeeze the excess moisture from the cauliflower through the muslin or tea towel, then transfer the cauliflower to a large bowl.

3. Use a fork to roughly mash the cannellini beans, then stir them into the cauliflower with the eggs and spring onions. Using your hands, divide the mixture into 4 even portions and place them, 2 apiece, on 2 of the lined trays. Shape each portion into an oval that is about 25 cm-long × 18 cm wide and just 4 mm thick. Lightly spray with olive oil.

4. Place the tomatoes on the third lined tray. Lightly spray with oil and season with freshly ground black pepper. Roast the cauliflower pizza bases and tomatoes for 15–20 minutes or until the pizza bases are firm to touch and the edges are golden, and the tomatoes have collapsed.

5. Top the pizza bases evenly with the zucchini, roasted tomatoes and crumbled ricotta. Bake for another 5 minutes or until the zucchini ribbons are wilted and the ricotta is lightly browned. Top with the salmon and drizzle with yoghurt. Serve with baby spinach, bread and lemon wedges on the side, if you like.

NUTRITIONAL ANALYSIS	ENERGY (KJ)	1768	CARBOHYDRATE (G)	34	SODIUM (MG)	880
TO SERVE 4 (PER SERVE)	PROTEIN (G)	34	SATURATED FAT (G)	4.7	FIBRE (G)	11

Lamb souvlaki wrap with garlic sauce

The garlic sauce in this recipe is a bit of a hybrid of hummus and tzatziki, and so it makes a delicious dip, too. Marinating the lamb is not essential, but will add a little more flavour. If this is for a packed lunch, simply chill the lamb before slicing and assembling to keep all the elements fresh.

SERVES 4
PREP TIME 20 MINUTES, PLUS 1 HOUR MARINATING
COOKING TIME 5 MINUTES, PLUS 5 MINUTES RESTING

300 g lamb backstrap
finely grated zest and juice of 1 lemon
1 clove garlic, crushed
1 teaspoon finely chopped oregano
4 multigrain wraps
3 large ripe tomatoes, sliced
1 baby cos lettuce, sliced lengthways into thin wedges
1 large red capsicum (pepper), seeded, membranes
    removed, cut into thin strips
lemon wedges, to serve (optional)

GARLIC SAUCE (MAKES ABOUT 300 ML)
1 × 400 g tin low-salt chickpeas, drained and rinsed
⅓ cup (95 g) reduced-fat natural Greek-style yoghurt
1 tablespoon flat-leaf parsley, chopped
2 teaspoons lemon juice
2 teaspoons hulled tahini
½ small clove garlic
1 Lebanese (short) cucumber, grated, with excess liquid
    squeezed out

1. Place the lamb, lemon zest and juice, garlic and oregano in a large zip-lock bag. Place in the fridge for 1 hour to marinate.

2. For the garlic sauce, blend half of the chickpeas (reserve the other half for filling the wraps), yoghurt, parsley, lemon juice, tahini and garlic in a blender or food processor until smooth. Transfer to a bowl, stir in the grated cucumber, cover with plastic film and refrigerate until required.

3. Heat a chargrill or heavy-based frying pan over medium–high heat. Remove the lamb from the marinade, shaking off the excess marinade, and cook for 2–3 minutes on each side for medium–rare – or simply cook to your liking. Remove the lamb from the pan, cover loosely with foil and leave to rest for 5 minutes. When rested, carve into slices.

4. Place each wrap on a plate, then top with one-quarter of all the elements: the garlic sauce, the remaining chickpeas, tomatoes, lettuce, red capsicum and sliced lamb. Roll the wraps, ready for eating, and serve immediately with lemon wedges, if desired.

NUTRITIONAL ANALYSIS	ENERGY (KJ)	1931	CARBOHYDRATE (G)	42	SODIUM (G)	552
TO SERVE 4 (PER SERVE)	PROTEIN (G)	31	SATURATED FAT (G)	5.6	FIBRE (G)	8

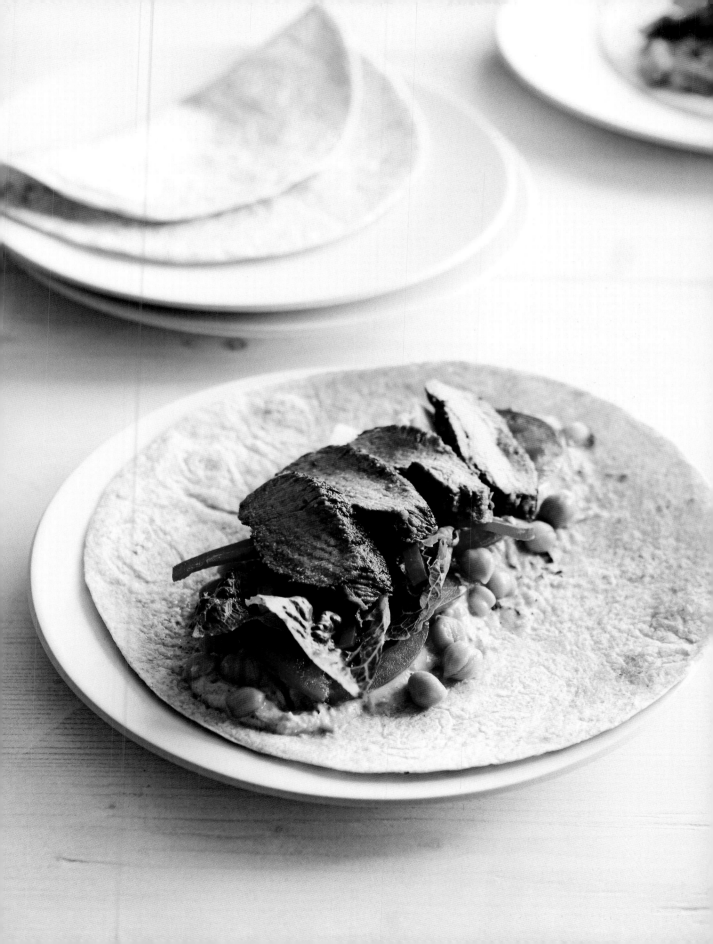

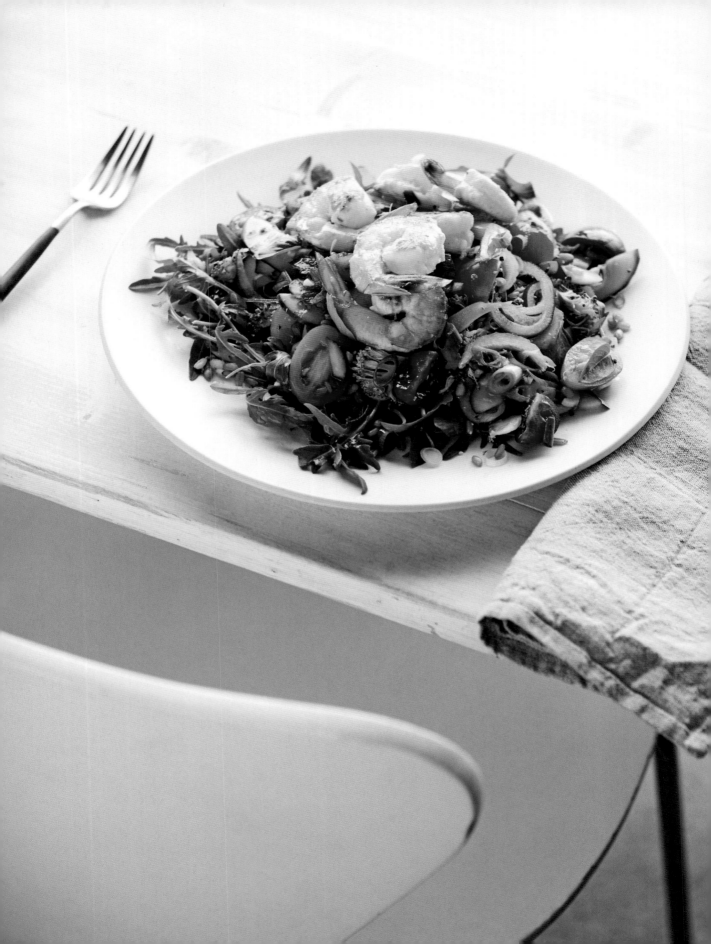

Freekeh salad with chargrilled prawns

Freekeh is a roasted wheat grain that has been harvested early, while it is still green. This helps it to keep more of its nutritional value than matured grains, packing this salad with nutritional punch.

SERVES 4
PREP TIME 20 MINUTES
COOKING TIME 30 MINUTES

400 g raw prawns, peeled and cleaned with tails intact
finely grated zest and juice of 1 lemon
2 cloves garlic, very thinly sliced
1 teaspoon olive oil
1 cup (180 g) cracked freekeh
1 small red onion, thinly sliced
2 tablespoons apple cider vinegar
olive oil spray, for cooking
400 g small mixed tomatoes, halved (quartered if large)
2 Lebanese (short) cucumbers, halved and sliced on the diagonal
200 g celery, thinly sliced
1¾ cups (150 g) broccoli florets, thinly sliced
4 spring onions, thinly sliced on the diagonal
1 large handful basil leaves, roughly torn
1 large handful flat-leaf parsley, roughly chopped
250 g rocket

LEMON AND GARLIC DRESSING
2 tablespoons lemon juice
1 tablespoon extra virgin olive oil
½ small clove garlic, crushed
pinch of caster sugar

1. Combine the lemon zest and juice, garlic and olive oil in a large bowl. Add the prawns, and set aside to marinate while you prepare the rest of the ingredients.

2. Bring 2 litres of water to the boil in a large heavy-based saucepan. Add the freekeh and return to the boil. Reduce the heat to medium, cover and simmer for 15–20 minutes or until the grains are just tender. Drain the freekeh in a sieve, then rinse under cold running water and drain well again. Set aside to cool.

3. Combine the sliced onion and apple cider vinegar in a small bowl. Set aside.

4. Heat a chargrill pan or barbecue hotplate over high heat. Drain the prawns, shaking off any excess marinade, then spray lightly with oil and cook for 2–3 minutes on each side or until just cooked through. Cook the prawns in 2–3 batches if necessary.

5. For the lemon and garlic dressing, you need a jar with a lid. Place the lemon juice, oil, garlic and caster sugar in the jar. Season to taste with sea salt and freshly ground black pepper. Seal with the lid, then shake until combined.

6. Meanwhile, toss the cooled freekeh, tomatoes, cucumbers, celery, broccoli, spring onions and herbs together in a large bowl. Add the dressing and toss to combine.

7. Drain the onion, discarding the vinegar. Divide the rocket among 4 plates and top evenly with the dressed freekeh mixture, prawns and drained onion.

NUTRITIONAL ANALYSIS	ENERGY (KJ)	1651	CARBOHYDRATE (G)	41	SODIUM (MG)	551
TO SERVE 4 (PER SERVE)	PROTEIN (G)	36	SATURATED FAT (G)	1.2	FIBRE (G)	13

Mexican chicken wrap

Poaching chicken is a wonderfully easy way to get a moist and tender breast that melts in your mouth. And including coriander stalks in the poaching liquid gives the chicken a subtle, fragrant flavour that beautifully complements the spicy bean salad.

SERVES 4
PREP TIME 20 MINUTES
COOKING TIME 15 MINUTES

1 × 200 g skinless chicken breast fillet
1 onion, roughly chopped
1 small handful coriander, stalks chopped and leaves left whole
2 cloves garlic, peeled and bruised
1 × 400 g tin low-salt kidney beans, drained and rinsed
finely grated zest of 1 lime
1 tablespoon lime juice
½ teaspoon ground coriander
½ teaspoon ground cumin
¼ teaspoon chipotle chilli powder (optional)
4 multigrain wraps
1 avocado, stone removed, peeled and roughly chopped
2 large tomatoes, sliced
250 g rocket
2 Lebanese (short) cucumbers, coarsely grated, excess liquid squeezed out
1 carrot, unpeeled and coarsely grated
2 tablespoons pepitas (roasted pumpkin seed kernels)
2 tablespoons sunflower seed kernels

1. Score the chicken breast three times in the thickest part of the fillet, to a depth of about 1 cm. Place the chicken, onion, chopped coriander stalks and garlic in a heavy-based saucepan, and add just enough water to cover the chicken. Bring to the boil over medium heat, then reduce the heat to low and simmer for 8–10 minutes or until the chicken is just cooked through. Transfer the chicken to a plate and set aside to rest. Discard the cooking liquid mixture.

2. Meanwhile, place the kidney beans in a bowl and roughly mash them with a fork. Add the lime zest and juice, spices and coriander leaves, and stir to combine. Set aside for the flavours to mingle and develop.

3. Spread each wrap with one-quarter of the avocado, then top with one-quarter of the bean salad, tomatoes, rocket, cucumbers and carrots. Thinly slice the cooked chicken on the diagonal, then add to the wrap fillings. Sprinkle with the seeds, then roll up tightly and serve immediately.

NUTRITIONAL ANALYSIS	ENERGY (KJ)	1976	CARBOHYDRATE (G)	37	SODIUM (G)	586
TO SERVE 4 (PER SERVE)	PROTEIN (G)	27	SATURATED FAT (G)	5.4	FIBRE (G)	11

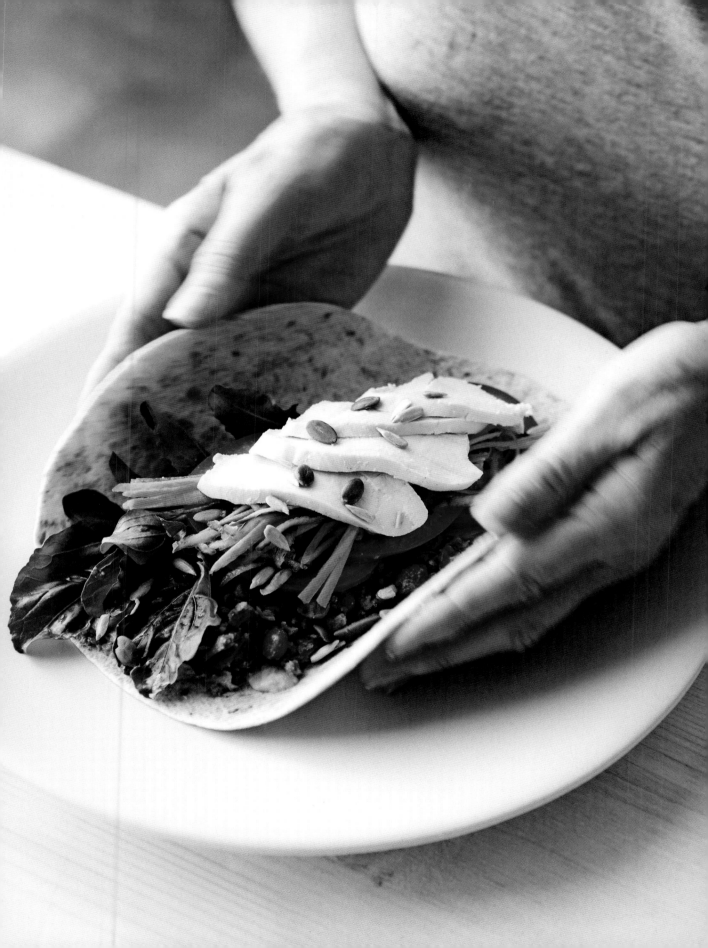

Baked ricotta with roasted cherry tomatoes

The fluffy creaminess of a baked ricotta always feels indulgent, yet it is so easy to make, and so versatile; you can easily swap ingredients in and out of the recipe, and it can be served warm or at room temperature, and reheated the next day if you fail to devour it in one go.

SERVES 4
PREP TIME 20 MINUTES
COOKING TIME 40 MINUTES

olive oil spray, for cooking
2 tablespoons homemade dukkah or nut-free dukkah
   (see page 293)
2½ cups (500 g) reduced-fat fresh, firm ricotta
2 eggs
3 spring onions, finely chopped
½ teaspoon red chilli flakes or 1 small fresh red chilli,
   seeded and finely chopped
8 (400 g) portobello (flat field) mushrooms,
   cut into quarters
400 g truss cherry tomatoes
1 small handful oregano sprigs
2 teaspoons olive oil
1 large handful baby spinach leaves or rocket
1 cup homemade baba ganoush (see page 262)
12 wholegrain rye crispbreads

1. Preheat the oven to 180°C (160°C fan-forced).

2. Lightly spray one 500 ml shallow ovenproof dish or two 1-cup (250 ml) ramekins with oil. Add the dukkah and tilt the dish or ramekins to cover the bases and sides. Leave any excess dukkah in the base.

3. Mash the ricotta in a bowl with a fork. Add the eggs, spring onions and chilli, and mix well. Season lightly with freshly ground black pepper. Spoon the mixture into the shallow dish or ramekins, smooth the surface with the back of the spoon, and bake for 35–40 minutes for the single dish or 25–30 minutes for the ramekins, until golden and set in the centre.

4. Meanwhile, place the mushroom quarters, gill-side up, in a large baking dish. Top evenly with the tomatoes and oregano sprigs. Drizzle with the oil and season with freshly ground black pepper. Roast in the oven with the ricotta for 25–30 minutes or until tender.

5. When the ricotta is cooked set it aside for 10 minutes to cool slightly. Then loosen the edge of the baked ricotta and turn it out onto a chopping board or plate. Divide the ricotta, mushrooms, tomatoes, baba ganoush and baby spinach or rocket among 4 plates. Serve with rye crispbread.

NUTRITIONAL ANALYSIS	ENERGY (KJ)	1802	CARBOHYDRATE (G)	31	SODIUM (MG)	449
TO SERVE 4 (PER SERVE)	PROTEIN (G)	28	SATURATED FAT (G)	6.5	FIBRE (G)	7

Carrot, zucchini and chickpea slice

This delicious slice is simple to make, and comforting to eat fresh from the oven while your kitchen is filled with those gratifying baking smells. Make light work of grating the zucchinis and carrots by using the fine-grating attachment on a food processor.

SERVES 4
PREP TIME 20 MINUTES
COOKING TIME 55 MINUTES

1 tablespoon olive oil
1 leek, white part only, well washed and thinly sliced
2 cloves garlic, crushed
5 large eggs
2 zucchinis (courgettes), coarsely grated
2 carrots, coarsely grated
400 g tin low-salt chickpeas or kidney beans, drained and rinsed
3 spring onions, finely chopped
½ cup (75 g) plain flour
1 teaspoon baking powder
150 g low-fat fresh, firm ricotta, crumbled
250 g cherry tomatoes, halved
1 handful baby spinach leaves or rocket
1 tablespoon homemade classic salad dressing (see page 289)

1. Preheat the oven to 180°C (160°C fan-forced). Line a 30 cm × 20 cm baking tin with baking paper, overhanging on two sides so that it is easy to remove the cooked slice from the tin.

2. Heat the oil in a large, heavy-based, non-stick frying pan over low–medium heat. Add the leek and garlic and cook, stirring occasionally, for 10 minutes or until tender. Transfer to a large bowl and set aside to cool.

3. Add the eggs, vegetables, chickpeas or kidney beans and spring onions to the leek mixture. Stir until well combined, then sift the flour and baking powder and fold into the mixture until just combined.

4. Spoon the mixture into the lined tin, smooth the surface with the back of the spoon to ensure it cooks evenly, and scatter the crumbled ricotta over the top. Lightly press the ricotta into the top of the mixture. Bake for 40–45 minutes or until lightly browned and set in the centre.

5. Leave the slice to cool in the tin for 10 minutes. Use the overhanging paper to lift the slice out of the tin onto a chopping board, then cut into 4 portions.

6. Toss the tomatoes and salad leaves with the dressing. Serve alongside the warm slice.

NUTRITIONAL ANALYSIS	ENERGY (KJ)	1524	CARBOHYDRATE (G)	29	SODIUM (MG)	754
TO SERVE 4 (PER SERVE)	PROTEIN (G)	20	SATURATED FAT (G)	4.8	FIBRE (G)	6

Spicy fish tacos

For an easy supply of fresh, homemade flour tortillas, make them in advance and freeze them – then simply thaw before warming them in a frying pan or on the barbecue. If you prefer small tacos or are making these for children's small hands, you can make the tortillas half-size and allow two per serve.

SERVES 4
PREP TIME 25 MINUTES
COOKING TIME 25 MINUTES

1 × 300 g blue-eye trevalla fillet
1 teaspoon ground cumin
½ teaspoon mild chilli powder
1 tablespoon lime juice
1 cob sweetcorn, husk and silks removed
olive oil spray, for cooking
4 cups (320 g) finely shredded red cabbage
1 baby cos lettuce, shredded
1 red onion, thinly sliced
2 handfuls coriander leaves, coarsely chopped
4 flour tortillas (see page 292)
½ quantity black bean dip (see page 262)

BAJA SAUCE
½ cup (140 g) reduced-fat natural Greek-style yoghurt
2 teaspoons lime juice
¼ teaspoon mild chilli powder, or to taste
pinch of salt

1. Sprinkle the fish all over with the cumin and chilli powder. Place in a glass bowl and add the lime juice. Set aside for 10–15 minutes to marinate.

2. Meanwhile, heat a barbecue flat-plate or heavy-based frying pan over high heat. Spray the corn lightly with oil and cook on the flat-plate or frying pan, turning occasionally, for 8–10 minutes or until the kernels are lightly charred and tender. Transfer to a plate to cool slightly. Leave the flat-plate or frying pan over a low heat, ready for cooking the fish.

3. Remove the fish from the marinade, shake off any excess liquid, then lightly spray the fillet with oil. Cook on the barbecue flat-plate or frying pan over medium heat for 3–4 minutes on each side or until browned and cooked through. (The cooking time will depend on the thickness of the fillet.) Using a sharp knife, cut the fish into 4 equal portions.

4. Using a large, sharp knife, carefully cut the corn kernels from your cooked cob. Toss the cabbage, lettuce, onion and coriander in a large bowl. Sprinkle with the corn and set aside.

5. For the Baja sauce, combine the yoghurt, lime juice, chilli powder and salt in a small bowl. Cover and set aside until required.

6. Meanwhile, warm the tortillas briefly on the barbecue flat-plate or in a dry non-stick frying pan. Wrap in a clean tea towel to keep them warm and pliable.

7. Top each tortilla with one-quarter of the black bean dip, 1 portion of fish and a dollop of Baja sauce. Add a heaped spoonful of the salad, then fold the tortilla in half and serve immediately with any remaining salad and sauce on the side.

NUTRITIONAL ANALYSIS	ENERGY (KJ)	1290	CARBOHYDRATE (G)	29	SODIUM (G)	334
TO SERVE 4 (PER SERVE)	PROTEIN (G)	28	SATURATED FAT (G)	2.2	FIBRE (G)	10

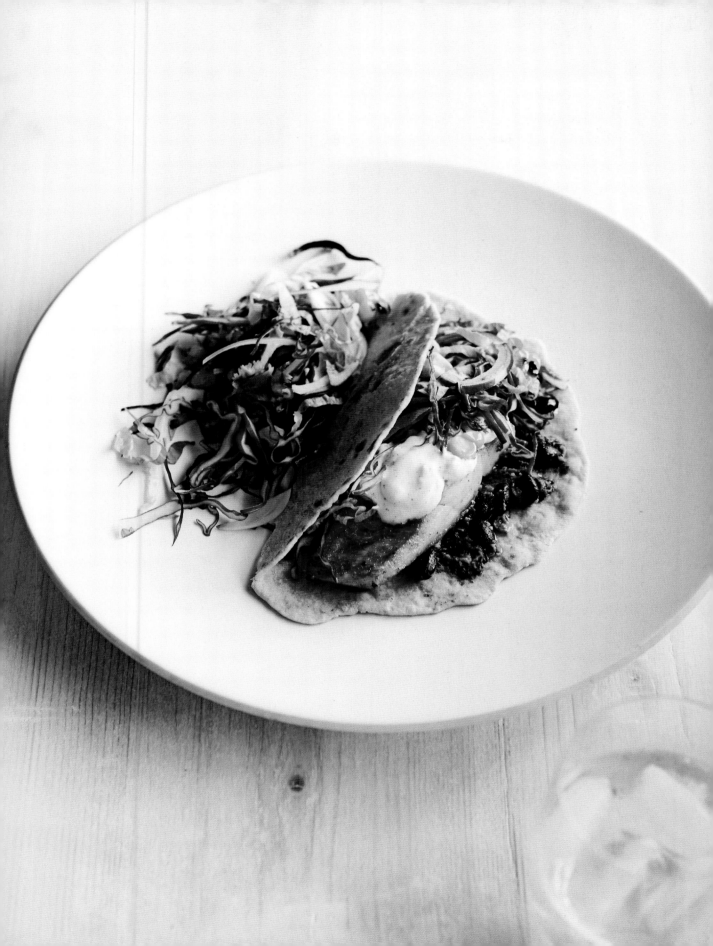

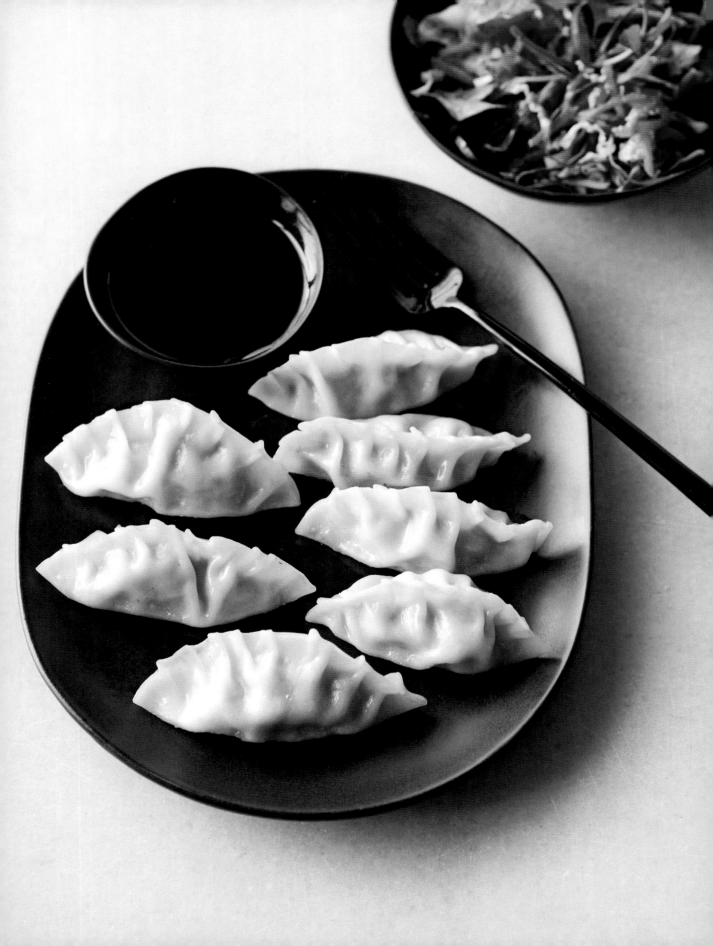

Prawn and mushroom pot stickers

Pot stickers are a real crowd pleaser – the steaming process keeps the filling beautifully moist and juicy while the frying gives the dumplings a pleasing stickiness and crisp finish. The salty soy-based dressing complements the sweetness of the prawn filling, and the Asian slaw provides that satisfying crunch to complete the dish.

SERVES 4
PREP TIME 30 MINUTES
COOKING TIME 20 MINUTES

5 teaspoons peanut oil
1 cup (50 g) shredded Chinese cabbage
50 g shiitake mushrooms, sliced
1 small clove garlic, finely chopped
200 g raw prawns peeled and cleaned,
    half coarsely chopped
1 free-range egg white
1 spring onion, finely chopped
½ teaspoon finely grated ginger
½ teaspoon sesame oil
28 gow gee wrappers

SOY AND BLACK VINEGAR DRESSING
1 spring onion, thinly sliced
1 tablespoon Chinese black vinegar
1 tablespoon sesame oil
1 tablespoon salt-reduced soy sauce
1 tablespoon water
2 teaspoons honey
1 clove garlic, crushed

ASIAN SLAW
2 cups (160 g) finely shredded red cabbage
2 cups (100 g) finely shredded Chinese cabbage (wombok)
2 carrots, coarsely grated
100 g watercress, leaves picked
1 tablespoon sesame seeds
1 tablespoon pepitas (roasted pumpkin seed kernels)
1 small fresh red chilli, thinly sliced (optional)

1. For the dressing, place all the ingredients in a screw-top jar. Seal with the lid and shake until emulsified. Season with a little freshly ground white pepper to taste. Set aside.

2. For the Asian slaw, combine all the ingredients in a large bowl. Set aside.

3. Heat 1 teaspoon of the peanut oil in a heavy-based non-stick frying pan over medium heat. Add the cabbage, mushrooms and garlic and cook, stirring, for 2–3 minutes or until the cabbage is wilted. Transfer to a bowl and set aside to cool.

4. Place the whole prawns, egg white, spring onions, ginger and sesame oil in a food processor, and process to form a paste. Add to the cooled cabbage mixture along with the chopped prawns, and mix well.

5. Working in batches, place the gow gee wrappers on a clean work surface. Place 2 teaspoons of the prawn mixture in the centre of each wrapper. Brush the wrapper edges lightly with water. Fold over, pleating and pinching one side of the wrapper to the other (this helps give the dumpling the classic curved shape) to seal. Place on a baking tray and cover with plastic film to keep the dumplings from drying out as you work.

6. Heat 2 teaspoons of the remaining peanut oil in a large, heavy-based non-stick frying pan over medium heat. Add ½ cup (125 ml) water to the pan and arrange half the dumplings in the pan in a single layer, seam-side-up. Cover the pan with a tight-fitting lid and steam the dumplings for 5 minutes. Remove the lid and cook until the water evaporates, around 2–3 minutes then cook for a further 2 minutes or until the dumplings are golden and crunchy on the bottom. Transfer to a plate and cover with foil to keep warm. Repeat with the remaining peanut oil and dumplings.

7. Meanwhile, toss the Asian slaw with half of the dressing. Divide the remaining dressing among 4 small bowls. Serve the dumplings with the dressing for dipping and the Asian slaw on the side.

NUTRITIONAL ANALYSIS	ENERGY (KJ)	2139	CARBOHYDRATE (G)	57	SODIUM (MG)	605
TO SERVE 4 (PER SERVE)	PROTEIN (G)	24	SATURATED FAT (G)	3.2	FIBRE (G)	8

Thai turkey omelette wrap

Adding water to the eggs increases the steam that rises through the eggs as they cook, creating light and fluffy omelettes. To lessen your knife work, pulse the turkey in a food processor.

SERVES 4
PREP TIME 30 MINUTES
COOKING TIME 25 MINUTES

100 g rice vermicelli
4 large eggs
olive oil spray, for cooking
1 teaspoon peanut oil
1 onion, finely chopped
1 teaspoon Thai red curry paste
1 handful coriander stalks and leaves, separated
250 g skinless turkey breast fillet, finely chopped
3 cups (160 g) shredded Chinese cabbage (wombok)
2 cups (160 g) bean sprouts
2 teaspoons lime juice
1 teaspoon salt-reduced soy sauce
1 handful mint leaves
1 tablespoon roasted unsalted peanuts, roughly chopped
lime wedges, to serve (optional)

BEAN, CAPSICUM AND CUCUMBER SALAD
150 g green beans, thinly sliced on the diagonal
1 large red capsicum (pepper), seeded, membrane removed, cut into long thin strips
2 Lebanese (short) cucumbers, halved lengthways and sliced on the diagonal
1 carrot, unpeeled and coarsely grated
1 teaspoon sesame oil
2 teaspoons salt-reduced soy sauce
2 tablespoons sesame seeds, toasted

1. Place the vermicelli noodles in a heatproof bowl, cover with boiling water and set aside to soak for 5 minutes or until tender. Then drain well.

2. For the salad, toss all the ingredients together in a large bowl. Set aside for the flavours to develop.

3. In a jug, measure ¼ cup (60 ml) water. Add the eggs and whisk until combined. Spray a non-stick frying pan lightly with oil and place over medium–high heat. Pour one-quarter of the egg mixture into the hot pan and cook for 1 minute or until lightly browned and the edge is starting to lift. Turn the omelette over carefully, peeling and lifting it from the pan with your fingertips or a spatula. Cook for a further 30 seconds or until set, then transfer to a plate. Repeat with the remaining egg mixture to make 4 omelettes.

4. Heat the peanut oil in a heavy-based frying pan over low–medium heat. Add the onion and curry paste and cook, stirring, for 5–6 minutes or until the onion has softened; add a splash of water if it starts to stick.

5. Chop the coriander stalks. Increase the heat to medium–high and add the turkey and stalks. Cook, stirring, for 3–4 minutes or until the turkey is lightly coloured and just cooked through. Add the Chinese cabbage and drained noodles, and cook, stirring, for 3–4 minutes or until the cabbage has wilted. Remove from the heat. Add the bean sprouts, lime juice, soy sauce, mint and coriander leaves, and toss to combine.

6. Top each omelette with one-quarter of the turkey mixture and sprinkle with the chopped peanuts. Roll up the omelette to enclose the filling, if desired. Serve with one-quarter of the salad on the side and lime wedges, if desired.

NUTRITIONAL ANALYSIS	ENERGY (KJ)	1742	CARBOHYDRATE (G)	30	SODIUM (G)	457
TO SERVE 4 (PER SERVE)	PROTEIN (G)	34	SATURATED FAT (G)	3.6	FIBRE (G)	7

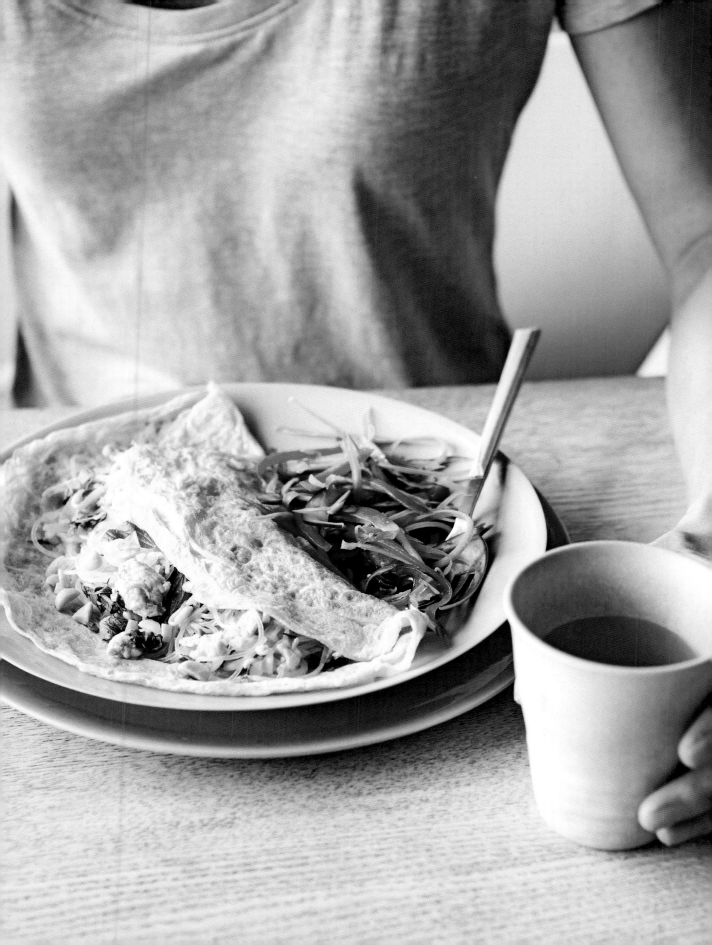

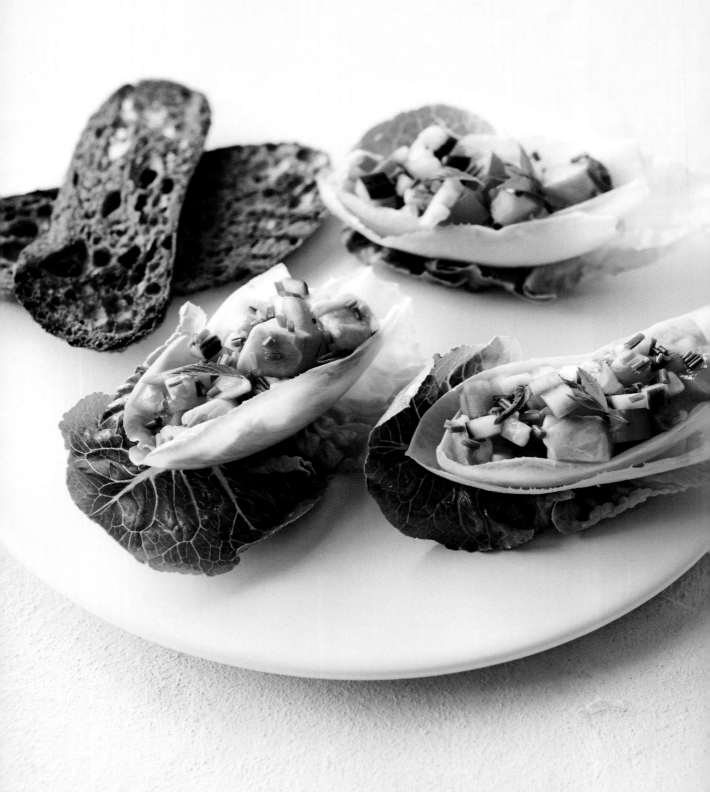

Salmon ceviche with witlof salad

The acid of the lime juice 'cooks' the fish in this wonderfully refreshing and simple dish.
The herbs and salad elements elegantly balance the citrus and chilli flavours,
and the leafy bowls are simply fun to plate and eat!

SERVES 4
PREP TIME 15 MINUTES
COOKING TIME 30 MINUTES

1 × 300 g skinless salmon fillet, pin-boned and
    cut into 1 cm dice
⅓ cup (80 ml) lime juice
8 thin slices wholegrain sourdough bread
olive oil spray, for cooking
4 tomatoes, diced
1 telegraph (long) cucumber, diced
1 avocado, stone removed, peeled and sliced
1 handful mint leaves
1 handful chives, chopped
1 small fresh red chilli, thinly sliced
1 baby cos lettuce, leaves separated
2 witlof, leaves separated
lime wedges, to serve (optional)

1. Place the salmon in a large glass or ceramic bowl
   with the lime juice, and stir gently to coat the
   salmon well. Cover with plastic film and refrigerate
   for 30 minutes to marinate.

2. Meanwhile, heat a chargrill pan over high heat.
   Spray the sourdough lightly with oil on both sides
   and chargrill for 2–3 minutes on each side or until
   toasted and crisp. Set aside.

3. Drain the excess lime juice from the salmon.
   Add the tomato, cucumber, avocado, herbs and
   chilli, and toss gently to combine. Lightly season
   with freshly ground white pepper.

4. Divide the lettuce leaves among 4 serving plates
   in a single layer and top with the witlof. Pile
   the salmon mixture into each witlof 'cup'. Serve
   with the chargrilled sourdough and lime wedges,
   if desired.

NUTRITIONAL ANALYSIS	ENERGY (KJ)	1851	CARBOHYDRATE (G)	21	SODIUM (MG)	306
TO SERVE 4 (PER SERVE)	PROTEIN (G)	29	SATURATED FAT (G)	5.4	FIBRE (G)	7

Scallop and noodle lettuce cups

Scallops are so delicious but can be expensive so mussels can be substituted, if preferred. To do this, place 2 kg freshly bearded mussels in a large saucepan with 1 cup (250 ml) water. Cover and cook, shaking the pan occasionally, for 3 minutes. Use tongs to transfer the opened mussels to a large bowl. Cook the remaining mussels, covered, for a further 1–2 minutes. Add the opened mussels to the bowl and discard any unopened mussels. Remove the mussel meat from the shells, and add them with the ginger and garlic to the frying pan in step 3. Then continue with the recipe as indicated. It is useful to note that 1 kg Australian blue mussels yields 170 g cooked mussel meat.

SERVES 4

PREP TIME 25 MINUTES

COOKING TIME 10 MINUTES

100 g rice vermicelli, broken into short lengths

2 baby cos lettuces, leaves separated

1 telegraph (long) cucumber, cut into thin strips

2 cups (160 g) bean sprouts

150 g snow peas (mangetout), cut lengthways into thin strips

1 handful mint leaves

1 handful coriander sprigs

¼ cup (35 g) dry roasted unsalted peanuts, roughly chopped

1 small fresh red chilli, finely chopped or thinly sliced

2 teaspoons peanut oil

400 g scallop meat (without roe), cut in half widthways

1 clove garlic, crushed

1 teaspoon finely grated ginger

1 tablespoon salt-reduced soy sauce

1 tablespoon hoisin sauce

lime wedges, to serve (optional)

1. Place the vermicelli in a heatproof bowl, cover with boiling water and leave to soak for 5 minutes or until tender. Then drain well.

2. Divide the lettuce, cucumber, bean sprouts, snow peas and herbs among 4 plates, creating separate piles. Do the same with the peanuts and chilli, or place them in separate little serving bowls.

3. Heat the peanut oil in a large, heavy-based non-stick frying pan or wok over medium–high heat. Add the scallops and stir-fry for 1–2 minutes or until just coloured. Add the garlic and ginger and stir-fry for a further minute. Add the sauces and drained noodles and stir-fry for about 2 minutes until heated through.

4. Divide the scallop and noodle mixture among the plates and scatter with herbs, peanuts and chilli; the idea is for people to assemble their own lettuce cups. Serve with lime wedges to the side, if using.

NUTRITIONAL ANALYSIS	ENERGY (KJ)	1824	CARBOHYDRATE (G)	30	SODIUM (MG)	661
TO SERVE 4 (PER SERVE)	PROTEIN (G)	30	SATURATED FAT (G)	3.7	FIBRE (G)	4

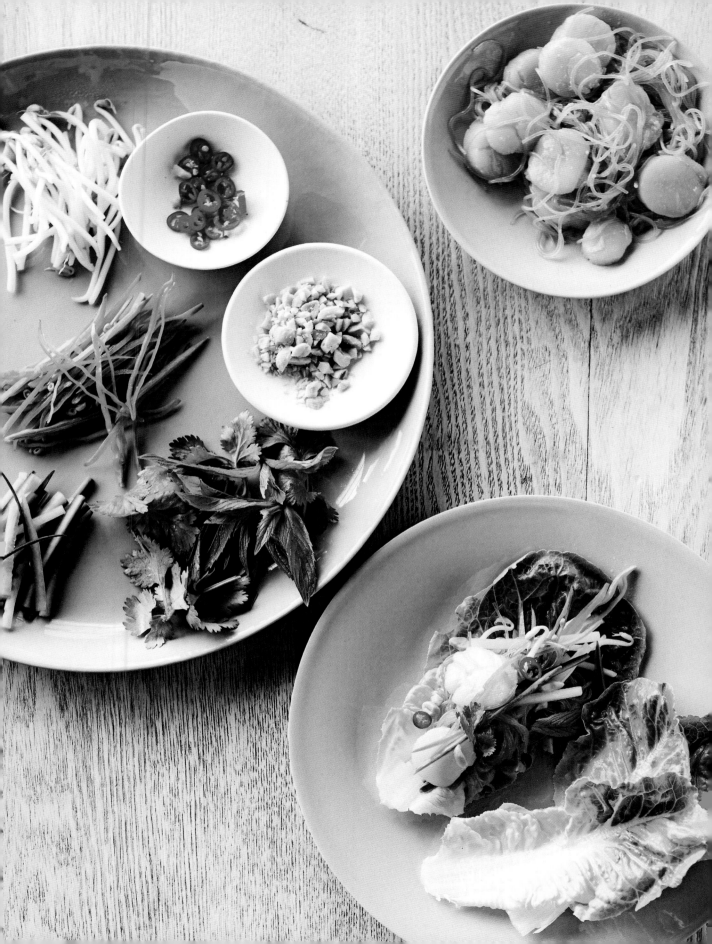

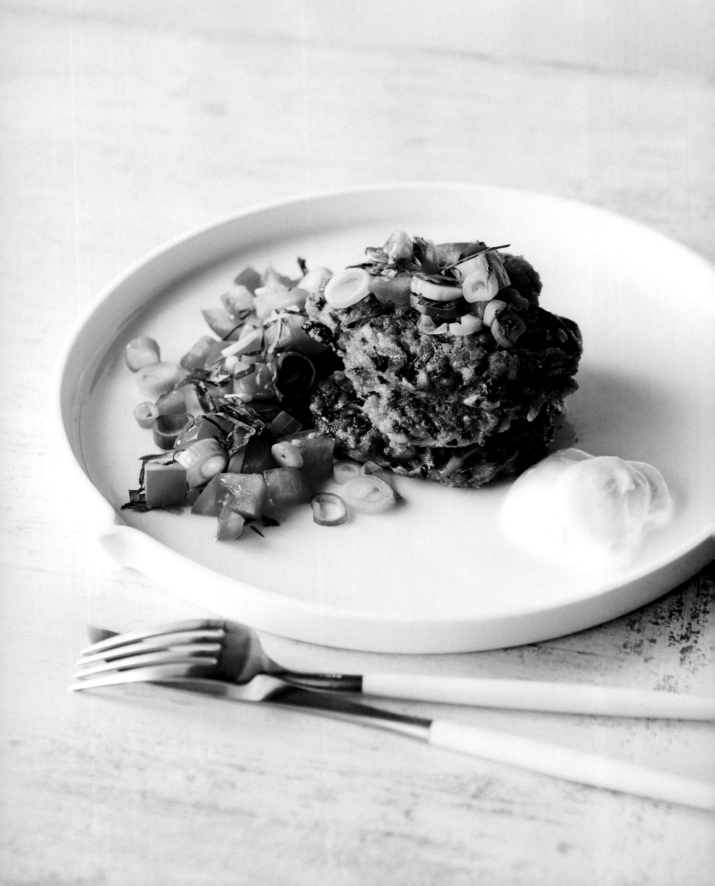

Spinach and chickpea pakoras
with tomato sambal

The spices in these traditional Indian fritters are wonderfully aromatic. Enjoy them as a finger food dipped in yoghurt, or plate up to relish with a hefty serving of sambal.

SERVES 4
PREP TIME 20 MINUTES
COOKING TIME 20 MINUTES

250 g baby spinach leaves
4 cups (1 litre) boiling water
1 × 400 g tin low-salt chickpeas, drained and rinsed
2 potatoes (400 g), peeled and grated
½ cup (75 g) chickpea (besan) flour, sifted
2 teaspoons baking powder
2 teaspoons finely grated ginger
2 teaspoons garam masala
1 teaspoon ground turmeric
1 teaspoon cumin seeds
4 large eggs, lightly beaten
light olive oil spray, for cooking
½ cup (140 g) reduced-fat natural Greek-style yoghurt

TOMATO SAMBAL
4 ripe tomatoes, cut into wedges
3 spring onions, thinly sliced
1 handful mint leaves, shredded
1 tablespoon lemon juice
1 small fresh red chilli, thinly sliced (optional)

1. Place the spinach in a colander and pour over the boiling water until the leaves have wilted. Drain and cool slightly, then squeeze out the excess water and roughly chop.

2. Place the chickpeas in a large bowl and roughly mash with a fork or potato masher. Add the chopped spinach to the chickpeas along with the potatoes, flour, baking powder, ginger and spices. Mix well, then stir in the beaten eggs.

3. Preheat the oven to 100°C (80°C fan-forced). Line a baking tray with baking paper.

4. Heat a large, heavy-based non-stick frying pan over low–medium heat. Working in batches, spray the pan lightly with oil and pour in three or four ¼ cup (60 ml) measures of your chickpea batter to the pan. Gently tilt the pan to spread the batter until each pakora is about 1 cm thick. Cook for 3–4 minutes on each side or until golden and cooked through.

5. Transfer to the lined tray, cover loosely with foil and keep warm in the oven while you cook the remaining pakoras. You should get around 12 pakoras in total.

6. Meanwhile, for the tomato sambal, combine the tomatoes, spring onions, mint and lemon juice in a small bowl and sprinkle with the chilli, if using.

7. Divide the pakoras among 4 plates, topped with one-quarter of the sambal alongside a dollop of yoghurt.

NUTRITIONAL ANALYSIS	ENERGY (KJ)	1674	CARBOHYDRATE (G)	47	SODIUM (MG)	1113
TO SERVE 4 (PER SERVE)	PROTEIN (G)	23	SATURATED FAT (G)	3.4	FIBRE (G)	8

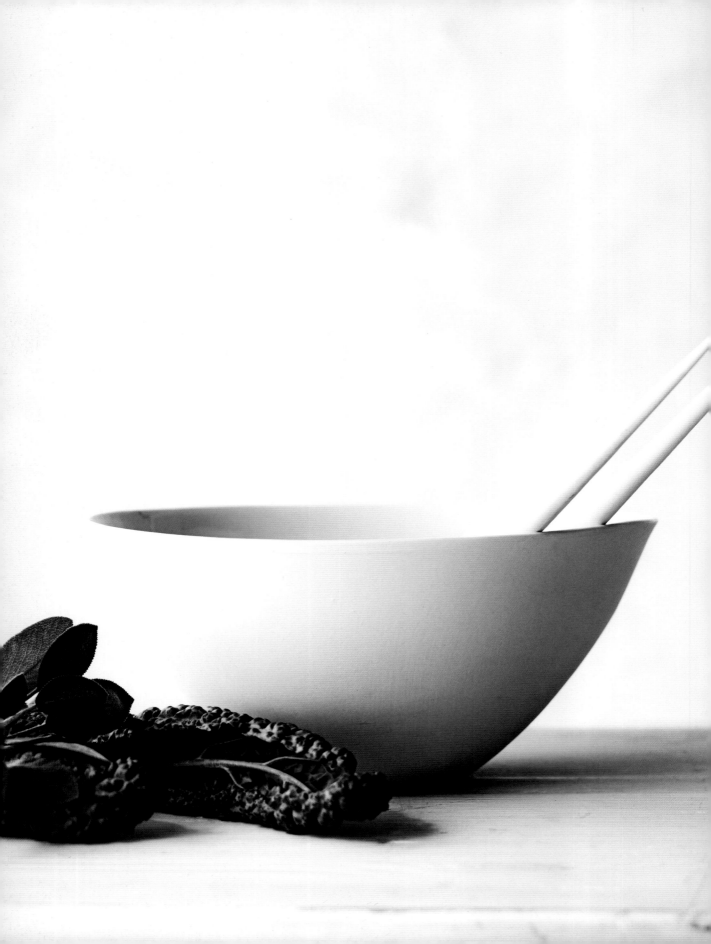

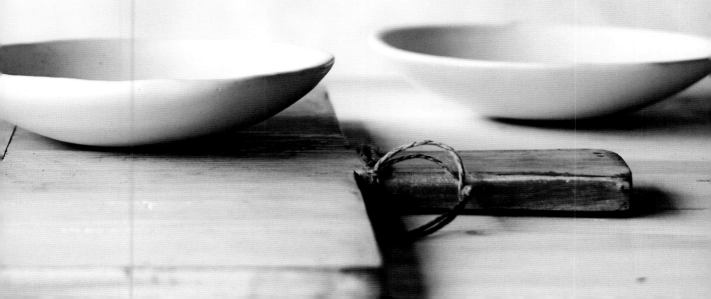

SALADS

Asian slaw with poached turkey

You can make this salad as hot or as mild as you like; simply remove the seeds
from the chilli for a milder chilli hit, or omit it all together, if preferred.

SERVES 4
PREP TIME 20 MINUTES
COOKING TIME 10 MINUTES

300 g skinless turkey breast fillet steaks
1 stalk lemongrass, pale section only, finely chopped
4 kaffir lime leaves, finely shredded
1½ cups (225 g) frozen shelled edamame (soybeans)
   or frozen double-peeled broad beans
6½ cups (350 g) shredded Chinese cabbage (wombok)
2 baby bok choy, thinly sliced widthways
1 small daikon, cut into thin strips
1 large handful mint leaves
1 large handful coriander leaves
1 long fresh red chilli, thinly sliced (optional)
lime wedges, to serve (optional)

SESAME-LIME DRESSING
2 tablespoons lime juice
1 tablespoon sesame oil
1 tablespoon salt-reduced soy sauce
2 teaspoons shaved palm sugar
1 small clove garlic, crushed

1. Place the turkey, lemongrass and half of the shredded lime leaves in a heavy-based saucepan and add just enough water to cover the turkey. Bring to the boil over medium heat, then reduce the heat to low and simmer for 4–5 minutes or until the turkey is just cooked through. Transfer the turkey to a plate and set aside to cool slightly.

2. Strain the cooking liquid into a small heavy-based saucepan, discarding the solids. Bring the liquid to the boil over high heat, then add the edamame or broad beans, and cook for 3–4 minutes or until the beans are tender. Drain, discarding the cooking liquid, and refresh the beans in a large bowl of cold water. Drain well and place the beans back in the bowl. Add the Chinese cabbage, bok choy, daikon, herbs and chilli (if using), as well as the remaining shredded lime leaves, and toss to combine.

3. Using 2 forks, shred the turkey, then transfer to a bowl and leave to cool completely.

4. For the dressing, place all the ingredients with 1 tablespoon water in a screw-top jar. Seal with the lid and shake until emulsified. Pour 1 tablespoon of the dressing over the cooled turkey and toss to coat.

5. Just before serving, add the turkey and half the remaining dressing to the slaw salad and toss to combine. Serve with the remaining dressing on the side and lime wedges, if desired.

NUTRITIONAL ANALYSIS	ENERGY (KJ)	1628	CARBOHYDRATE (G)	34	SODIUM (MG)	747
TO SERVE 4 (PER SERVE)	PROTEIN (G)	34	SATURATED FAT (G)	1.8	FIBRE (G)	11

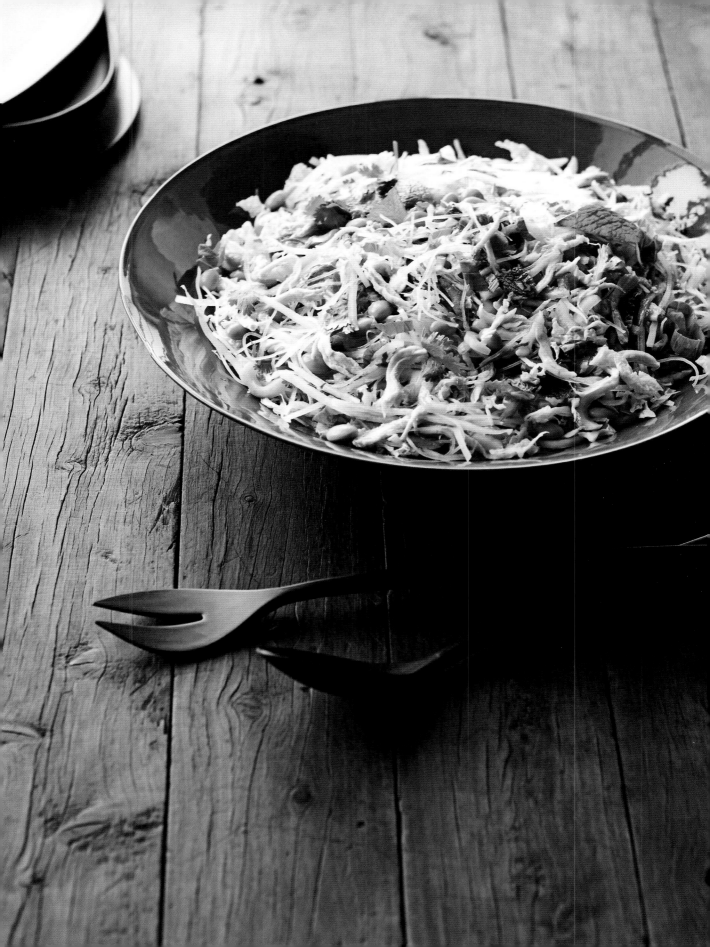

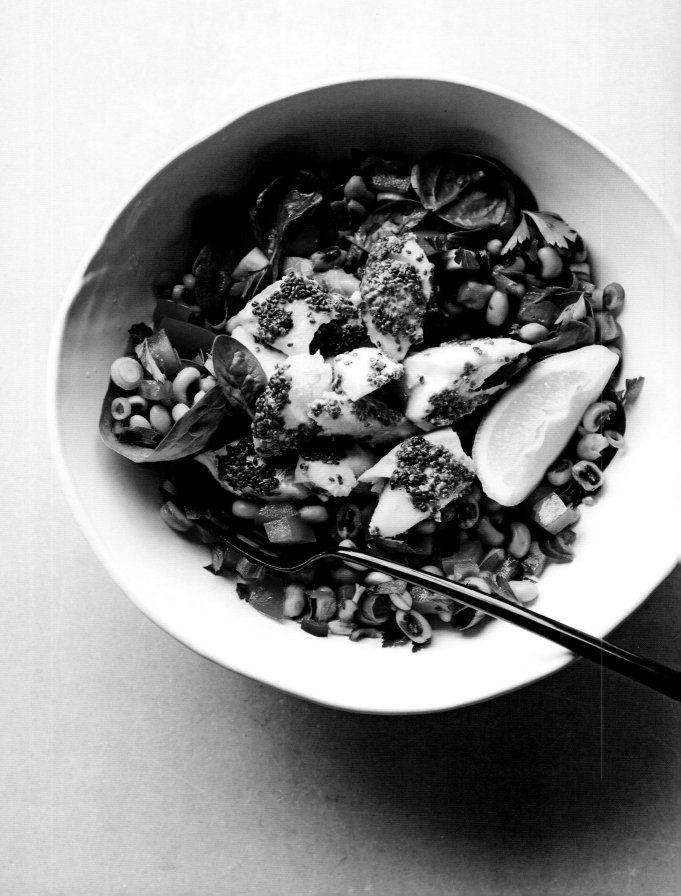

Black-eyed bean salad with flaked chia flathead

This is a delicious and simple salad that is particularly good when served warm. Remember that you will need to put the beans in water the night before you cook this dish, so that they can soak overnight.

SERVES 4

PREP TIME 15 MINUTES, PLUS OVERNIGHT SOAKING

COOKING TIME 30 MINUTES

1 cup (200 g) dried black-eyed beans
1 onion, quartered, leaving the root intact
2 tablespoons black chia seeds
500 g flathead fillets
olive oil spray, for cooking
2 tablespoons olive oil
4 tomatoes, chopped
2 spring onions, thinly sliced
1 long fresh green chilli, finely chopped (optional)
1 handful flat-leaf parsley, finely chopped
80 g baby spinach leaves
¼ cup (60 ml) lemon juice
lemon wedges, to serve

1. Place the beans in a large bowl, cover with plenty of cold water and soak overnight. Then drain well.

2. Place the beans, onion and 6 cups (1.5 litres) water in a large heavy-based saucepan and bring to the boil over high heat. Reduce the heat to low–medium and simmer for 20–25 minutes or until the beans are tender, topping up with extra boiling water from the kettle if necessary.

3. Meanwhile, place the chia seeds on a plate. Pat the fish fillets dry with paper towel and press into the seeds to lightly coat all over. Heat a large heavy-based non-stick frying pan over medium heat and spray lightly with oil. Cook the fish for 2–3 minutes or until golden. Turn the fillets and cook for a further 1–2 minutes or until just cooked through. Transfer to a plate to rest.

4. Drain the beans, discarding the onion and liquid. Transfer the beans to a large serving bowl, drizzle with the olive oil and stir gently to coat. Add the tomatoes, spring onions, chilli (if using), parsley, spinach and lemon juice and toss gently until well combined. Flake the fish, removing any bones, then scatter over the salad.

5. Serve immediately or at room temperature, with lemon wedges on the side.

NUTRITIONAL ANALYSIS	ENERGY (KJ)	1548	CARBOHYDRATE (G)	14	SODIUM (MG)	175
TO SERVE 4 (PER SERVE)	PROTEIN (G)	42	SATURATED FAT (G)	2.3	FIBRE (G)	9

Broccolini, broccoli and tofu salad

Tinned soybeans are not stocked in all supermarkets – look for them in the health food aisle, or try a health food store instead. Alternatively, you can cook your own: soak 1½ cups (300 g) dried soybeans overnight in cold water, then drain and boil for 90 minutes or until tender. Alternatively, use another type of bean – just about any other legume would work just as well.

SERVES 4
PREP TIME 20 MINUTES
COOKING TIME 15 MINUTES

1 × 400 g tin soybeans, drained and rinsed
3 spring onions, thinly sliced
1 teaspoon peanut oil
250 g firm tofu, cut into 2 cm cubes
2 teaspoons sesame seeds
½ teaspoon ground turmeric
olive oil spray, for cooking
350 g broccolini, trimmed and halved lengthways
2½ cups (200 g) broccoli florets
2 tablespoons pepitas (roasted pumpkin seed kernels)
4 homemade wholemeal yoghurt flatbreads (see page 290)
lime wedges, to serve (optional)

GINGER-SESAME DRESSING
1 tablespoon black sesame seeds, toasted
1 teaspoon finely grated ginger
½ small clove garlic, crushed
1 tablespoon mirin
3 teaspoons sesame oil
2 teaspoons salt-reduced soy sauce
1 teaspoon peanut oil
1 teaspoon lime juice

1. For the dressing, whisk all the ingredients with 2 tablespoons water in a medium bowl. Add the soybeans and spring onions to the dressing, stir to mix well and set aside.

2. Heat the oil in a large heavy-based non-stick frying pan over medium heat. Gently toss the cubed tofu with the sesame seeds and turmeric to coat, then cook for 4–5 minutes or until lightly browned and slightly crispy on the edges. Add to the soybean mixture.

3. Working in batches using the same frying pan and spraying the pan with oil as needed, cook the broccolini over medium heat, turning occasionally, for 4–5 minutes or until just tender and slightly browned in spots.

4. Meanwhile, steam the broccoli florets in a steamer basket over a saucepan of boiling water for 3 minutes or until tender but still slightly crisp. Set aside to cool slightly.

5. Arrange the broccolini and broccoli on a large platter or divide evenly among 4 bowls. Top with the soybean and tofu mixture, including all the dressing. Sprinkle with the pepitas. Serve warm or at room temperature with the flatbreads, and lime wedges if desired.

NUTRITIONAL ANALYSIS	ENERGY (KJ)	1552	CARBOHYDRATE (G)	9	SODIUM (MG)	135
TO SERVE 4 (PER SERVE)	PROTEIN (G)	31	SATURATED FAT (G)	3	FIBRE (G)	13

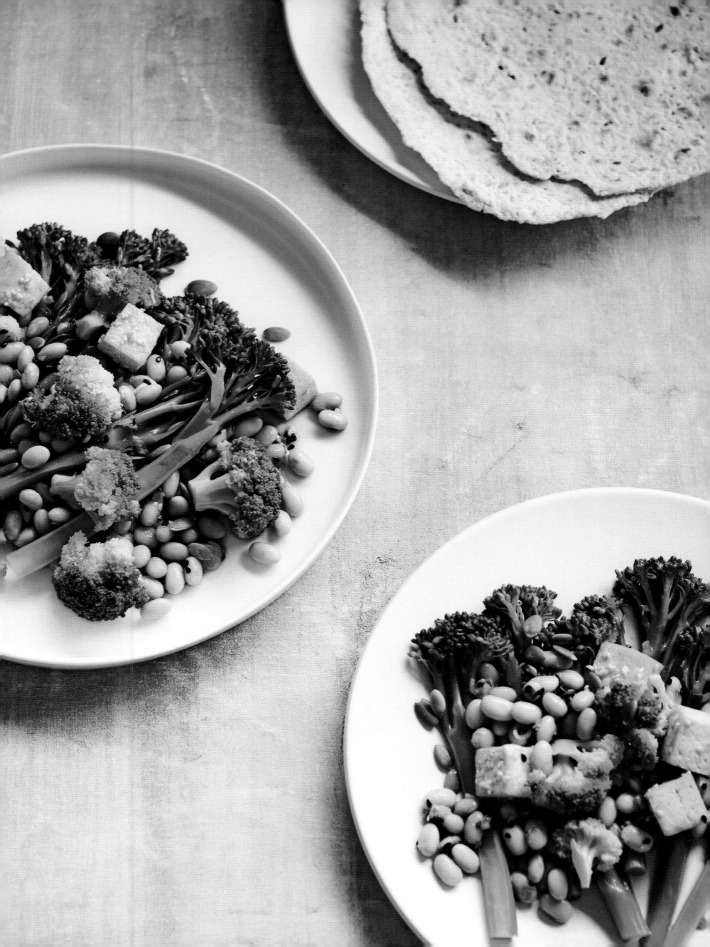

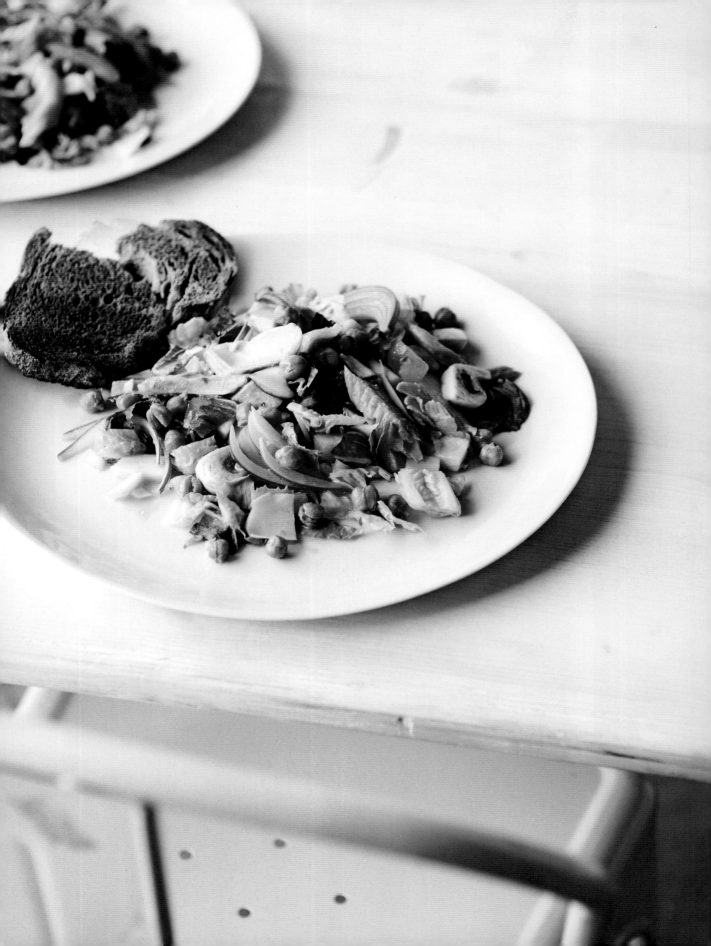

Chopped salad with smoked rainbow trout

Roasting chickpeas makes them pleasingly crunchy and salty and the perfect 'crouton' for a salad. Chop all the ingredients into bite-size chunks, including the lettuce, for an easy-to-eat salad.

SERVES 4
PREP TIME 20 MINUTES
COOKING TIME 20 MINUTES

1 × 400 g tin low-salt chickpeas, drained and rinsed
olive oil spray, for cooking
1 small red onion, thinly sliced
2 tablespoons malt vinegar
⅓ cup (80 ml) homemade classic salad dressing
    (see page 289)
2 teaspoons chopped tarragon
2 baby cos lettuces, cut into bite-sized pieces
1 small radicchio, cut into bite-sized pieces
1 small bulb fennel, base trimmed and cut into
    bite-sized pieces
5 button mushrooms, trimmed and cut into
    bite-sized pieces
5 radishes, cut into bite-sized pieces
150 g baby carrots, scrubbed and cut into
    bite-sized pieces
150 g flaked smoked trout, skin and bones removed
4 slices wholegrain sourdough bread,
    toasted or chargrilled

1. Preheat the oven to 200°C (180°C fan-forced). Line a large baking tray with baking paper.

2. Pat the chickpeas dry with paper towel, then spread over the lined tray and spray lightly with oil. Roast for 10 minutes, then stir and roast for a further 5–10 minutes, until dry and crisp.

3. Place the sliced onion in a small bowl with the vinegar and set aside. Combine the salad dressing and tarragon in a separate small bowl and set aside.

4. Place the chopped lettuce and vegetables in a large bowl. Drain the onion, discarding the vinegar, and add to the vegetables. Add the dressing and tarragon mixture, and toss to combine.

5. Divide the salad among 4 plates or place on a large platter. Top with the flaked trout (or toss through, if preferred), then scatter with the roasted chickpeas. Serve with the toasted bread.

NUTRITIONAL ANALYSIS	ENERGY (KJ)	1604	CARBOHYDRATE (G)	32	SODIUM (MG)	683
TO SERVE 4 (PER SERVE)	PROTEIN (G)	19	SATURATED FAT (G)	2.9	FIBRE (G)	8

Gado gado

Smearing the bowls with a little of the peanut sauce and piling the ingredients on top – with more of the sauce – ensures you get a hit of its nutty, crunchy, salty flavours with every mouthful, and makes for an interesting presentation.

SERVES 4
PREP TIME 20 MINUTES
COOKING TIME 20 MINUTES

8 baby new potatoes (320 g), scrubbed
2 teaspoons white vinegar
4 large eggs, at room temperature
2 baby bok choy, trimmed, leaves separated
2 carrots, scrubbed and thinly sliced on the diagonal
200 g green beans, trimmed and halved or cut into bite-sized lengths
160 g shredded Chinese cabbage (wombok)
160 g bean sprouts, trimmed
1 tablespoon white sesame seeds (optional)
1 tablespoon roasted black sesame seeds (optional)
lime wedges, to serve

SPICY PEANUT SAUCE (MAKES ABOUT ¾ CUP (225 g))
1 teaspoon peanut oil
1 onion, finely chopped
1 small clove garlic, crushed
1 tablespoon shaved palm sugar
1 small fresh red chilli, finely chopped
¼ cup (35 g) dry-roasted unsalted peanuts, finely chopped
2 tablespoons lime juice
1 tablespoon crunchy natural peanut butter
2 teaspoons salt-reduced soy sauce

1. Boil or steam the potatoes for 15 minutes or until tender. Drain and leave until cool enough to handle, then cut in half.

2. Meanwhile, for the sauce, heat the peanut oil in a small heavy-based saucepan over medium heat. Add the onion and garlic, and cook, stirring, for 2–3 minutes or until lightly caramelised and tender. Add the palm sugar, chilli and ¼ cup (60 ml) water, and cook, stirring, for 1–2 minutes or until the sugar dissolves. Remove from the heat and whisk in the peanuts, lime juice, peanut butter and soy sauce. Set aside to cool. Blend for a slightly smoother sauce, if you like.

3. Bring a small saucepan of water to the boil and add the vinegar. Using a spoon, carefully lower the 4 eggs into the boiling water. Reduce the heat to medium and cook for 6 minutes. Drain and cool the eggs under cold running water. Peel and set aside.

4. Bring a second saucepan of water to the boil and submerge the bok choy leaves for 2 minutes or until tender but still crisp, then refresh them in a bowl of cold water. Drain well.

5. Spread a spoonful of the spicy peanut sauce around the side of 4 wide serving bowls. Divide the potatoes, bok choy and chopped raw salad ingredients evenly among the bowls. Cut the eggs in half and add to the bowls. Spoon over the remaining sauce, and pour any leftover sauce into a small serving bowl. Serve with lime wedges on the side.

NUTRITIONAL ANALYSIS	ENERGY (KJ)	1440	CARBOHYDRATE (G)	23	SODIUM (MG)	437
TO SERVE 4 (PER SERVE)	PROTEIN (G)	21	SATURATED FAT (G)	4.1	FIBRE (G)	9

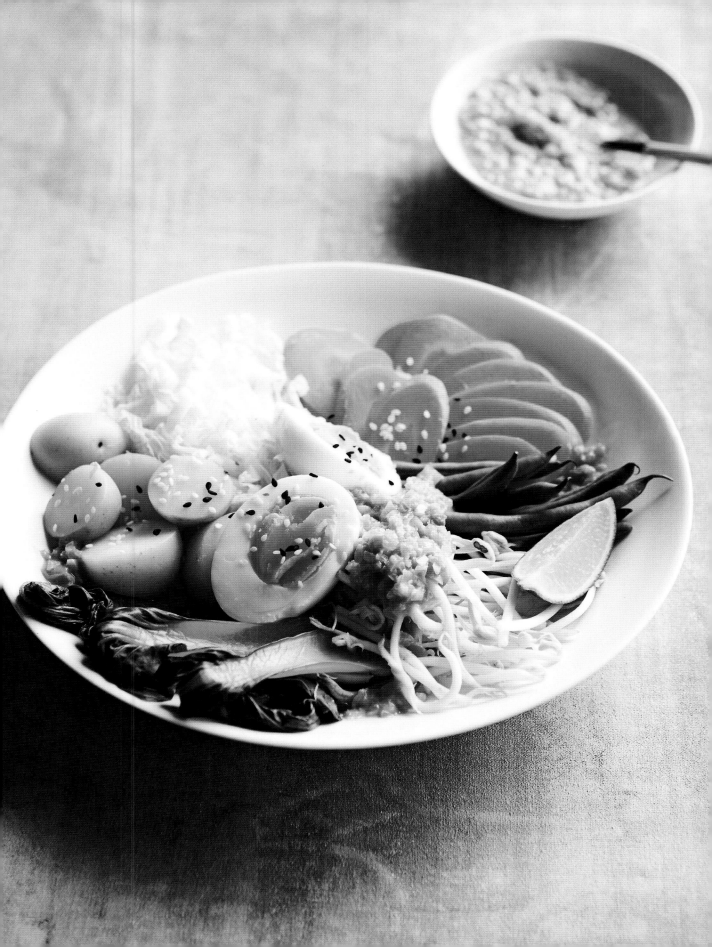

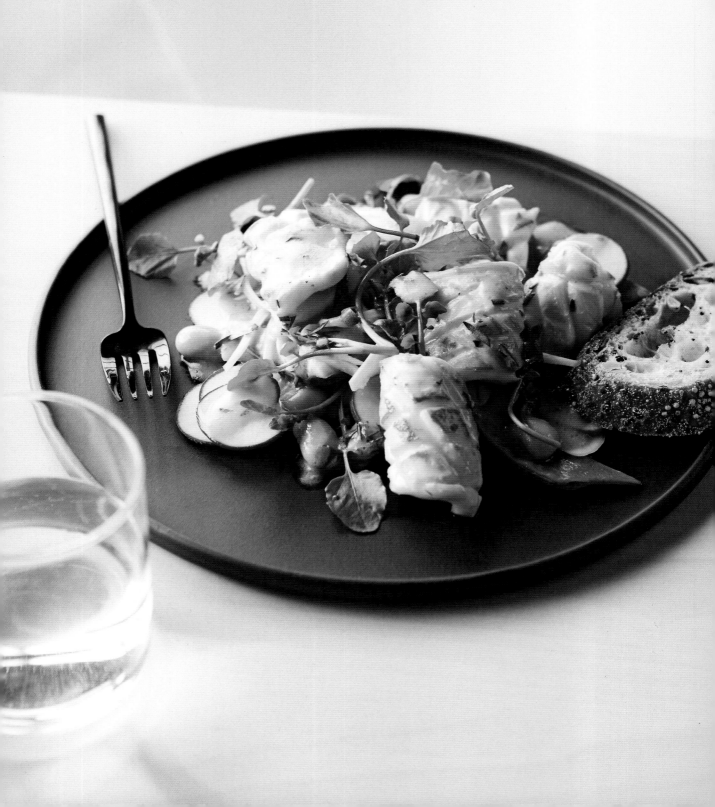

Pan-seared squid with tarragon dressing

Using a mandoline, if you have one, to thinly slice the fennel and radishes makes putting this salad together a breeze. You could toast or chargrill the bread, if you prefer more crunch.

SERVES 4
PREP TIME 25 MINUTES
COOKING TIME 15 MINUTES

1 bulb fennel, thinly sliced
¼ cup (60 ml) white balsamic condiment
2 teaspoons honey
500 g cleaned squid hoods
olive oil spray, for cooking
¼ cup (60 ml) homemade classic salad dressing
    (made with lemon juice, see page 289)
2 teaspoons chopped French tarragon, plus extra leaves
    to serve
2 × 400 g tins low-salt butter beans, drained and rinsed
200 g snow peas (mangetout), trimmed and halved
    on the diagonal
200 g watercress or rocket
8 radishes, thinly sliced
4 slices wholegrain sourdough bread

1. Combine the fennel, balsamic and honey in a medium-sized bowl, stirring until the honey has dissolved. Set aside for the fennel to lightly pickle, stirring occasionally.

2. Wash the squid under running water, then remove the shell – the hard, clear quill – from inside the hood. Then, using a very sharp knife cut the hood in half lengthways and score the inside in a crisscross pattern. Pat the squid dry with paper towel, then cut into 3 cm-wide strips. Spray with oil to coat.

3. Heat a large heavy-based non-stick frying pan over high heat. Working in 3 batches, pan-fry the squid, turning occasionally, for 3–4 minutes or until curled and just cooked through. Transfer to a bowl and loosely cover with foil to keep warm.

4. Drain the fennel, reserving 2 tablespoons of the balsamic mixture. Place the reserved balsamic mixture in a screw-top jar and add the salad dressing and French tarragon. Seal with the lid and shake until emulsified. Pour half of the dressing over the squid and toss to combine.

5. Place the pickled fennel, butter beans, snow peas, watercress or rocket and radishes in a large bowl. Toss to combine, then arrange on a large platter. Top with the squid and all the juices from the bowl. Drizzle with the remaining dressing and serve with the bread on the side.

NUTRITIONAL ANALYSIS	ENERGY (KJ)	1601	CARBOHYDRATE (G)	29	SODIUM (MG)	603
TO SERVE 4 (PER SERVE)	PROTEIN (G)	32	SATURATED FAT (G)	2.1	FIBRE (G)	7

Roasted cauliflower and black lentil salad

Roasting cauliflower caramelises its natural sugars, bringing out a sweetness in its flavour which, when combined with the creamy tahini dressing, makes this salad extremely moreish.

SERVES 4
PREP TIME 20 MINUTES
COOKING TIME 30 MINUTES

1 cup (220 g) black or green (Puy) lentils, rinsed
1 small cauliflower, cut into small florets
1 onion, cut into thin wedges
olive oil spray, for cooking
2 teaspoons soft brown sugar
2 tablespoons red wine vinegar
1 cup (80 g) shredded red cabbage
80 g rocket
¼ cup (40 g) raw almonds, roughly chopped

TAHINI DRESSING
½ cup (140 g) reduced-fat natural Greek-style yoghurt
2 teaspoons lemon juice
3 teaspoons hulled tahini
½ small clove garlic, crushed (optional)

1. Preheat the oven to 220°C (200°C fan-forced). Line 1 large or 2 small baking trays with baking paper.

2. Place the lentils and 6 cups (1.5 litres) water in a large heavy-based saucepan and bring to the boil over high heat. Reduce the heat to low and simmer for 20–25 minutes or until just tender (do not over-cook the lentils or they will be mushy). Top up the pan with extra boiling water if necessary. Drain.

3. Meanwhile, spread the cauliflower florets and onion over the lined tray/s and spray lightly with oil. Roast for 15–20 minutes, stirring after 10 minutes, until the cauliflower is lightly browned around the edges. Set aside to cool slightly.

4. Bring the brown sugar, red wine vinegar and ⅓ cup (80 ml) water to the boil in a small heavy-based saucepan over high heat. Remove from the heat and add the cabbage. Set aside to cool, stirring occasionally, then drain, discarding the liquid.

5. Meanwhile, for the dressing, whisk all the ingredients together in a bowl. Add a little cold water, if necessary, to bring the dressing to a pouring consistency. Season with freshly ground white pepper, then cover with plastic film and refrigerate until required.

6. Toss the lentils, cauliflower mixture and rocket in a large bowl. Transfer to a serving platter or divide among 4 bowls. Top with the drained cabbage and scatter with the almonds. Drizzle with the dressing and serve immediately.

| NUTRITIONAL ANALYSIS | ENERGY (KJ) | 1653 | CARBOHYDRATE (G) | 39 | SODIUM (MG) | 120 |
| TO SERVE 4 (PER SERVE) | PROTEIN (G) | 26 | SATURATED FAT (G) | 2.5 | FIBRE (G) | 17 |

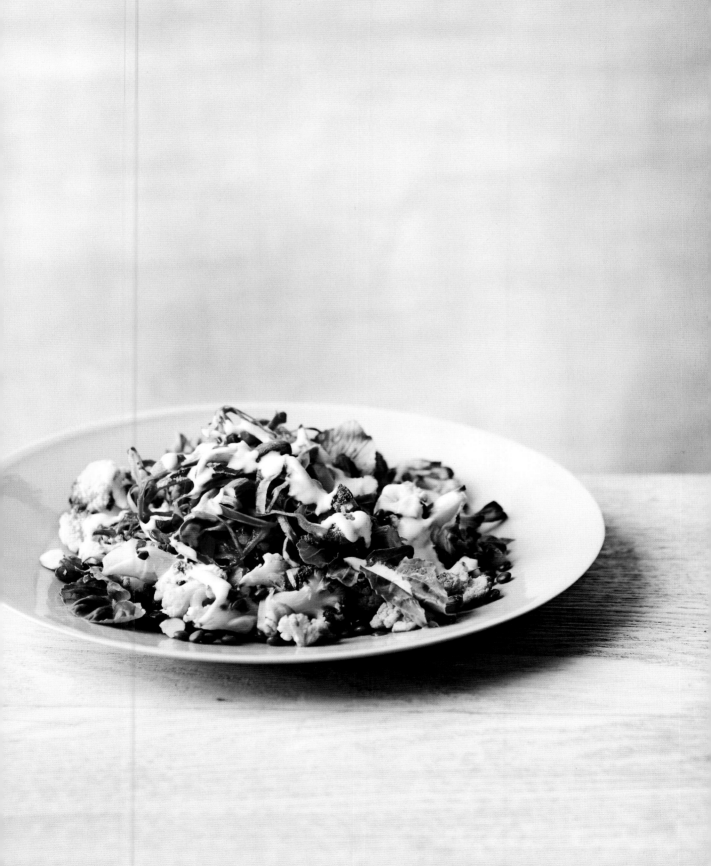

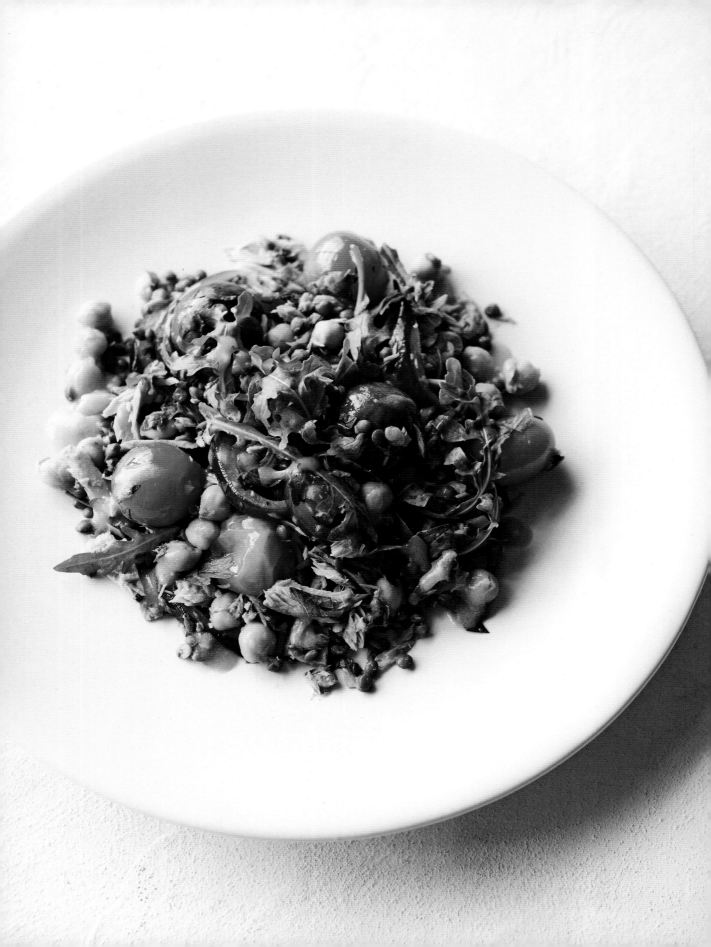

Tuna, tomato, lentil and chickpea salad

This salad is delicious when warm and when chilled, and so you can prepare it in advance for a quick and easy meal, or take it as a packed lunch for eating on the go.

SERVES 4
PREP TIME 15 MINUTES
COOKING TIME 15 MINUTES

1 teaspoon olive oil
500 g mixed cherry tomatoes
½ red onion, cut into thin wedges
1 × 400 g tin low-salt brown lentils, drained and rinsed
1 × 400 g tin low-salt chickpeas, drained and rinsed
¼ cup (60 ml) homemade classic salad dressing
   (see page 289)
160 g rocket or baby spinach leaves
1 × 425 g tin tuna in springwater, drained
1 large handful roughly chopped flat-leaf parsley
lemon wedges, to serve (optional)

1. Heat the oil in a large heavy-based non-stick frying pan over medium heat. Add the tomatoes and onion and cook, shaking the pan occasionally, for 3–5 minutes or until the tomatoes begin to soften and split, releasing some of their juices. Add the lentils, chickpeas and 1 tablespoon of the dressing and cook, stirring, for 2–3 minutes or until heated through.

2. Remove from the heat and fold in the rocket or spinach leaves, tuna, parsley and remaining dressing. Season with pepper to taste, and serve immediately with lemon wedges on the side, if using.

NUTRITIONAL ANALYSIS	ENERGY (KJ)	1178	CARBOHYDRATE (G)	18	SODIUM (MG)	520
TO SERVE 4 (PER SERVE)	PROTEIN (G)	36	SATURATED FAT (G)	1.3	FIBRE (G)	6

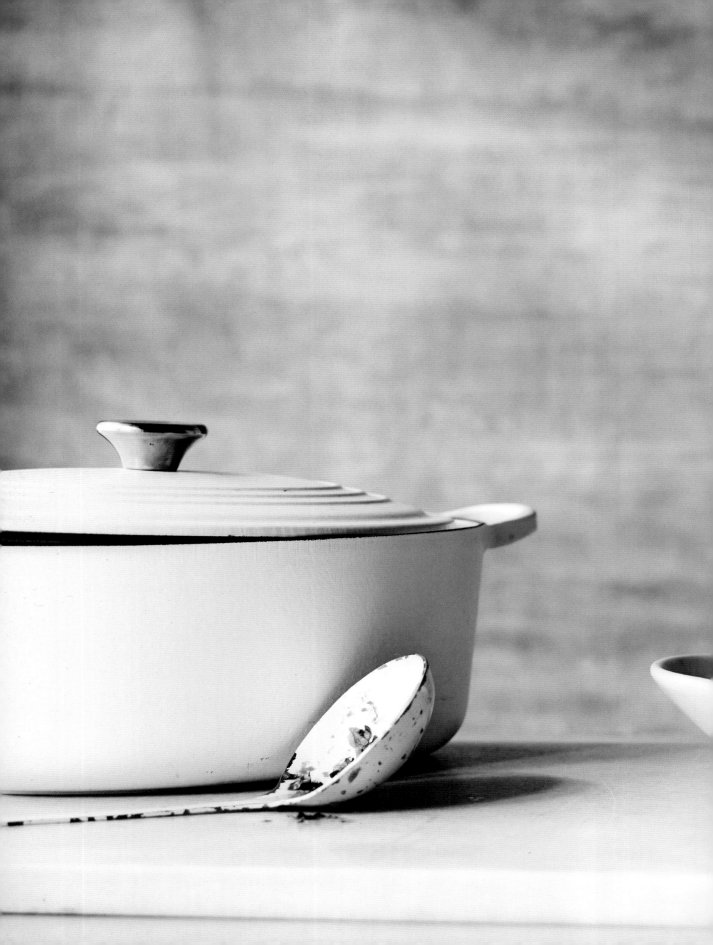

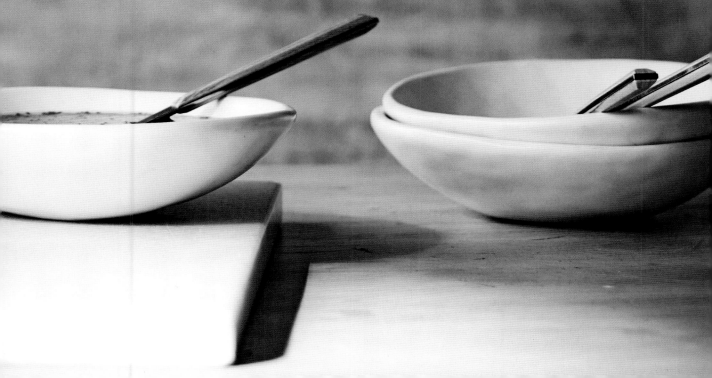

SOUPS

Broccoli and pea soup with scallops

The scallops are a wonderfully indulgent element in this tasty soup, which is the perfect winter warmer for those cold and rainy days. Serve with crusty or toasted bread to up the comfort factor.

SERVES 4
PREP TIME 15 MINUTES
COOKING TIME 25 MINUTES

1 tablespoon olive oil

1 onion, finely chopped

2 cloves garlic, crushed

4 cups (1 litre) homemade chicken stock (see page 288) or salt-reduced chicken stock

1 × 400 g tin low-salt cannellini or butter beans, drained and rinsed

4 cups (340 g) chopped broccoli

2 cups (240 g) frozen peas

1 cup (150 g) frozen shelled edamame (soybeans), thawed

100 g scallop meat (without roe)

1 tablespoon dukkah (see page 293)

4 slices wholegrain sourdough bread (optional)

1. Heat 3 teaspoons of the oil in a large heavy-based saucepan over low–medium heat. Cook the onion and garlic for 5 minutes or until tender but not coloured.

2. Add the stock and beans, and bring to the boil over high heat. Add the broccoli and peas; reduce the heat to medium and cook for 10 minutes or until the broccoli is very tender. Set aside to cool slightly, then use a stick blender to blend until smooth. Return the pan over medium heat to heat through. (Alternatively, leave to cool further and use a blender or food processor to puree the soup, in batches if necessary, until smooth. Then return to the pan to heat through.)

3. Meanwhile, heat the remaining oil in a large heavy-based non-stick frying pan over medium heat. Add the edamame and stir-fry for 2–3 minutes or until just starting to lightly brown. Push the edamame to the side of the pan, add the scallop meat to the centre and cook for 1–2 minutes or until the scallops are browned and just cooked through.

4. Ladle the soup evenly into 4 bowls, then top each one with one-quarter of the scallop and edamame mixture. Sprinkle with the dukkah, and serve with the bread, if desired.

NUTRITIONAL ANALYSIS	ENERGY (KJ)	1642	CARBOHYDRATE (G)	29	SODIUM (MG)	1495
TO SERVE 4 (PER SERVE)	PROTEIN (G)	27	SATURATED FAT (G)	2.1	FIBRE (G)	11

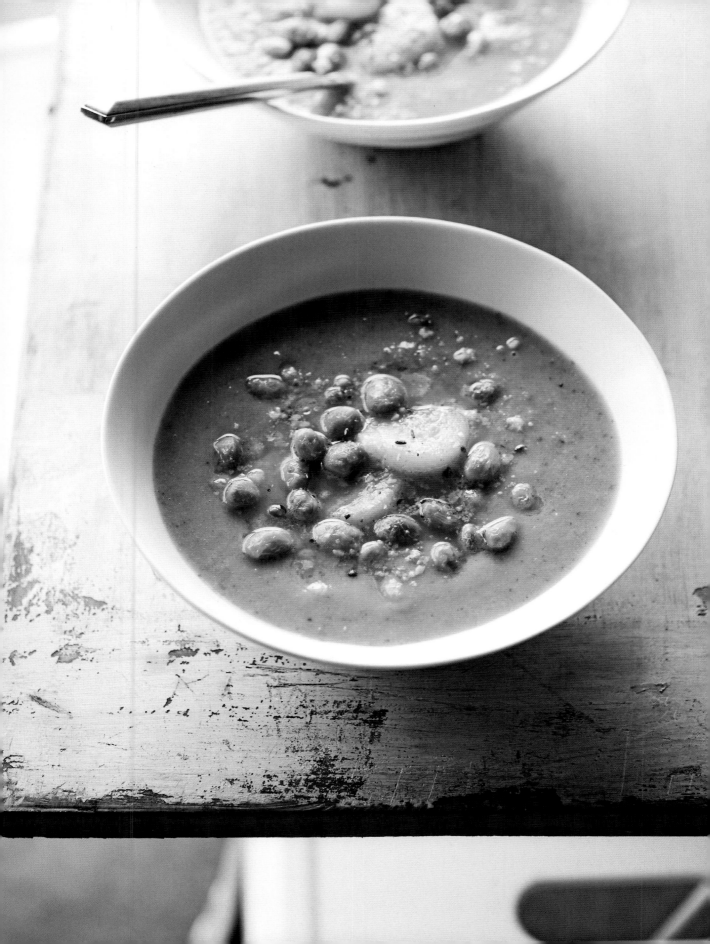

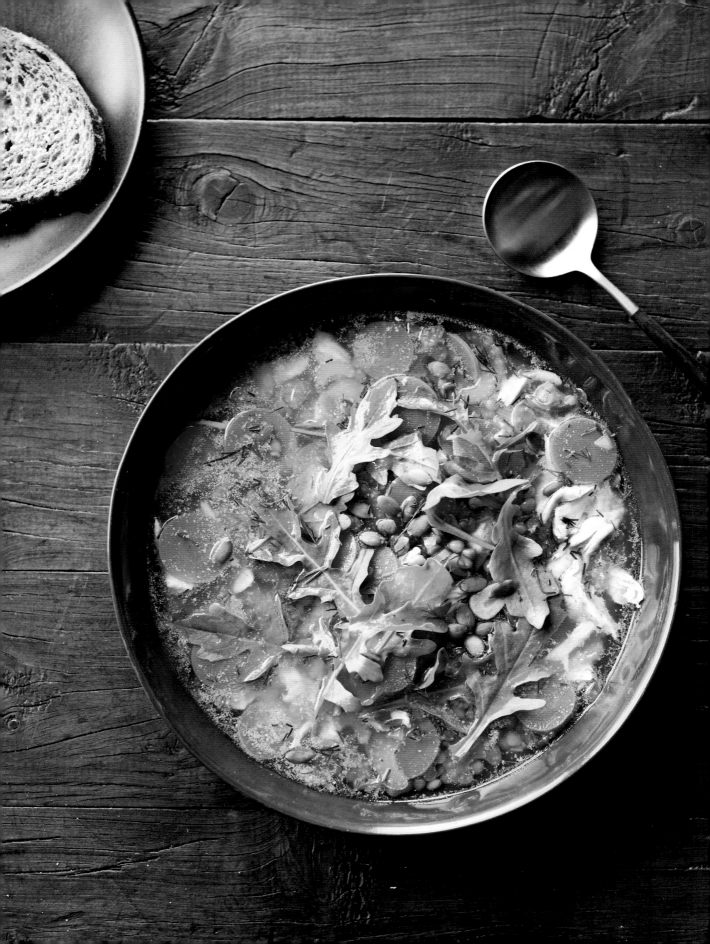

Chicken, lemon and dill soup

Good stock is the key ingredient of tasty soup. However, if you are low on homemade stock or don't have time to make it first, then a shop-bought salt-reduced stock will do just fine.

SERVES 4
PREP TIME 20 MINUTES
COOKING TIME 35 MINUTES

1 tablespoon olive oil
1 onion, finely chopped
3 stalks celery, including leaves, bases trimmed, thinly sliced
3 carrots, scrubbed and thinly sliced
2 cloves garlic, thinly sliced
200 g skinless chicken breast tenderloins
4 cups (1 litre) homemade chicken stock (see page 288) or salt-reduced chicken stock
1 × 400 g tin low-salt brown lentils, drained and rinsed
¼ cup (60 ml) lemon juice
2 tablespoons chopped dill
60 g rocket
2 tablespoons pepitas (roasted pumpkin seed kernels)
4 slices wholegrain sourdough bread

1. Heat the olive oil in a large heavy-based saucepan and cook the onion, celery and carrot over low–medium heat for 10–15 minutes or until tender and just starting to colour. Add the garlic and cook, stirring, until fragrant.

2. Add the chicken and enough stock to just cover. Bring slowly to the boil over low–medium heat, then reduce the heat to low and poach the chicken for 5–6 minutes or until just cooked through. Using tongs, transfer the chicken to a plate and set aside.

3. Add the lentils and remaining stock to the pan and bring to the boil, then reduce the heat to low and simmer for 10 minutes or until the vegetables are very tender.

4. Meanwhile, use 2 forks to shred the chicken. Remove the pan from the heat and stir in the chicken, lemon juice and dill. Season with freshly ground black pepper.

5. Ladle the soup evenly into 4 bowls. Top each with one-quarter of the rocket and pepitas, and serve with the bread on the side.

NUTRITIONAL ANALYSIS	ENERGY (KJ)	1435	CARBOHYDRATE (G)	28	SODIUM (MG)	1283
TO SERVE 4 (PER SERVE)	PROTEIN (G)	25	SATURATED FAT (G)	2.3	FIBRE (G)	6

Chunky beetroot, farro and vegetable soup

The beetroot not only fills your bowl with nutritional goodness and antioxidants, it also makes this soup a beautifully vibrant ruby-red colour. Leaving the ingredients chunky adds texture to the silky smooth liquid of this delicious soup.

SERVES 4
PREP TIME 20 MINUTES
COOKING TIME 55 MINUTES

2 tablespoons olive oil
1 leek, white section only, sliced
2 beetroots, peeled and diced
1 parsnip, peeled and diced
2 carrots, scrubbed and diced
4 cloves garlic, thinly sliced
2 teaspoons caraway seeds
2 bay leaves
½ cup (100 g) cracked farro (or barley)
4 cups (1 litre) homemade chicken stock (see page 288)
    or salt-reduced vegetable stock
1 × 400 g tin low-salt red kidney beans, drained and rinsed
2 cups (160 g) finely shredded red cabbage
½ cup (140 g) reduced-fat natural Greek-style yoghurt
2 tablespoons dill sprigs

1. Heat the oil in a large heavy-based saucepan over low–medium heat. Add the leek, beetroots, parsnip, carrots, garlic, caraway seeds and bay leaves and cook, stirring, for 10 minutes or until the vegetables start to soften.

2. Add the farro or barley to the stock and bring to the boil over high heat, then reduce the heat to low and simmer, covered, for 30 minutes or until the farro or barley is almost tender. Stir in the kidney beans and cabbage, adding a little water if you prefer a thinner soup, then simmer, covered, for a further 10 minutes or until the vegetables and farro or barley are tender.

3. Season the soup with freshly ground black pepper and ladle evenly into 4 large bowls, removing the bay leaves. Top with a spoonful of yoghurt and sprinkle with sprigs of dill, then serve.

NUTRITIONAL ANALYSIS	ENERGY (KJ)	1817	CARBOHYDRATE (G)	54	SODIUM (MG)	1256
TO SERVE 4 (PER SERVE)	PROTEIN (G)	16	SATURATED FAT (G)	3.4	FIBRE (G)	17

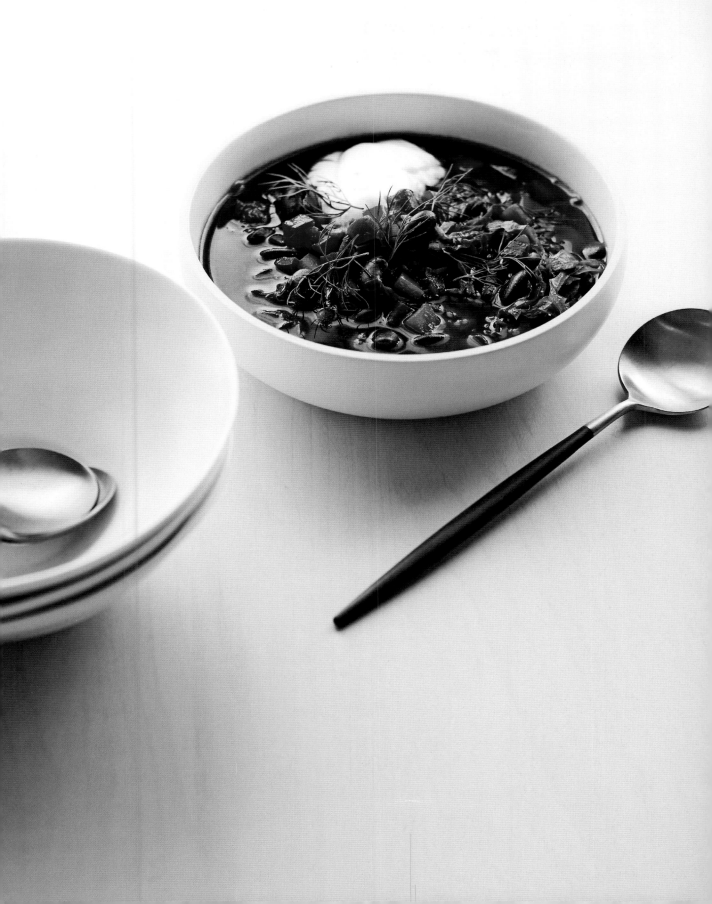

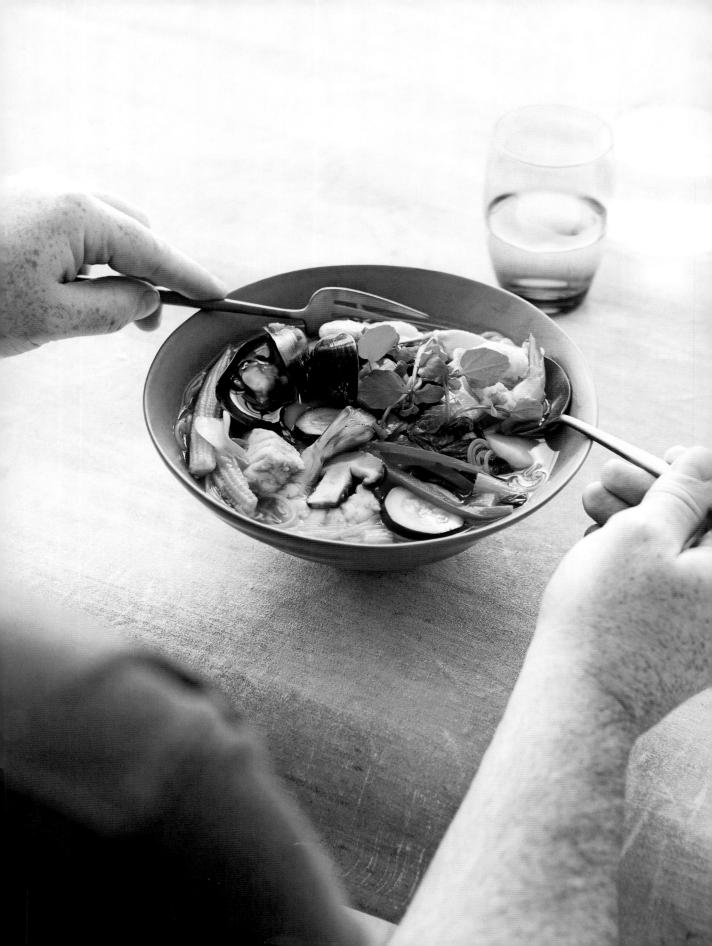

Hot and sour seafood soup

This mouth-watering prawn broth, filled to the brim with fresh seafood, noodles and vegetables, is wonderfully fragrant and aromatic, with a subtle heat from the red curry paste that is balanced by the citrus flavour from the lime. This soup gives you hot and sour, sweet and salty, all in one dish.

SERVES 4
PREP TIME 30 MINUTES
COOKING TIME 40 MINUTES

150 g raw prawns, peeled and cleaned with tails intact, shells reserved
1 teaspoon peanut oil
2 teaspoons Thai red curry paste
4 kaffir lime leaves
1 stalk lemongrass, pale part only, roughly chopped
150 g bean-thread vermicelli (glass noodles)
½ small daikon, cut into thin strips
1 red capsicum (pepper), seeded, membrane removed, cut into long thin strips
230 g baby corn, halved lengthways
50 g shiitake mushrooms, sliced
2 baby bok choy, trimmed and cut into 1 cm-thick slices
2 zucchinis (courgettes), thinly sliced
1 × 200 g mackerel fillet, cut into 3 cm cubes
100 g scallop meat (without roe), cut in half widthways
500 g black mussels, bearded and scrubbed
2–3 tablespoon lime juice, to taste
1 teaspoon salt-reduced soy sauce
1 teaspoon grated palm sugar or soft brown sugar
50 g watercress

1. Place the prawns on a plate, cover with plastic film and refrigerate until required.

2. Heat the oil in a heavy-based saucepan over high heat. Add the prawn shells and heads and cook, stirring frequently, for 4–5 minutes or until the shells turn orange. Add the curry paste and cook, stirring, for 30 seconds or until aromatic; add a splash of water if the paste is sticking to the pan. Add 6 cups (1.5 litres) water, the lime leaves and lemongrass and bring to the boil. Reduce the heat to low–medium and simmer, covered, for 20 minutes or until the stock is well flavoured.

Strain the prawn stock through a fine-mesh sieve into a large heavy-based saucepan, discarding the solids caught in the sieve.

3. Meanwhile, bring a large heavy-based saucepan of water to the boil over high heat. Add the vermicelli and cook for 6–8 minutes or until just tender (or follow the packet directions). Drain and refresh under cold water.

4. Bring the prawn stock to the boil over medium heat. Add the vegetables and return to a simmer. Add the prawns, mackerel, scallops and mussels and cook for 3–4 minutes or until they are just cooked through. Stir in lime juice to taste, along with the soy sauce and sugar.

5. Divide the noodles among 4 large bowls. Ladle the soup into the bowls, ensuring the vegetables and seafood are divided evenly among them. Top with the watercress and serve.

NUTRITIONAL ANALYSIS	ENERGY (KJ)	1995	CARBOHYDRATE (G)	29	SODIUM (MG)	1095
TO SERVE 4 (PER SERVE)	PROTEIN (G)	55	SATURATED FAT (G)	3.2	FIBRE (G)	6

Moroccan pumpkin and lentil soup
with dukkah-dusted rainbow trout

Pumpkin is always a pleasing staple for a soup, and the Moroccan flavours from the ras el hanout perfectly complement the pumpkin's sweetness and nutty crumb on the trout.

SERVES 4
PREP TIME 20 MINUTES
COOKING TIME 35 MINUTES

1 tablespoon olive oil
1 onion, finely chopped
2 cloves garlic, thinly sliced
1.5 kg kent or butternut pumpkin (squash), peeled, seeded and cut into chunks
½ cup (100 g) red split lentils, well rinsed
1 teaspoon ras el hanout
4 cups (1 litre) homemade chicken stock (see page 288) or salt-reduced vegetable stock or water
1 tablespoon homemade dukkah or nut-free dukkah (see page 293)
1 × 200 g rainbow trout fillet
½ cup (140 g) reduced-fat natural Greek-style yoghurt
coriander leaves, to serve

1. Heat the oil in a large heavy-based saucepan over low–medium heat. Cook the onion and garlic, stirring occasionally, for 8 minutes or until softened.

2. Increase the heat to medium and add the pumpkin, lentils and ras el hanout, then cook, stirring, for 3 minutes. Add the stock and bring to the boil, then reduce the heat to low and simmer, covered, for 15–20 minutes or until the pumpkin and lentils are tender, stirring every 5 minutes or so to prevent the lentils sticking to the base of the pan.

3. Meanwhile, spread the dukkah over a small plate. Pat the fish dry with paper towel and press one side firmly in the dukkah to coat it. Heat a non-stick frying pan over medium heat and spray lightly with oil. Cook the trout, dukkah-side down, for 2–3 minutes or until golden. Turn and cook for a further 1–2 minutes or until just cooked through. Transfer to a plate to rest.

4. Using a potato masher, crush the pumpkin in the soup – this will result in a chunky soup. (Use a stick blender to blend the soup if you prefer a smooth consistency.)

5. Flake the trout, removing and discarding the skin and any bones. Using a ladle, share the soup between 4 large bowls. Top with the flaked trout, a spoonful of yoghurt and coriander leaves, then serve.

NUTRITIONAL ANALYSIS	ENERGY (KJ)	1923	CARBOHYDRATE (G)	52	SODIUM (MG)	1074
TO SERVE 4 (PER SERVE)	PROTEIN (G)	24	SATURATED FAT (G)	3.6	FIBRE (G)	11

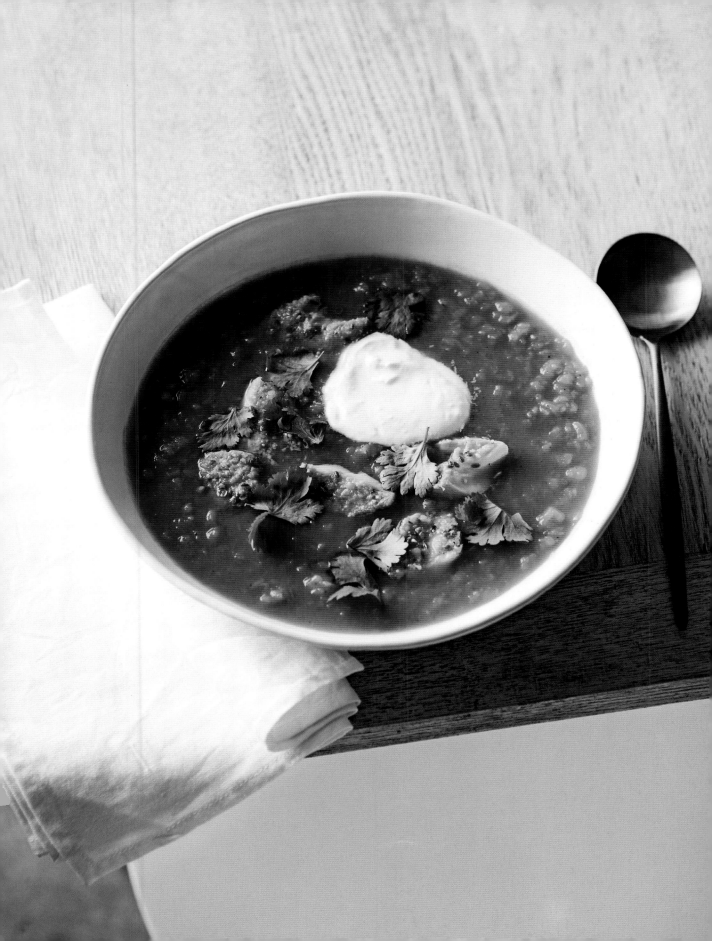

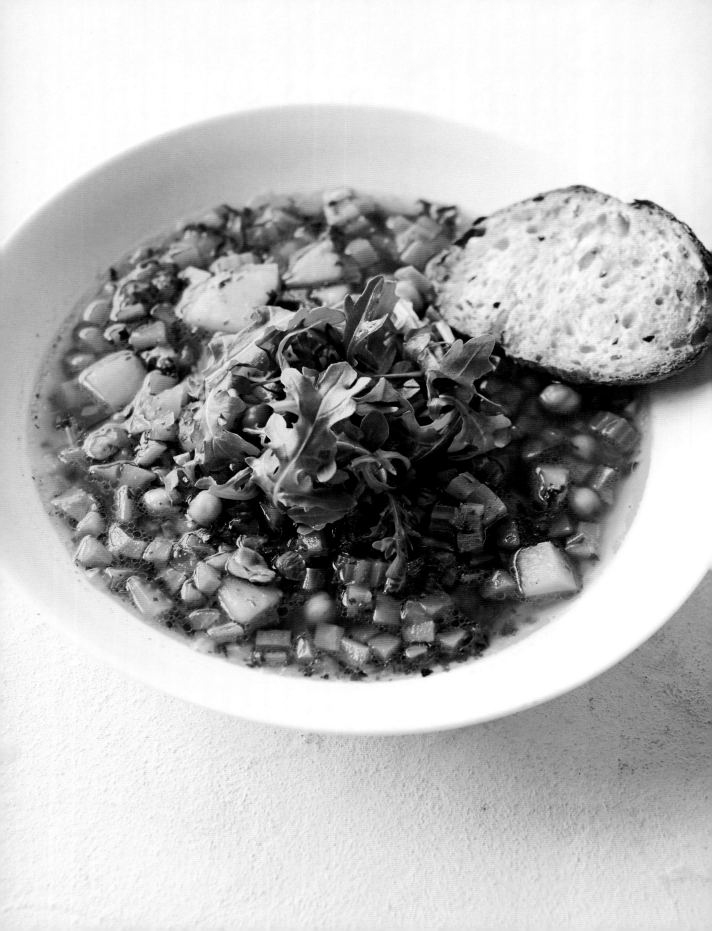

Rocket, potato and chickpea soup

Pureeing rocket intensifies its rich, peppery flavour to give this soup
a taste of summer alongside the wintry root vegetables.

SERVES 4
PREP TIME 15 MINUTES
COOKING TIME 35 MINUTES

1 tablespoon olive oil

1 onion, finely chopped

2 stalks celery, including leaves, bases trimmed,
    thinly sliced

3 carrots, scrubbed and diced

2 potatoes (400 g), diced

2 cloves garlic, crushed

5 cups (1.25 litres) homemade vegetable or chicken stock
    (see page 288) or salt-reduced vegetable or chicken
    stock

1 × 400 g tin low-salt chickpeas, drained and rinsed

¼ cup (40 g) blanched almonds

200 g rocket

4 slices wholegrain sourdough bread, toasted or
    chargrilled if desired

1. Heat the oil in a large heavy-based saucepan over
   low–medium heat and cook the onion, celery
   and carrots, covered, stirring occasionally, for
   10–15 minutes or until tender and starting to
   caramelise. Add all the potato and garlic to the pan
   and cook, stirring, until the potato starts to colour.

2. Add the stock and chickpeas and bring to the boil
   over high heat. Reduce the heat to low and simmer,
   covered, for 15–20 minutes or until the vegetables
   are very tender and some of the potato starts to
   break down.

3. Meanwhile, toast the almonds in a small heavy-
   based frying pan over medium heat for 5 minutes
   or until fragrant. Transfer to a bowl to cool,
   then roughly chop.

4. Place three-quarters of the rocket on top of the
   soup and, without stirring, blanch for 30 seconds.
   Use a slotted spoon to carefully remove the rocket
   and puree in a blender or food processor until
   smooth; if necessary, add a little of the broth to
   help it process. Add the rocket puree to the soup
   and stir well, then season with white pepper.

5. Ladle the soup into 4 bowls. Top with the chopped
   almonds and remaining rocket. Serve with bread
   or toast alongside.

NUTRITIONAL ANALYSIS	ENERGY (KJ)	1666	CARBOHYDRATE (G)	45	SODIUM (MG)	1584
TO SERVE 4 (PER SERVE)	PROTEIN (G)	18	SATURATED FAT (G)	1.7	FIBRE (G)	8

Ocean trout ramen

What could be better than a big bowl of noodles in a yummy broth? The marinated trout brings bucket-loads of flavour to this already flavoursome soup, and the cucumber and spinach add freshness and supply the crunch to make it a fully satisfying, well-rounded meal.

SERVES 4

PREP TIME 20 MINUTES, PLUS 1 HOUR MARINATING

COOKING TIME 15 MINUTES

4 × 80 g ocean trout fillets

100 g ramen noodles

2 cloves garlic, crushed

4 cups (1 litre) homemade chicken stock (see page 288) or salt-reduced chicken stock

1 teaspoon salt-reduced soy sauce

3 carrots, scrubbed and cut into thin strips

2 baby bok choy, trimmed and quartered lengthways

150 g green beans, trimmed and halved lengthways

150 g baby spinach leaves

1 telegraph (long) cucumber, cut into thin strips

coriander leaves, to serve

GINGER-SOY MARINADE

1 teaspoon grated ginger

2 teaspoons mirin

2 teaspoons salt-reduced soy sauce

1. For the marinade, combine the ingredients in a glass bowl. Add the ocean trout. Turn the fish to coat it well and refrigerate for 1 hour to marinate.

2. Meanwhile, bring a large heavy-based saucepan of water to the boil over high heat. Add the noodles and cook for 2 minutes or until just tender (or follow the packet instructions). Drain and refresh under cold water.

3. Place the garlic, stock, 2 cups (500 ml) water and the soy sauce in a large heavy-based saucepan. Bring to the boil over medium heat. Add the trout and its marinade, then simmer, covered, over low heat for 3 minutes. Add the carrots, bok choy and beans and simmer for a further 1–2 minutes or until the trout is just cooked. Remove the trout and set aside on a plate, covered with foil to keep it warm. Season the broth with a little white pepper, if necessary.

4. Divide the noodles, spinach leaves and cucumber strips among 4 bowls. Ladle over the soup, ensuring each bowl gets an equal share of vegetables, noodles and broth. Top with the trout and scatter with coriander leaves, then serve.

NUTRITIONAL ANALYSIS	ENERGY (KJ)	1070	CARBOHYDRATE (G)	16	SODIUM (MG)	1347
TO SERVE 4 (PER SERVE)	PROTEIN (G)	24	SATURATED FAT (G)	1.9	FIBRE (G)	7

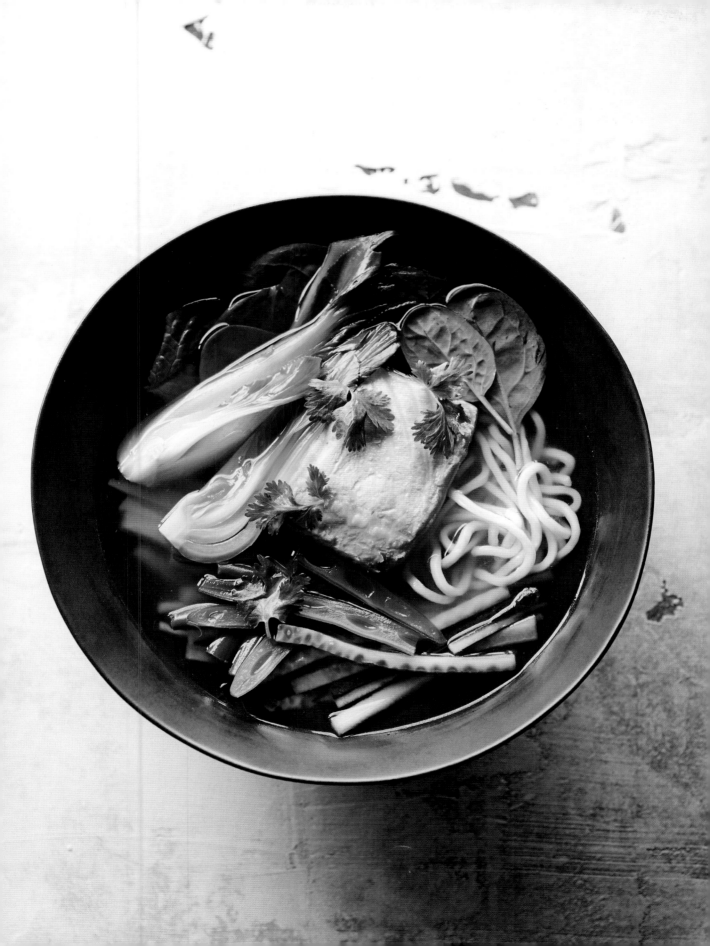

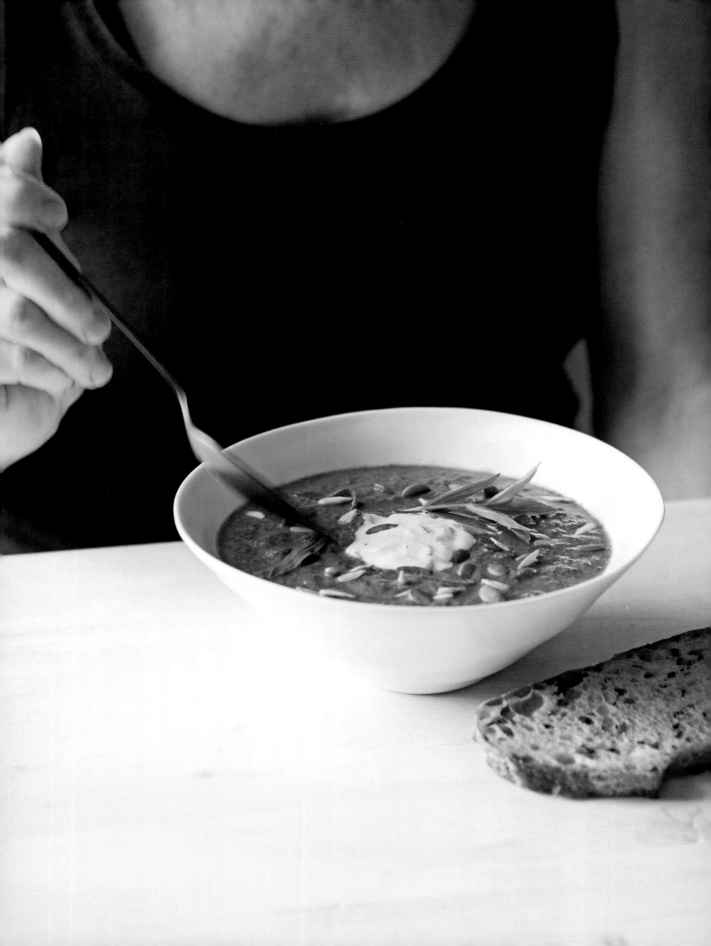

Super greens soup

If you want to add some heat, a splash of sriracha chilli sauce
or tabasco goes really well with this soup.

SERVES 4

PREP TIME 20 MINUTES

COOKING TIME 35 MINUTES

1 tablespoon olive oil

1 leek, white section only, well washed and thinly sliced

1 bunch silverbeet (about 1 kg), leaves and stalks separated
and thinly sliced

2 cloves garlic, crushed

1 bunch curly kale (about 350 g), stalks removed,
leaves chopped

2 × 400 g tins low-salt butter beans, drained and rinsed

5 cups (1.25) litres homemade vegetable stock
(see page 288) or salt-reduced vegetable stock

½ cup (140 g) reduced-fat natural Greek-style yoghurt

2 teaspoons chopped French tarragon, plus extra leaves
to serve

2 tablespoons lemon juice

2 tablespoons pepitas (roasted pumpkin seed kernels)

2 tablespoons sunflower seeds

4 slices wholegrain sourdough bread

1. Heat the oil in a large heavy-based saucepan
and cook the leek and silverbeet stalks over low–
medium heat for 10 minutes or until softened and
starting to colour. Add the garlic, silverbeet leaves
and kale leaves and cook, stirring, until the garlic
is fragrant; you may need to add the leaves in
batches if the saucepan isn't large enough – wait
for one batch to wilt before adding the next.

2. Add the beans and stock and bring to the boil over
high heat, then reduce the heat to low and simmer,
covered, for 10 minutes or until the vegetables are
very tender. Set aside to cool slightly.

3. Using a stick blender, blend the soup until smooth,
then return the pan to medium heat to warm
through. (Alternatively, leave to cool further and
use a blender or food processor to puree the soup,
in batches if necessary, until smooth. Return to
the pan to heat through.)

4. Combine the yoghurt and chopped French
tarragon in a small bowl. Set aside.

5. Remove the pan from the heat, stir in the lemon
juice and season with freshly ground pepper. Ladle
the soup evenly into 4 bowls. Top each one with
one-quarter of the tarragon yoghurt and sprinkle
with one-quarter of the seeds and extra tarragon
leaves. Serve with the bread.

NUTRITIONAL ANALYSIS	ENERGY (KJ)	1548	CARBOHYDRATE (G)	35	SODIUM (MG)	10
TO SERVE 4 (PER SERVE)	PROTEIN (G)	18	SATURATED FAT (G)	3.4	FIBRE (G)	1885

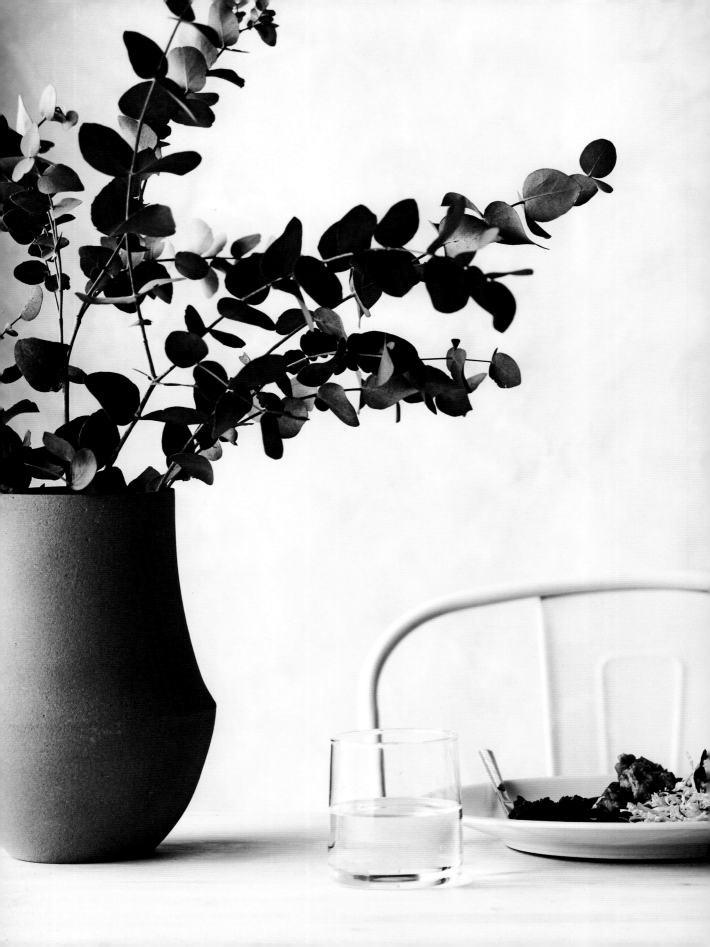

EVERYDAY

MAINS

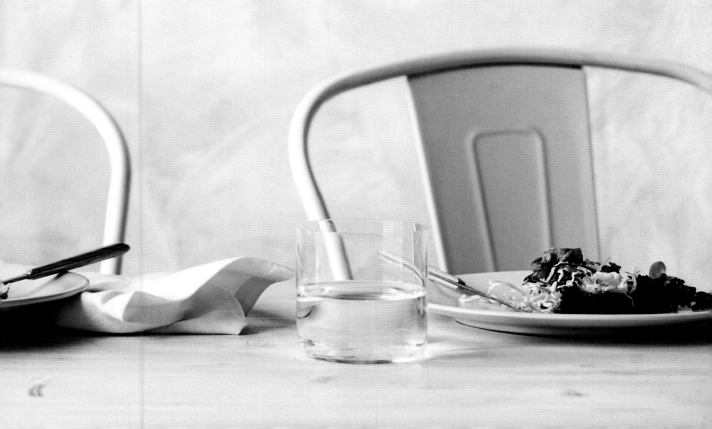

Roast beef with cauliflower 'steaks' and salsa verde

Store any leftover beef in an airtight container in the fridge for up to two days, and use in sandwiches or salads along with any remaining salsa verde for a delicious accompaniment.

SERVES 4
PREP TIME 20 MINUTES
COOKING TIME 1 HOUR, PLUS 15 MINUTES RESTING

1 × 800 g beef bolar roast, visible fat trimmed, tied into an even shape with kitchen string
olive oil spray, for cooking
4 sprigs rosemary
4 cloves garlic, lightly bruised
1 small cauliflower, trimmed with stalk left intact
2 small orange-fleshed sweet potatoes, scrubbed and cut into 2 cm-thick rounds
2 carrots, peeled, cut into batons
340 g asparagus, bases trimmed

SALSA VERDE
1 small handful curly parsley, finely chopped
1 small handful French tarragon, finely chopped
2 tablespoons capers in vinegar, rinsed and finely chopped
4 anchovy fillets, finely chopped
2 teaspoons finely grated lemon zest
1 tablespoon lemon juice
1½ tablespoons extra virgin olive oil

1. Preheat the oven to 180°C (160°C fan-forced). Line 2 roasting pans with baking paper.

2. Heat a large heavy-based non-stick frying pan over high heat. Spray the beef lightly with oil and sear in the pan for 6–8 minutes, turning the beef until it is browned all over. Place the rosemary sprigs and garlic in 1 of the lined pans and top with the beef. Roast for 50 minutes or until cooked but still a little rare in the centre (or continue until cooked to your liking).

3. Meanwhile, place the cauliflower on a chopping board, stem-side down. Cut into 1.5 cm-thick slices. Spray the cauliflower lightly with oil. Heat the same frying pan that was used to sear the beef over high heat and cook the cauliflower (including any incomplete slices) for 2 minutes on each side or until golden. Transfer to the second lined roasting pan, add the sweet potato and place in the oven once the beef has been roasting for 20 minutes. Roast the vegetables with the beef until tender; they may need to roast for a few more minutes once you've removed the beef.

4. For the salsa verde, place all the ingredients in a small bowl. Stir to mix well and set aside.

5. When the beef is cooked to your liking, transfer to a warm plate or cutting board. Cover loosely with foil and set aside for 15 minutes to rest. Scoop up the roasted garlic cloves from the roasting pan and squeeze out the soft flesh, discarding the skins. Mash, then stir into the salsa verde.

6. Steam the carrots and asparagus in a steamer basket over a saucepan of simmering water for 3–5 minutes or until cooked to your liking.

7. Carve the beef into slices, then serve 80 g beef per person with one-quarter of the vegetables and the salsa verde on the side.

NUTRITIONAL ANALYSIS	ENERGY (KJ)	2374	CARBOHYDRATE (G)	38	SODIUM (MG)	537
TO SERVE 4 (PER SERVE)	PROTEIN (G)	53	SATURATED FAT (G)	5.4	FIBRE (G)	15

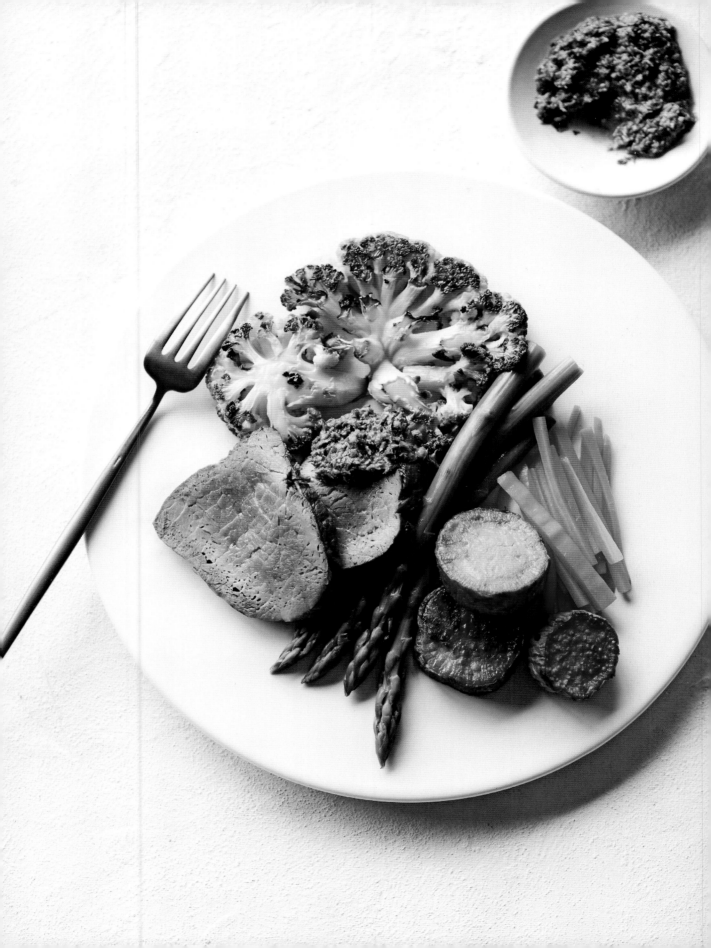

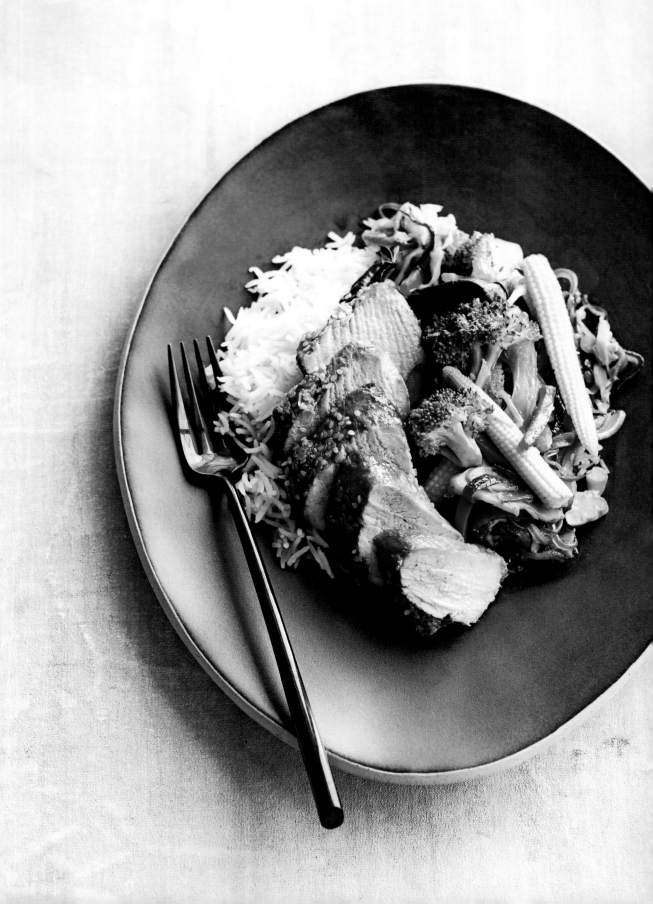

Maple and soy-glazed pork with vegetable stir-fry

The sweetness of the maple syrup and saltiness of the soy sauce are a classic combination of flavours that beautifully complement the juicy roast pork. Including the broccoli stalk as well as the florets in the vegetable stir-fry helps you get the most from your vegetables. Make sure you peel the stalk first.

SERVES 4
PREP TIME 20 MINUTES
COOKING TIME 40 MINUTES, PLUS 10 MINUTES RESTING

1 tablespoon sesame seeds
1 clove garlic, crushed
2 tablespoons salt-reduced soy sauce
1½ tablespoons pure maple syrup
1 × 400 g pork tenderloin (fillet)
olive oil spray, for cooking
¾ cup (150 g) basmati rice
2 teaspoons peanut oil
1 red onion, halved and thinly sliced
3 teaspoons finely shredded ginger
2 stalks celery, trimmed and sliced on the diagonal
2 cups (160 g) shredded cabbage
300 g broccoli, stalk peeled and sliced, and head cut into florets
500 g choy sum, trimmed and cut into 6 cm lengths
125 g baby corn, halved lengthways
1 large red capsicum (pepper), seeded, membrane removed, cut into thin strips
¼ cup (60 ml) shao hsing rice wine
2 teaspoons sesame oil

1. Preheat the oven to 180°C (160°C fan-forced). Line a roasting pan with baking paper.

2. Combine the sesame seeds, garlic, soy sauce and maple syrup in a large glass or ceramic bowl. Add the pork and turn to coat. Set aside for 5 minutes to marinate.

3. Heat a heavy-based, non-stick frying pan over medium heat.

4. Remove the pork from the marinade, shaking off the excess; reserve the marinade. Lightly spray the pork with oil and pan-fry, turning occasionally, for 4–5 minutes or until golden all over. Transfer to the lined roasting pan and roast in the oven for 10 minutes. Brush with a little of the reserved marinade and roast for a further 15–20 minutes or until the pork is just cooked through. Transfer to a warm plate or cutting board. Cover loosely with foil and set aside for 10 minutes to rest. Reserve the pan juices.

5. Meanwhile, place the rice and 1¼ cups (310 ml) water in a heavy-based saucepan. Bring to the boil over high heat, then cover and reduce the heat to low. Cook for 10 minutes, then remove from the heat and set aside, still covered, for a further 10 minutes. Just before serving, stir with a fork to loosen the grains.

6. Meanwhile, heat the peanut oil in a large wok or deep non-stick frying pan over high heat until the surface shimmers slightly. Add the onion and ginger and stir-fry for 1 minute. Add the vegetables, in batches if necessary, and stir-fry for 3 minutes or until they start to soften. Add the rice wine, sesame oil, any pan juices from the pork and the reserved marinade. Bring to the boil and stir-fry for a further 1–2 minutes or until the vegetables are tender yet still slightly crisp.

7. Cut the pork into thick slices and divide among 4 plates, along with the vegetable stir-fry and steamed rice.

| NUTRITIONAL ANALYSIS | ENERGY (KJ) | 1817 | CARBOHYDRATE (G) | 46 | SODIUM (MG) | 518 |
| TO SERVE 4 (PER SERVE) | PROTEIN (G) | 35 | SATURATED FAT (G) | 1.5 | FIBRE (G) | 9 |

Burghul pilaf with spiced fish

Cooking the fish with the skin on keeps it in one piece while it cooks on top of the pilaf. Once cooked, it is easy to remove the skin and flake the harissa-spiced flesh into the dish, ready for eating.

SERVES 4
PREP TIME 20 MINUTES
COOKING TIME 35 MINUTES

2 teaspoons harissa paste
1 × 400 g boneless mackerel fillet, skin-on

BURGHUL PILAF
3½ cups (350 g) roughly chopped cauliflower
1 tablespoon olive oil
1 red onion, thinly sliced
1 clove garlic, very thinly sliced
1 eggplant (aubergine), cut into 2 cm pieces
1 stick cinnamon
3 cardamom pods, bruised
¾ cup (120 g) burghul (cracked wheat), rinsed
1 × 400 g tin chopped tomatoes
1½ cups (375 ml) homemade chicken stock (see page 288), or salt-reduced chicken stock or water
1 × 400 g tin low-salt chickpeas, drained and rinsed
200 g baby spinach leaves
1 tablespoon thinly sliced dried apricots
2 teaspoons rinsed and thinly sliced preserved lemon rind
1 tablespoon roughly chopped unsalted pistachio kernels
1 handful mint leaves

1. In a small bowl spread the harissa paste over the mackerel so that it is completely covered, and set aside.

2. For the pilaf, working in 2 batches, process the cauliflower in a food processor until it resembles grains of rice.

3. Heat the oil in a large heavy-based saucepan over medium heat. Add the onion and garlic and cook, stirring occasionally, for 4–5 minutes or until the onion is soft. Add the eggplant, cinnamon and cardamom and cook for a further 5 minutes or until the eggplant is lightly browned. Stir in the processed cauliflower, burghul, tomatoes and stock or water. Bring to the boil, then place the mackerel on top of the mixture. Reduce the heat to low and cook, covered, for 15–20 minutes or until the burghul and fish are cooked and the stock is almost completely absorbed. (There will be more liquid at the top of the pilaf than the bottom.) Remove from the heat.

4. Transfer the mackerel to a plate. Cover to keep warm. Stir the chickpeas, spinach leaves and apricots into the pilaf. Cover and set aside for 2 minutes or until the spinach is wilted.

5. Remove the skin (it should come away easily) from the fish and gently flake the flesh.

6. Divide the pilaf and fish among serving plates, scatter with the preserved lemon, pistachios and mint, and serve.

NUTRITIONAL ANALYSIS	ENERGY (KJ)	2267	CARBOHYDRATE (G)	44	SODIUM (MG)	1011
TO SERVE 4 (PER SERVE)	PROTEIN (G)	39	SATURATED FAT (G)	4.1	FIBRE (G)	9

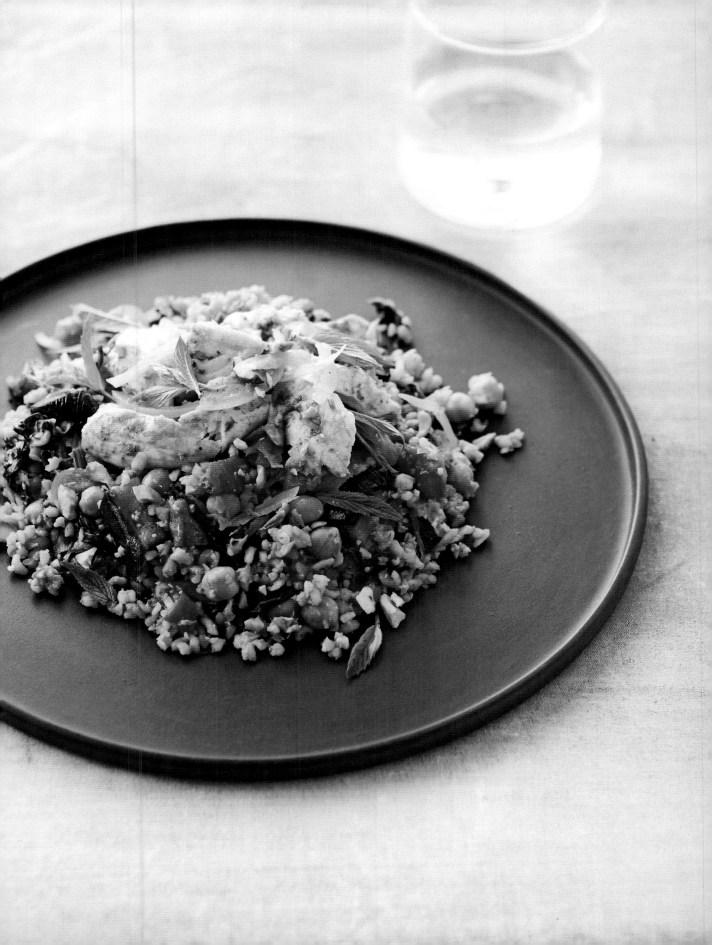

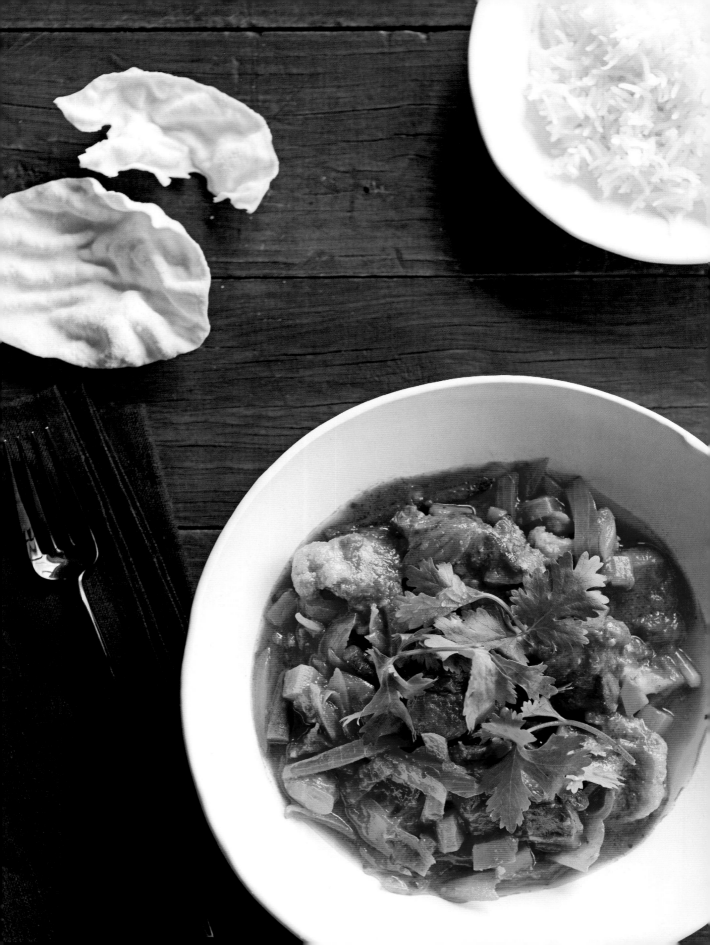

Beef and vegetable curry

Oyster blade is a versatile shoulder-cut of beef that can be cooked in a number of ways, and it is deliciously tender when braised. Cooking it on a low heat for two hours in this tasty and spicy sauce ensures it cooks slowly and perfectly and absorbs all those delicious flavours.

SERVES 4

PREP TIME 20 MINUTES

COOKING TIME 2 HOURS

1 teaspoon peanut oil

2 onions, cut into thin wedges

2 carrots, peeled and chopped

2 teaspoons finely grated ginger

2 tablespoons tikka masala curry paste

1 × 600 g beef oyster blade, visible fat trimmed, cut into 3 cm pieces

1 × 400 g tin chopped tomatoes

2 cardamom pods

1 stick cinnamon

2 cups (200 g) small cauliflower florets

200 g green beans, cut into 3 cm lengths

1 cup (120 g) frozen peas

¾ cup (150 g) basmati rice

1 handful coriander leaves

8 × large poppadums

1. Heat the peanut oil in a large heavy-based non-stick saucepan over medium heat. Add the onions, carrots and ginger and cook for 4–5 minutes or until the onion just begins to soften. Add the curry paste and cook, stirring, for 2–3 minutes or until fragrant; take care not to burn the spices.

2. Add the beef and cook for 2–3 minutes, stirring until browned all over. Add the tomatoes and spices and bring to the boil. Reduce the heat to low and simmer, covered, for 1½ hours or until the beef is tender.

3. When the curry has been simmering for about 45 minutes, place the rice and 1¼ cups (310 ml) water in a heavy-based saucepan. Bring to the boil over high heat, then cover and reduce the heat to low. Cook for 10 minutes, then remove from the heat and set aside, covered, for a further 10 minutes.

4. When the beef is tender, add the cauliflower and cook, covered, for 10 minutes, then add the beans and peas and cook, covered, for a further 5 minutes or until the cauliflower is tender.

5. Meanwhile, cook the poppadams in the microwave, without oil, following the packet instructions.

6. Stir the rice with a fork to loosen the grains. Divide the curry among 4 bowls and sprinkle with the coriander. Serve the poppadams and rice on the side.

NUTRITIONAL ANALYSIS	ENERGY (KJ)	1692	CARBOHYDRATE (G)	30	SODIUM (MG)	381
TO SERVE 4 (PER SERVE)	PROTEIN (G)	40	SATURATED FAT (G)	3.7	FIBRE (G)	9

Lamb cutlets with fattoush and baba ganoush

Bahārāt means 'spice' in Arabic, and the same-named spice mix is simply a Middle Eastern all-purpose seasoning that is the perfect flavouring to accompany the lamb in this yummy dish.

SERVES 4
PREP TIME 20 MINUTES, PLUS 5-10 MINUTES MARINATING
COOKING TIME 10 MINUTES

8 × 60 g French-trimmed lamb cutlets, visible fat removed
1 clove garlic, crushed
1 teaspoon finely grated lemon zest
2 teaspoons lemon juice
1 small red onion, thinly sliced
1 tablespoon malt vinegar
2 teaspoons sumac
1 teaspoon baharat spice mix
olive oil spray, for cooking
2 tablespoons dukkah or nut-free dukkah (see page 293), to serve
1 cup baba ganoush (see page 262), to serve
lemon cheeks, to serve

FATTOUSH
1 × 85 g wholemeal pita bread
3 Lebanese (short) cucumbers, cut into 1 cm cubes
3 tomatoes, cut into 1 cm cubes
1 large red capsicum (pepper), seeded, membrane removed, cut into 1 cm pieces
1 × 400 g tin low-salt chickpeas, drained and rinsed
1 large handful mint leaves
1 large handful coriander leaves
2 tablespoons classic salad dressing (see page 289)

1. Place the lamb, garlic, lemon zest and juice in a zip-lock bag. Seal and set aside for 5-10 minutes to marinate.

2. Combine the onion, vinegar and a pinch of the sumac in a small bowl and set aside, stirring occasionally.

3. Heat a chargrill pan, heavy-based frying pan or barbecue grill-plate over medium–high heat. Drain the lamb, shaking off the excess marinade, then sprinkle with the baharat and spray lightly with oil. Cook the lamb for 2–3 minutes on each side for medium–rare or until cooked to your liking. Transfer to a plate, sprinkle with the remaining sumac, cover loosely with foil and set aside for 5 minutes to rest.

4. For the fattoush, warm the pita bread in the same pan you cooked your lamb in or on the barbecue for 1–2 minutes on each side or until golden and crisp. Remove and set aside to cool, then break into 5 cm pieces.

5. Combine the cucumbers, tomatoes, capsicum, chickpeas, mint, coriander and dressing in a large bowl. Drain the onion, discarding the liquid, and add to the salad with the pita, then gently toss to combine.

6. Divide the fattoush and lamb evenly among 4 plates and sprinkle with the dukkah. Serve with the baba ganoush and lemon cheeks.

NUTRITIONAL ANALYSIS	ENERGY (KJ)	2349	CARBOHYDRATE (G)	33	SODIUM (MG)	545
TO SERVE 4 (PER SERVE)	PROTEIN (G)	29	SATURATED FAT (G)	10	FIBRE (G)	14

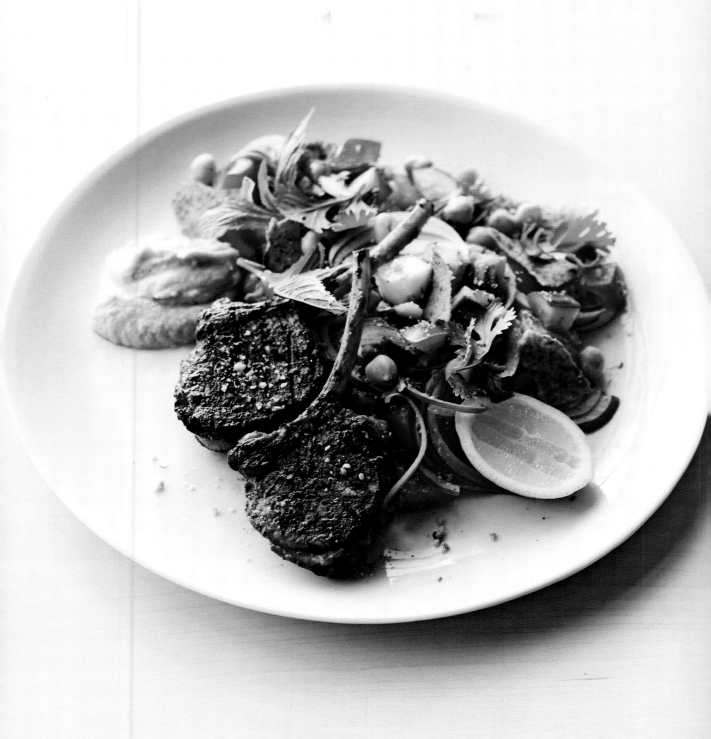

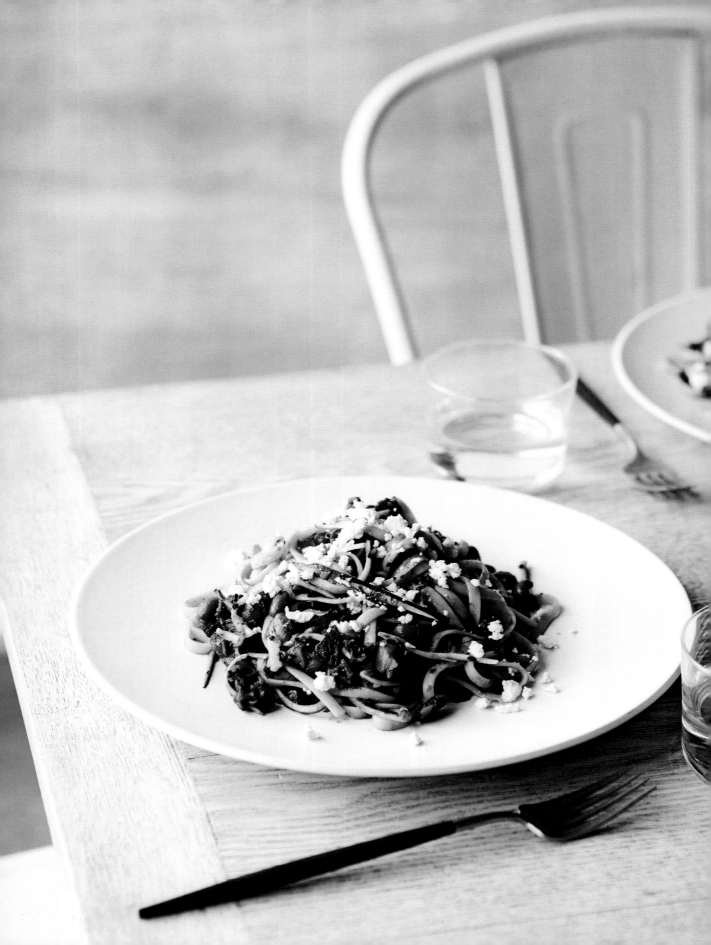

Mushroom bolognese

The portobello mushrooms bring a meaty texture to this tasty take on spaghetti bolognese, and the dried porcini mushrooms pack the sauce full of flavour. Top the dish with crumbled feta for a healthy alternative to parmesan.

SERVES 4
PREP TIME 20 MINUTES
COOKING TIME 30 MINUTES

15 g dried porcini mushrooms, rinsed
1 onion, roughly chopped
1 carrot, peeled and roughly chopped
3 cloves garlic, peeled
1 tablespoon olive oil
10 portobello (flat field) mushrooms (500 g), stems trimmed, roughly chopped
2 tablespoons low-salt tomato paste
½ cup (125 ml) dry red wine
1 × 400 g tin chopped tomatoes
1 × 400 g tin low-salt kidney beans, drained and rinsed
½ cup (125 ml) homemade vegetable stock (see page 288) or salt-reduced vegetable stock or water
2 teaspoons salt-reduced soy sauce
150 g linguine
2 zucchinis (courgettes)
100 g reduced-fat feta, crumbled, to serve

1. Place the porcini mushrooms in a small bowl and cover with warm water. Set aside for 15 minutes to soften. Drain, reserving the soaking liquid, then finely chop the mushrooms.

2. Meanwhile, process the onion, carrot and garlic in a food processor and pulse until finely chopped, but not a paste. Heat the oil in a large heavy-based saucepan over medium heat. Add the processed onion mixture and cook, partially covered, stirring occasionally, for 5 minutes or until soft.

3. Meanwhile, working in batches if necessary, pulse the portobello mushrooms in a food processor to pieces no larger than 1 cm.

4. Add the portobello mushrooms to the pan, stir in well and cook, covered, stirring occasionally, for 5 minutes or until the mushrooms release their liquid. Add the porcini mushrooms, increase the heat to medium–high and cook, stirring frequently, for 5 minutes or until the mixture is quite dry. Add the tomato paste and cook, stirring, for 1 minute. Stir in the wine and simmer for 2 minutes or until it has nearly evaporated.

5. Add the tomatoes, beans, stock, soy sauce and reserved mushroom soaking liquid, then bring to a simmer. Reduce the heat to medium and simmer for 10 minutes or until the sauce has slightly thickened.

6. Meanwhile, bring a large heavy-based saucepan of water to the boil over high heat. Add the linguine and cook for 10–12 minutes or until al dente. Then drain.

7. While the pasta is cooking, use a 'spiral cutter' or julienne peeler to cut the zucchinis into long strands. (Alternatively, use a knife to cut lengthways into very thin slices, then into long, thin strands.)

8. Add the zucchinis to the drained pasta and toss to combine. Add to the sauce and gently toss to coat the pasta. Season with freshly ground black pepper to taste. Divide evenly among 4 plates or bowls, scatter with the feta and serve.

NUTRITIONAL ANALYSIS	ENERGY (KJ)	1726	CARBOHYDRATE (G)	49	SODIUM (MG)	651
TO SERVE 4 (PER SERVE)	PROTEIN (G)	23	SATURATED FAT (G)	3.5	FIBRE (G)	9

Harissa fish with freekeh and cauliflower pilaf

Crunchy chargrilled vegetables bring a barbecue smokiness to this dish that goes well with the creamy sauce. Instead of rice, broken-down cauliflower and nutrient-rich freekeh create a light but filling pilaf that is the perfect accompaniment to the harissa-marinated fish.

SERVES 4
PREP TIME 20 MINUTES
COOKING TIME 35 MINUTES

4 × 150 g blue-eye trevalla fillets
2 teaspoons harissa paste
1 tablespoon lemon juice
olive oil spray, for cooking
2 ripe tomatoes, thickly sliced
2 zucchinis (courgettes), thinly sliced on the diagonal
1 large eggplant (aubergine), thinly sliced
1 large red capsicum (pepper), seeded, membranes
    removed, cut into thick strips

FREEKEH AND CAULIFLOWER PILAF
3½ cups (350 g) roughly chopped cauliflower
½ cup (90 g) cracked freekeh, rinsed
1 × 400 g tin low-salt chickpeas, drained and rinsed
1 handful flat-leaf parsley, roughly chopped
1 handful mint, shredded
1 tablespoon lemon juice

PARSLEY, LEMON AND GARLIC SAUCE
⅓ cup (95 g) low-fat natural Greek-style yoghurt
1 tablespoon chopped flat-leaf parsley
2 teaspoons lemon juice
2 teaspoons hulled tahini
½ small clove garlic, finely chopped

1. Combine the fish, harissa paste and lemon juice in a large zip-lock bag. Seal and refrigerate until required.

2. For the pilaf, working in 2 batches, process the cauliflower in a food processor and pulse until it resembles grains of rice. Bring 8 cups (2 litres) water to the boil in a large heavy-based saucepan.

Add the freekeh and return to the boil. Reduce the heat to medium, partially cover and simmer for 15–20 minutes or until the freekeh is tender but with some bite. Add the processed cauliflower and chickpeas and cook for a further 2 minutes or until the freekeh and cauliflower are tender. Drain well and return to the pan. Stir in the parsley, mint, lemon juice and freshly ground black pepper to taste. Cover to keep warm and set aside.

3. Meanwhile, heat a chargrill pan or barbecue grill-plate over medium–high heat. Working in batches, lightly spray the tomatoes, zucchinis, eggplant and capsicum with oil, and chargrill or barbecue for 3–4 minutes, turning often, until lightly charred and tender. (The tomatoes will take less time to cook than the firmer vegetables.) Transfer to a baking tray, cover with foil to keep warm and set aside.

4. Drain the fish, discarding the liquid and shaking off the excess marinade and cook on the same chargrill or barbecue grill-plate for 3–5 minutes on each side until just cooked through. Transfer to a plate, cover loosely with foil and leave to rest for 5 minutes.

5. For the sauce, stir all the ingredients together in a small bowl.

6. Divide the pilaf among 4 plates, top with the chargrilled vegetables and fish plus a dollop of sauce, then serve, with the remaining sauce in a small bowl on the side.

NUTRITIONAL ANALYSIS	ENERGY (KJ)	1786	CARBOHYDRATE (G)	39	SODIUM (MG)	324
TO SERVE 4 (PER SERVE)	PROTEIN (G)	36	SATURATED FAT (G)	2.2	FIBRE (G)	13

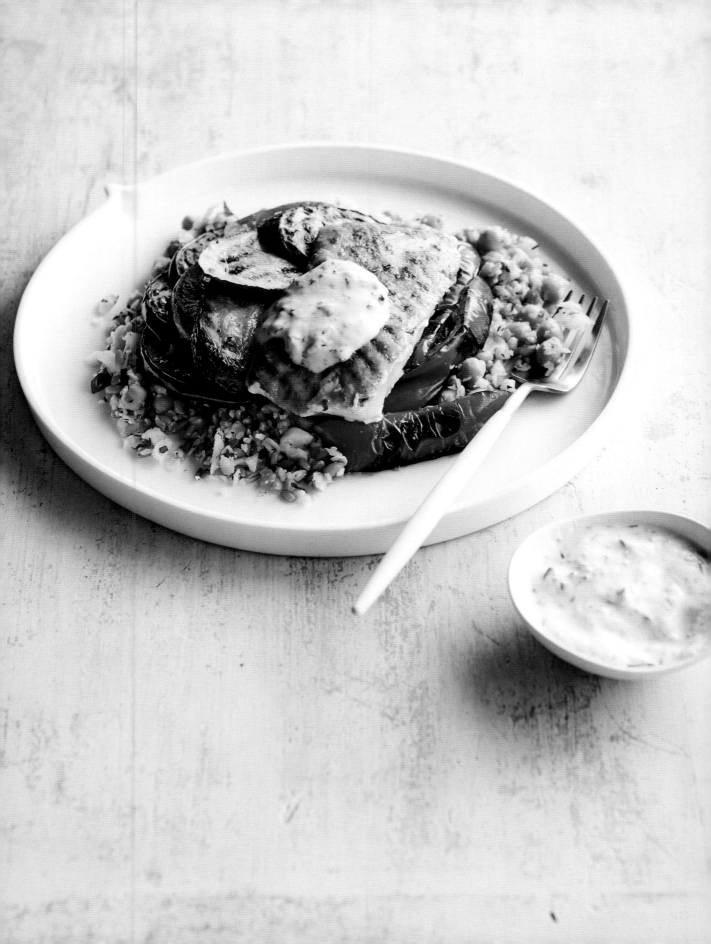

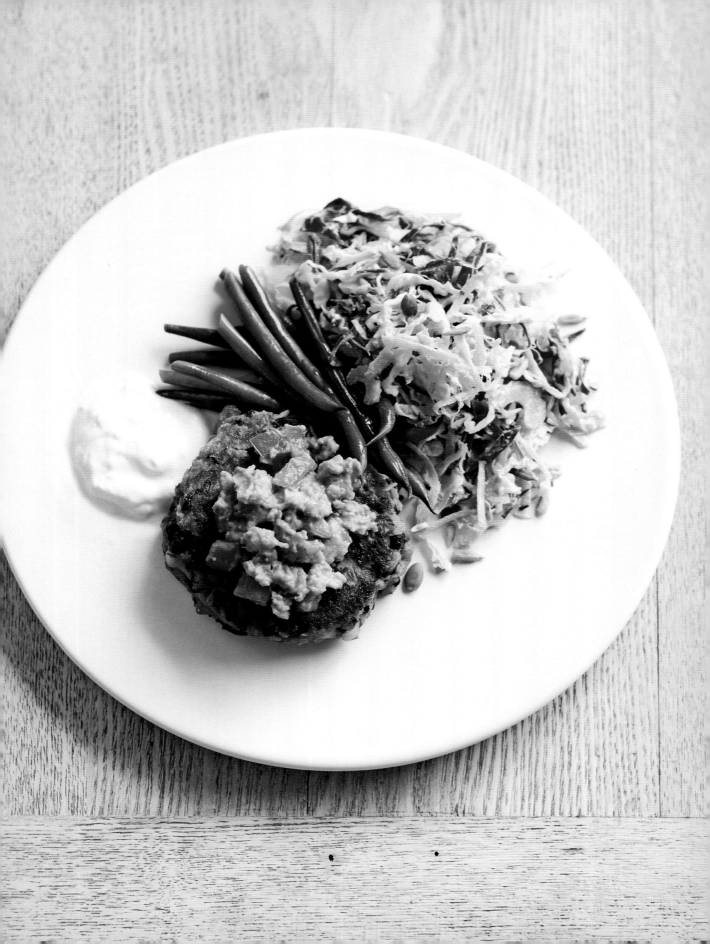

Black bean and jalapeño burgers
with avocado tomato salsa

Pickled jalapeños can be fantastically hot, so use smaller quantities if you prefer less heat or spice. The yoghurt is a refreshing and cooling side to the dish, while the creamy texture of the avocado salsa is the natural accompaniment to the Mexican flavours in the burger.

SERVES 4
PREP TIME 20 MINUTES + 15 MINUTES CHILLING
COOKING TIME 20 MINUTES

1 teaspoon olive oil
1 onion, finely chopped
2 cloves garlic, crushed
1 teaspoon ground cumin
1 teaspoon ground coriander
1 carrot, scrubbed and grated
2 × 400 g tins black beans, drained and rinsed well
1 large egg, lightly beaten
½ cup (35 g) fresh wholegrain breadcrumbs
2 tablespoons chickpea flour (besan)
1 tablespoon chopped pickled jalapeño chillies
olive oil spray, for cooking
200 g green beans, trimmed
½ cup (140 g) low-fat natural Greek-style yoghurt
homemade basic slaw (see page 291), to serve

AVOCADO TOMATO SALSA
½ avocado, halved, stone removed and peeled
1 tomato, cut into 5 mm dice
2 teaspoons lime juice

1. Heat the oil in a heavy-based non-stick frying pan over medium heat and cook the onion, stirring occasionally, for 6–8 minutes or until soft and golden. Add the garlic, cumin and coriander and cook, stirring, for 30 seconds or until fragrant. Add the carrot and cook, stirring, for 1–2 minutes or until softened. Transfer to a bowl and set aside to cool.

2. Roughly mash the black beans in a large bowl, and stir in the egg, breadcrumbs, chickpea flour, jalapeños and cooled carrot mixture. Mix well. Shape into 4 patties, place on a plate, cover with plastic film and refrigerate for 15 minutes to firm.

3. Heat a large heavy-based non-stick frying pan over medium heat. Lightly spray each burger with oil and cook for 3–5 minutes each side or until golden and heated through.

4. Steam the green beans in a steamer basket over a saucepan of boiling water for 3–4 minutes or until tender and cooked to your liking.

5. Meanwhile, for the salsa, roughly mash the avocado in a bowl. Stir in the tomato and lime juice and season with freshly ground black pepper.

6. Serve the patties topped with the salsa, with the beans, yoghurt and slaw arranged on the side.

NUTRITIONAL ANALYSIS	ENERGY (KJ)	1991	CARBOHYDRATE (G)	40	SODIUM (MG)	245
TO SERVE 4 (PER SERVE)	PROTEIN (G)	24	SATURATED FAT (G)	3.8	FIBRE (G)	21

Braised lentils and silverbeet with teff and poached eggs

Teff is a tiny, gluten-free grain that has a slightly nutty taste. It is packed with goodness and is an extremely effective prebiotic. It comes in a variety of colours, which differ slightly in taste, but the brown teff used here tends to be readily available from some large supermarkets and health food stores.

SERVES 4

PREP TIME 20 MINUTES, PLUS 30 MINUTES SETTING

COOKING TIME 35 MINUTES

1½ cups (375 ml) homemade vegetable stock (see page 288) or salt-reduced vegetable stock or water

2 tomatoes, chopped

⅔ cup (140 g) brown teff grain

olive oil spray, for cooking

8 large free-range eggs

100 g rocket

BRAISED LENTILS AND SILVERBEET

2 teaspoons olive oil

1 onion, thinly sliced

400 g silverbeet, bases trimmed, stalks thinly sliced and leaves shredded

2 cloves garlic, crushed

1¾ cups (430 ml) homemade vegetable stock (see page 288) or salt-reduced vegetable stock or water

¾ cup (165 g) Puy (French-style green) lentils, rinsed and drained

1 bay leaf

2 teaspoons sherry vinegar

1. Line the base of a 20 cm round cake tin with baking paper.

2. Place the stock or water and tomatoes in a heavy-based saucepan and bring to the boil. Add the teff and stir well, then return to the boil. Reduce the heat to low and simmer, partially covered, for 15 minutes or until the teff is tender and the mixture is thick. Pour into the lined tin, then press a round of baking paper on top to prevent the surface from drying out. Refrigerate for 30 minutes or until set.

3. Meanwhile, for the braised lentils and silverbeet, heat the oil in a large heavy-based saucepan and cook the onion and silverbeet stalks over low–medium heat for 10 minutes or until softened and starting to colour. Add the garlic and cook, stirring, for 30 seconds or until fragrant. Add the stock or water, lentils and bay leaf and bring to the boil. Reduce the heat to low and simmer, partially covered, stirring occasionally, for 25 minutes; add a little water if the mixture is drying out.

4. Meanwhile, once set, turn the round of teff out of the tin. Heat a large heavy-based non-stick frying pan over medium heat. Spray the teff lightly with oil and cook the whole piece for 3–5 minutes on each side or until a crust has formed and it is heated through. Remove from the pan and cut into wedges or quarters. Cover to keep warm.

5. When the lentils and silverbeet have been simmering for 25 minutes, add the silverbeet leaves and stir until wilted, then continue to cook, partially covered, for 5–10 minutes or until the silverbeet and lentils are tender. Remove from the heat, stir in the vinegar and season with freshly ground black pepper to taste. Cover to keep warm.

6. To poach the eggs, fill a deep, heavy-based frying pan or wide saucepan with water until about 7.5 cm deep, and bring to the boil. Carefully break each egg into a separate saucer or small ramekin. Stir the water to form a whirlpool, and quickly slide the eggs into the whirlpool (you can cook them one at a time if you prefer). Reduce the heat so the water is just simmering, and poach the eggs for 3–4 minutes or until the whites are set. Lift out the eggs with a slotted spoon and briefly drain on paper towel. (Alternatively, use an egg poacher if you have one.)

7. Divide the teff between 4 plates and top each with one-quarter of the braised lentils and silverbeet, plus 2 eggs. Share the rocket among the 4 plates, then serve.

NUTRITIONAL ANALYSIS	ENERGY (KJ)	1788	CARBOHYDRATE (G)	44	SODIUM (MG)	1144
TO SERVE 4 (PER SERVE)	PROTEIN (G)	26	SATURATED FAT (G)	3.9	FIBRE (G)	7

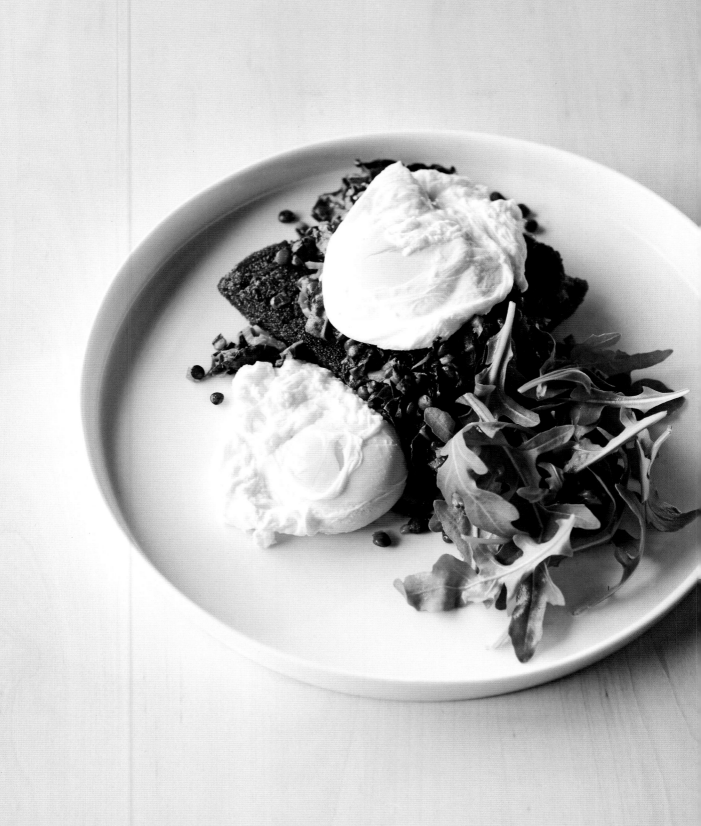

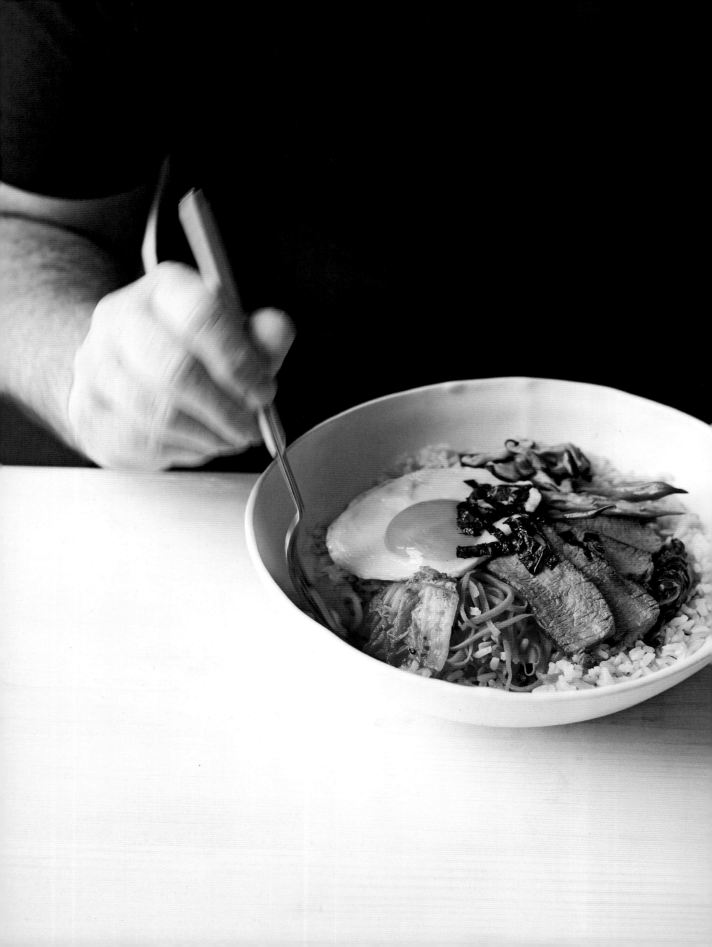

Bibimbap

For a vegetarian version of this Korean, mixed rice dish, replace the beef with firm tofu, which can be cut into slices and cooked in the same way. The idea is that you mix everything up as you eat, and the runny egg yolk forms the sauce. The Korean seasoned seaweed and chilli powder (gochugaru) can be bought in Asian grocery stores.

SERVES 4
PREP TIME 30 MINUTES
COOKING TIME 30 MINUTES, PLUS 5 MINUTES RESTING

¾ cup (150 g) long-grain brown rice or brown basmati rice
2 cups (160 g) bean sprouts
300 g baby spinach or trimmed spinach leaves
250 g rump steak, trimmed of all visible fat
olive oil spray, for cooking
3 carrots, shredded
100 g shiitake mushrooms, thinly sliced
4 large eggs
250 g green beans, trimmed and sliced lengthways
⅓ cup (80 g) kimchi
Korean seasoned seaweed, cut into strips with kitchen scissors (optional)
pinch of Korean chilli powder (gochugaru, optional)

SEASONING SAUCE
2 spring onions, finely chopped
1 clove garlic, crushed
2 teaspoons sesame seeds, toasted
1 tablespoon sesame oil
1 tablespoon salt-reduced soy sauce

1. Bring 8 cups (2 litres) water to the boil in a large heavy-based saucepan. Add the rice and return to the boil, then reduce the heat to medium and simmer for 25–30 minutes or until tender and slightly chewy. Drain well and return to the pan. Cover and set aside.

2. Meanwhile, for the seasoning sauce, combine all the ingredients in a small bowl and set aside.

3. Blanch the bean sprouts in a large saucepan of boiling water for 30 seconds, then drain and refresh in cold water, squeeze out the excess liquid and transfer to a bowl. Repeat this process with the spinach leaves. Add 1 tablespoon of the seasoning sauce to each vegetable and mix well. Set aside.

4. Heat a heavy-based non-stick frying pan over medium–high heat. Lightly spray the steak all over with oil and cook for 2–3 minutes on each side for medium. Spread half of the remaining seasoning sauce on top of the steak, then turn and cook the steak for a further 30 seconds. Spread the upper side with the remaining seasoning sauce, then turn and cook for a final 30 seconds, or continue to cook until done to your liking. Transfer to a plate, cover loosely with foil and set aside for 5 minutes to rest.

5. Meanwhile, leave the frying pan over medium heat and lightly spray it with olive oil. Cook the carrots, stirring, for 1–2 minutes, until just starting to soften. Transfer to a warm plate. Repeat with the mushrooms and transfer to a separate plate. Lightly spray the pan with oil, crack in the eggs and cook until the whites are just set. Don't overcook them as you want the yolks nice and runny.

6. Divide the rice among 4 deep bowls and top each with one-quarter of the bean sprouts, spinach leaves, carrots, mushrooms, green beans and kimchi. Slice the steak across the grain into thin strips and share between the plates. Top with a fried egg, and sprinkle with seaweed and chilli, if desired.

NUTRITIONAL ANALYSIS	ENERGY (KJ)	2072	CARBOHYDRATE (G)	38	SODIUM (MG)	456
TO SERVE 4 (PER SERVE)	PROTEIN (G)	41	SATURATED FAT (G)	4.9	FIBRE (G)	7

Kangaroo, lentil and eggplant moussaka

Kangaroo is one of the leanest meats around. It can be easy to overcook,
but using it minced and baking it in the moussaka sauce keeps it beautifully moist and tender.

SERVES 4
PREP TIME 20 MINUTES
COOKING TIME 50 MINUTES

4 eggplants (aubergines), cut lengthways into 1 cm-thick
    slices
olive oil spray, for cooking
1 orange fleshed sweet potato, cut into 5 mm-thick rounds
2 teaspoons olive oil
1 leek, white part only, well washed and thinly sliced
1 carrot, scrubbed and coarsely grated
2 cloves garlic, crushed
400 g kangaroo mince
¼ cup (70 g) low-salt tomato paste
1 × 400 g tin low-salt brown lentils, drained and rinsed
½ cup (125 ml) homemade chicken stock (see page 288)
    or salt-reduced chicken stock
1 large handful flat-leaf parsley, roughly chopped
2 tomatoes, sliced
175 g broccolini, stalks trimmed

1. Preheat the grill on high heat. Lightly spray the eggplant slices with oil and, working in batches, grill for 3–4 minutes on each side or until lightly browned.

2. Meanwhile, steam the sweet potato rounds in a steamer basket over a saucepan of boiling water for 10–12 minutes or until tender.

3. Heat the olive oil in a large heavy-based saucepan over low–medium heat. Add the leek, carrot and garlic and cook, covered, stirring occasionally, for 5 minutes or until soft. Increase the heat to high, remove the lid and cook, stirring, for 1 minute to colour the vegetables slightly. Add the kangaroo mince and cook, stirring to break up any lumps, for 5 minutes or until browned. Stir in the tomato paste and cook for another 2 minutes. Add the lentils, chicken stock and half the parsley. Bring to the boil, then reduce the heat to low and simmer for 5 minutes or until slightly thickened. Season with freshly ground black pepper and remove from the heat.

4. Preheat the oven to 180°C (160°C fan-forced).

5. Spray a 2 litre-capacity baking dish lightly with oil. Layer one-third of the grilled eggplant followed by a layer of half the sweet potato, then half the kangaroo mixture in the dish. Repeat with half the remaining eggplant, all the remaining sweet potato and kangaroo mixture, finishing with a layer of the remaining eggplant. Arrange the tomato slices on top and sprinkle with the remaining parsley.

6. Cover with foil and bake in the oven for 20 minutes, then remove the foil and bake for a further 10 minutes or until the moussaka is heated through and bubbling. Remove from the oven and set aside for 10 minutes to slightly cool.

7. Meanwhile, steam the broccolini in a steamer basket over a saucepan of boiling water for 3–4 minutes or until just tender.

8. Cut the moussaka into 4 pieces, then place a slice on each of 4 plates and serve with the broccolini alongside.

NUTRITIONAL ANALYSIS	ENERGY (KJ)	1641	CARBOHYDRATE (G)	38	SODIUM (MG)	246
TO SERVE 4 (PER SERVE)	PROTEIN (G)	35	SATURATED FAT (G)	1.1	FIBRE (G)	18

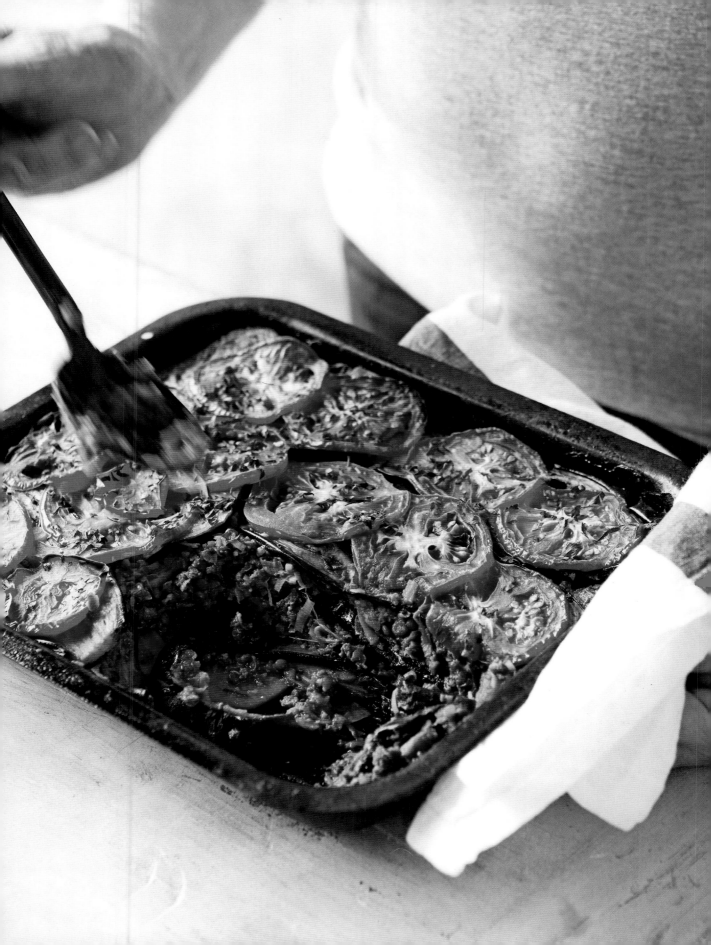

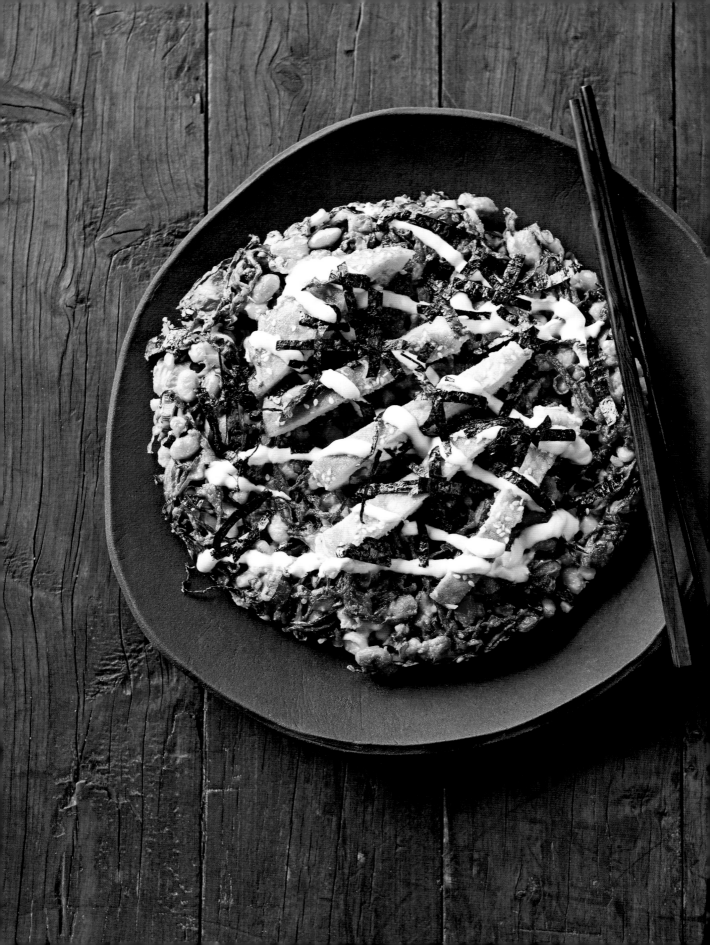

Okonomiyaki with pork leg steaks

Using chickpea flour (besan) instead of plain flour makes a slightly denser pancake – or okonomiyaki. If you are unable to find chickpea flour, though, just use plain flour instead. The creamy sauce can be put into a squeeze bottle, piping bag or sturdy sandwich bag with the corner snipped off and then squeezed onto the pancake in a zigzag pattern. If you have more than two large frying pans, you can cook two pancakes at a time and halve the cooking time.

SERVES 4

PREP TIME 30 MINUTES

COOKING TIME 50 MINUTES, PLUS 5 MINUTES RESTING

1 teaspoon olive oil

1 onion, finely chopped

2 cloves garlic, crushed

4 cups (320 g) shredded red cabbage

2 cobs sweetcorn, husks and silks removed, kernels cut from cob

1 cup (150 g) frozen shelled edamame (soybeans), blanched

1 × 400 g tin soybeans, drained and rinsed

3 spring onions, thinly sliced

⅔ cup (100 g) chickpea flour (besan)

2 teaspoons baking powder

4 large eggs, lightly whisked

olive oil spray, for cooking

1 tablespoon sesame seeds

1 tablespoon psyllium husks

2 × 120 g pork butterfly loin steaks, visible fat trimmed

1 sheet yaki nori (toasted seaweed), shredded with kitchen scissors

OKONOMIYAKI SAUCE

½ cup (140 g) low-fat natural Greek-style yoghurt

1 teaspoon reduced-salt soy sauce

½ teaspoon Worcestershire sauce

1. Preheat the oven to 100°C (80°C fan-forced). Line a baking tray with baking paper.

2. Heat the olive oil in a heavy-based non-stick frying pan over medium heat. Add the onion and garlic and cook, covered, stirring occasionally, for 4–5 minutes or until softened. Transfer to a large bowl and set aside to cool.

3. Add the cabbage, corn kernels, blanched edamame, soybeans and spring onions to the cooled onion mixture. Sift the flour and add the baking powder. Combine, then add the onion mixture. Stir to coat the vegetables in the flour. Add the egg and mix well.

4. Heat a large heavy-based non-stick frying pan over low–medium heat. Lightly spray the pan with oil and add one-quarter of the mixture, gently spreading it to make a large pancake about 1 cm thick. Cook for 4–5 minutes or until a golden crust has formed underneath. Carefully slide the pancake onto a plate. Lightly spray the pan with oil, then hold the pan upside down over the plate and carefully invert both the frying pan and plate so that the pancake drops back into the pan. Remove the plate, and cook the pancake for a further 3–4 minutes or until golden and cooked through. Transfer to the lined tray, cover loosely with foil and keep warm in the oven while you cook the remaining okonomiyaki.

5. Heat another large heavy-based non-stick frying pan over medium heat. Combine the sesame seeds and psyllium husks, and rub them over both sides of the pork steaks, pressing them on so they stick. Lightly spray the coated pork steaks with oil and cook for 3–4 minutes on each side or until browned and just cooked through. Transfer to a warm plate, cover loosely with foil and set aside for 5 minutes to rest.

6. Meanwhile, for the sauce, place all the ingredients in a small bowl and mix until combined.

7. Thickly slice the pork across the grain. Place 1 okonomiyaki on each plate, top with one-quarter of the sliced pork drizzle generously with the sauce, and sprinkle with the shredded nori.

NUTRITIONAL ANALYSIS	ENERGY (KJ)	2344	CARBOHYDRATE (G)	38	SODIUM (MG)	1034
TO SERVE 4 (PER SERVE)	PROTEIN (G)	46	SATURATED FAT (G)	5.1	FIBRE (G)	15

Smoky braised pork and black beans

This yummy dish is basically a version of chilli con carne. It is quick and easy to cook, and is comfort food at its best. Brown rice adds a nutty flavour that complements the braised pork sauce. Squeeze a bit of lime juice over the top for a refreshing zing to the heavy flavours.

SERVES 4
PREP TIME 20 MINUTES
COOKING TIME 40 MINUTES

½ cup (100 g) long-grain brown rice or brown basmati rice
2 teaspoons olive oil
1 leek, white part only, well washed and thinly sliced
2 carrots, scrubbed and finely chopped
1 stalk celery, finely chopped
2 tablespoons low-salt tomato paste
2 cloves garlic, crushed
1 fresh long green chilli, finely chopped
1 teaspoon smoked paprika
1 teaspoon ground coriander
1 teaspoon ground cumin
400 g lean pork mince
4 tomatoes, chopped
1 × 400 g tin low-salt black beans, drained and rinsed
2 spring onions, thinly sliced
1 large handful coriander leaves
175 g broccolini, stalks trimmed, or 100 g green beans, trimmed
lime wedges and extra chilli, to serve (optional)

1. Bring 8 cups (2 litres) water to the boil in a large heavy-based saucepan. Add the rice and return to the boil. Reduce the heat to medium and simmer for 25–30 minutes or until tender and slightly chewy. Drain well and return to the pan. Cover and set aside.

2. Meanwhile, heat the olive oil in a large non-stick frying pan over medium heat. Add the leek, carrots and celery and cook, covered, stirring occasionally, for 10 minutes or until softened. Add the tomato paste, garlic, chilli and spices and cook, stirring, for 1–2 minutes or until aromatic.

3. Increase the heat to medium–high, add the pork mince and cook, stirring to break up any lumps, for 4–5 minutes or until browned. Add the tomatoes, black beans and 1 cup (250 ml) water. Cover and bring to the boil, then reduce the heat to low–medium and simmer, stirring occasionally, for 10 minutes. Remove the lid and cook for a further 5–10 minutes or until slightly thickened. Stir in the spring onions and coriander.

4. Meanwhile, steam the broccolini or beans in a steamer basket over a saucepan of boiling water for 3–4 minutes or until just tender.

5. Divide the rice among 4 plates and top with one-quarter of the pork and beans, along with the broccolini or beans. Serve with lime wedges and extra chilli, if desired.

NUTRITIONAL ANALYSIS	ENERGY (KJ)	1631	CARBOHYDRATE (G)	39	SODIUM (MG)	396
TO SERVE 4 (PER SERVE)	PROTEIN (G)	36	SATURATED FAT (G)	1.5	FIBRE (G)	13

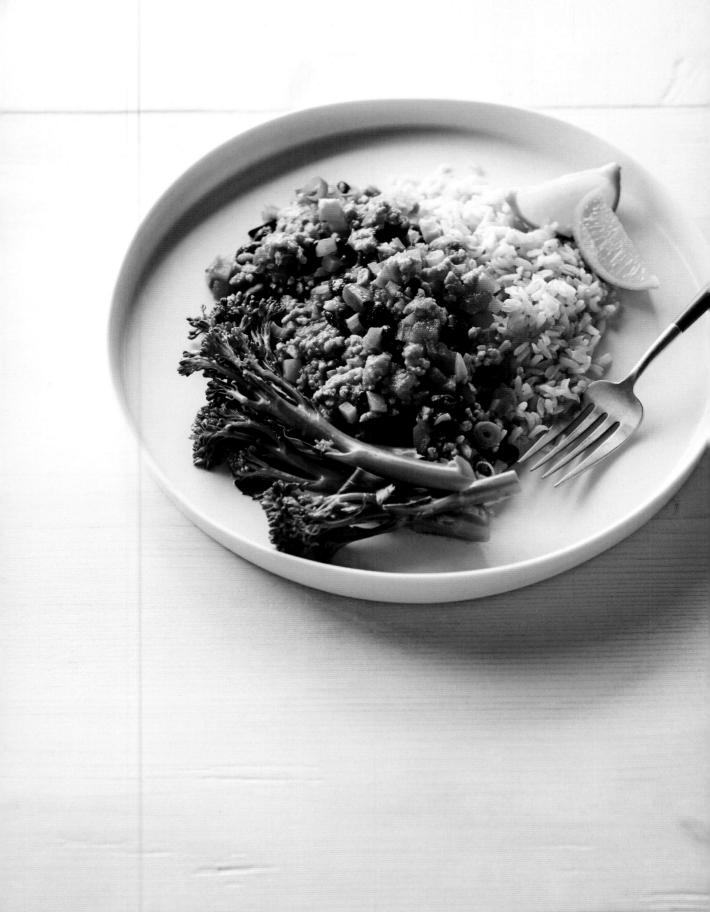

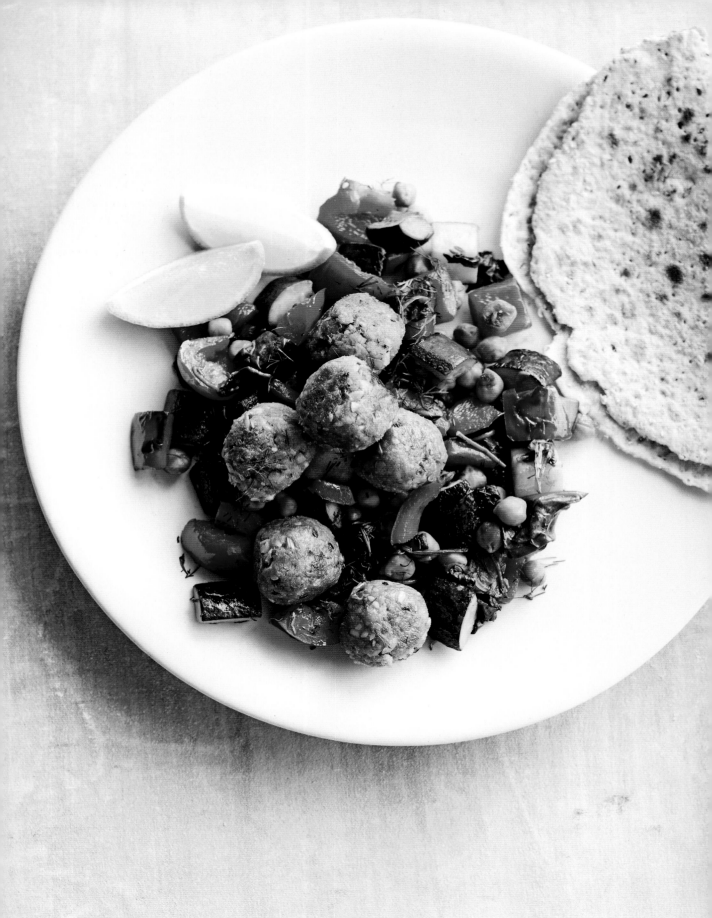

Tuna, lemon and herb 'meatballs'

The 'meatballs' and veggies in this dish are fantastic hot or cold, so you can refrigerate a couple of portions and enjoy them cold for an appetising fuss-free lunch the next day.

SERVES 4
PREP TIME 20 MINUTES
COOKING TIME 25 MINUTES

2 slices (70 g) wholegrain bread
1 × 425 g tin tuna in springwater, drained
¼ cup (35 g) sunflower seed kernels
1 tablespoon sesame seeds
2 large eggs
2 spring onions, finely chopped
finely grated zest of 1 lemon
olive oil spray, for cooking
2 large zucchinis (courgettes), cut into 1 cm pieces
2 red capsicums (peppers), seeded, membranes removed,
    cut into 1 cm pieces
1 × 400 g tin low-salt chickpeas, drained and rinsed
2 cloves garlic, thinly sliced
1 teaspoon cumin seeds
1 teaspoon ground coriander
200 g baby spinach leaves
1 tablespoon roughly chopped dill
4 homemade wholemeal yoghurt seeded flatbreads
    (see page 290)
lemon wedges, to serve

1. Line a baking tray with baking paper. Process the bread in a food processor to form breadcrumbs. Add the tuna, sunflower seeds, sesame seeds, eggs, spring onions and lemon zest and pulse until just combined. Shape tablespoonfuls of the mixture into balls and place on your lined tray.

2. Heat a large heavy-based non-stick frying pan over medium heat. Lightly spray the tuna meatballs with oil and cook for 5–6 minutes or until browned all over and cooked through. Transfer to a plate and cover loosely with foil to keep warm.

3. Reheat the frying pan over medium–high heat and spray lightly with olive oil. Add the zucchinis and capsicums and cook, stirring occasionally, for 8–10 minutes or until lightly browned and tender. Add the chickpeas, garlic, cumin and coriander and cook, stirring, until fragrant. Add the spinach leaves and cook, stirring, until wilted.

4. Divide the vegetable mixture among 4 serving plates and top with the tuna 'meatballs'. Scatter with dill and serve immediately with the flatbreads and lemon wedges on the side.

NUTRITIONAL ANALYSIS	ENERGY (KJ)	2137	CARBOHYDRATE (G)	41	SODIUM (MG)	705
TO SERVE 4 (PER SERVE)	PROTEIN (G)	45	SATURATED FAT (G)	3	FIBRE (G)	13

Turkey and zucchini kofte
with iceberg salad

Make the flatbreads in advance and store them in the freezer, ready to be pulled out and used. Thaw them first, and reheat briefly in a hot frying pan or under the grill. They are delicious just when dipped in the yoghurt-sumac sauce, so you can always take out extra flatbreads and make the sauce first for starter nibbles while you prepare the rest of the dish.

SERVES 4

PREP TIME 30 MINUTES

COOKING TIME 15 MINUTES

500 g lean turkey mince

3 spring onions, thinly sliced

3 tablespoons chopped mint

1 large egg

2 cloves garlic, crushed

1 teaspoon ground cumin

¼ teaspoon chilli flakes (optional)

1 × 400 g tin low-salt cannellini beans, rinsed and drained, roughly mashed

1 zucchini (courgette), coarsely grated, excess liquid squeezed out

2 tablespoons sesame seeds

olive oil spray, for cooking

4 wholemeal yoghurt seeded flatbreads (see page 290)

ICEBERG SALAD

½ iceberg lettuce, cut into wedges

4 tomatoes, cut into wedges

2 Lebanese (short) cucumbers, sliced

1 tablespoon classic salad dressing (see page 289)

YOGHURT-SUMAC SAUCE

½ cup (140 g) reduced-fat natural Greek-style yoghurt

1 tablespoon shredded mint

½ teaspoon finely grated lemon zest

1 teaspoon lemon juice

½ small clove garlic, crushed

1–2 teaspoons sumac, to taste, plus extra to sprinkle

1. Place the turkey, spring onions, mint, egg, garlic, cumin and chilli flakes (if using) in a large bowl. Using clean hands (or wear disposable kitchen gloves if you prefer), knead the mixture in the bowl for 5 minutes or until sticky. Stir in the mashed cannellini beans and zucchini (courgette). Divide the mixture into 16 equal portions and shape each into an oval kofte. Sprinkle all over with the sesame seeds, then lightly spray with oil.

2. Preheat the oven to 180°C (160°C fan-forced). Line a baking tray with baking paper.

3. Heat a large heavy-based non-stick frying pan over medium–high heat. Working in batches, if necessary, cook each kofte for 2–3 minutes on each side or until well browned. Take care, as they are a little delicate; don't try to turn them before they have formed a crust. Transfer to the lined tray and bake for 5–6 minutes or until cooked through.

4. Meanwhile, for the salad, combine all the ingredients in a large bowl and toss gently to coat in the dressing.

5. For the sauce, place all the ingredients in a small bowl and mix until combined.

6. Arrange the kofte, salad and flatbreads in equal portions on 4 plates. Add a generous dollop of sauce, and sprinkle with the remaining sumac.

NUTRITIONAL ANALYSIS	ENERGY (KJ)	1774	CARBOHYDRATE (G)	23	SODIUM (MG)	403
TO SERVE 4 (PER SERVE)	PROTEIN (G)	40	SATURATED FAT (G)	4.4	FIBRE (G)	9

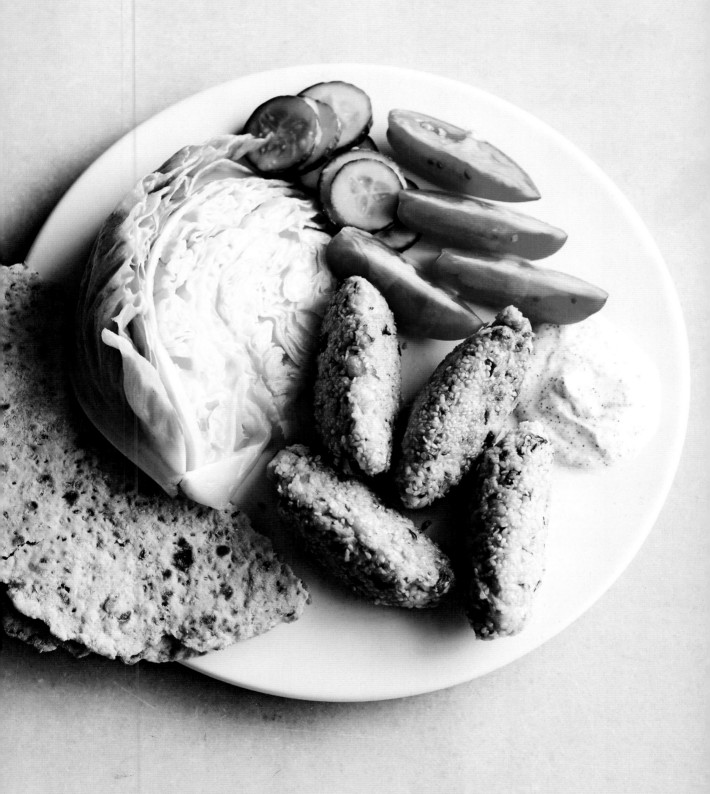

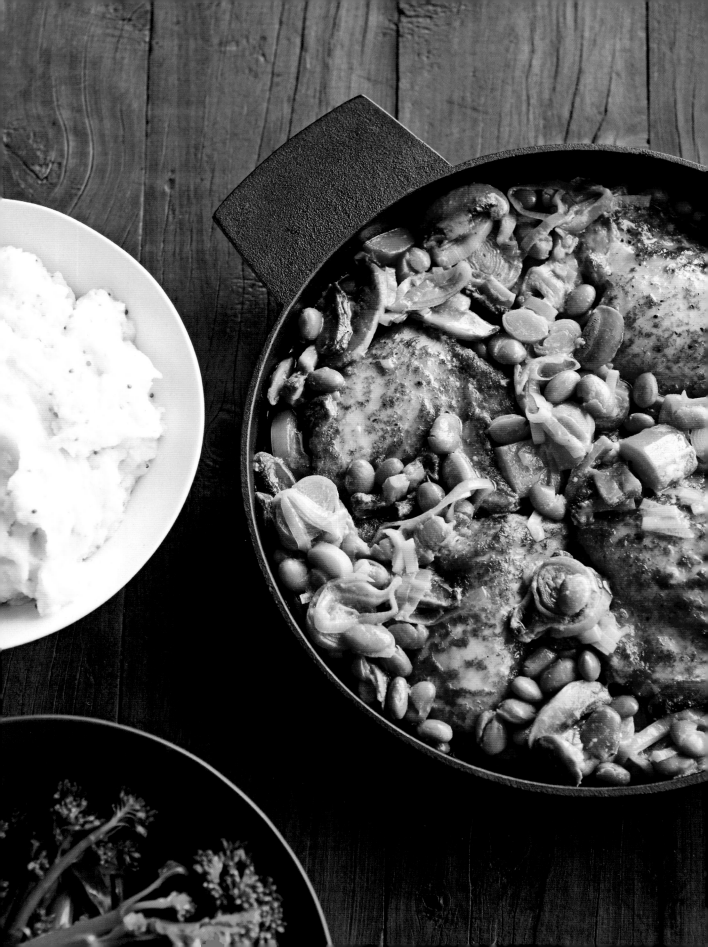

Tarragon chicken with celeriac-mustard mash

The creamy mash melts in the mouth in this comforting winter warmer. The tarragon-chicken casserole bursts with flavour, with tasty meat on the bone and a rich gravy that is filled with yummy goodness.

SERVES 4
PREP TIME 20 MINUTES
COOKING TIME 1 HOUR

4 × 150 g skinless chicken thigh cutlets on-the-bone (sold as 'lovely legs'), trimmed of visible fat
1 tablespoon psyllium husks
2 teaspoons olive oil
2 leeks, white part only, well washed and thinly sliced
350 g small portobello or Swiss brown mushrooms, sliced
2 carrots, peeled and cut into 2.5 cm pieces
1 tablespoon Dijon mustard
2 cups (500 ml) homemade chicken stock (see page 288) or salt-reduced chicken stock
1 tablespoon lemon juice
1 × 400 g tin low-salt borlotti beans, drained and rinsed
2 tablespoons roughly chopped French tarragon
350 g broccolini, trimmed and halved lengthways

CELERIAC-MUSTARD MASH
2 desiree (400 g) potatoes, peeled and chopped
1 celeriac with leaves and stalk removed (550 g), peeled and chopped
1 tablespoon wholegrain mustard
½ cup (125 ml) buttermilk
1 tablespoon lemon juice
pinch of white pepper

1. Preheat the oven to 200°C (180°C fan-forced).

2. Place the chicken and psyllium husks in a large zip-lock bag and shake to coat the chicken all over.

3. Heat the oil in a large flameproof roasting pan or enamelled cast-iron casserole dish over medium heat. Add the chicken and cook, turning occasionally, for 5–6 minutes or until browned all over. Transfer to a plate. Add the leeks, mushrooms and carrots and cook, stirring, for 6–8 minutes or until the leeks are tender. Stir in the Dijon mustard, stock and lemon juice and bring to the boil, stirring to scrape any residue off the base. Return the chicken to the pan or dish, then cover with foil or the lid and bake for 35 minutes.

4. Stir, then bake for a further 10 minutes or until the chicken is cooked through, the vegetables are tender and the sauce has slightly thickened. Stir in the borlotti beans and French tarragon.

5. Meanwhile, for the mash, steam the potatoes and celeriac in a steamer basket over a large saucepan of simmering water for 10–12 minutes or until very tender. Cool slightly, then transfer to a food processor. Add the wholegrain mustard, buttermilk and lemon juice and process until smooth. Season lightly with freshly ground white or black pepper. Empty the water from the steaming pan, and transfer your mash into the pan. Cover to keep warm.

6. Steam the broccolini in a steamer basket over a saucepan of simmering water for 3–4 minutes or until cooked to your liking.

7. Transfer the broccolini and mash into separate serving bowls, and place on the table next to your tarragon chicken for everyone to help themselves.

NUTRITIONAL ANALYSIS	ENERGY (KJ)	2769	CARBOHYDRATE (G)	41	SODIUM (MG)	1005
TO SERVE 4 (PER SERVE)	PROTEIN (G)	43	SATURATED FAT (G)	3.1	FIBRE (G)	17

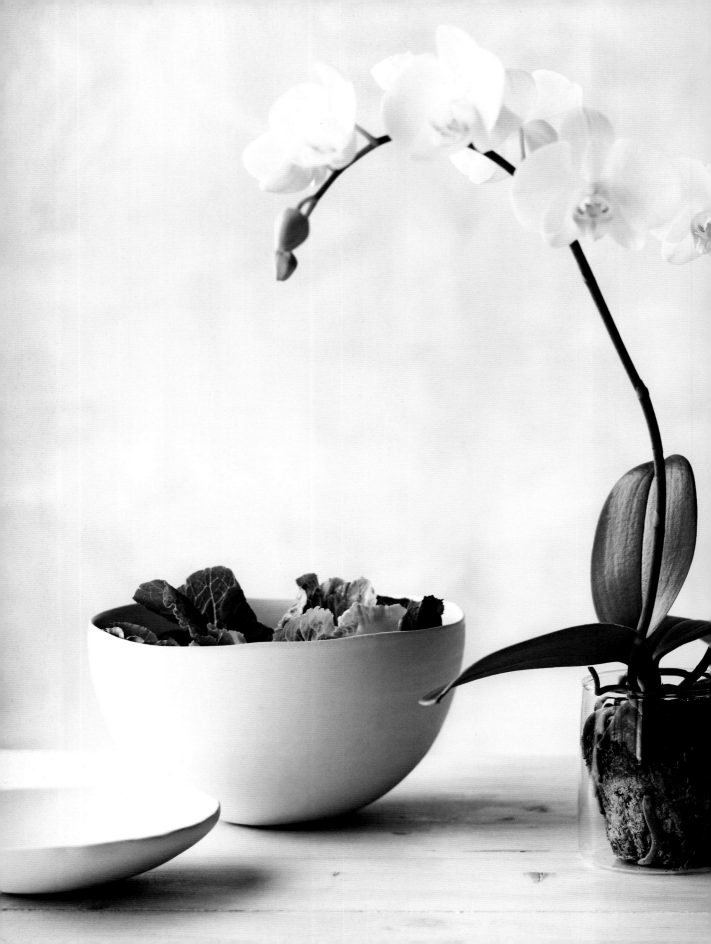

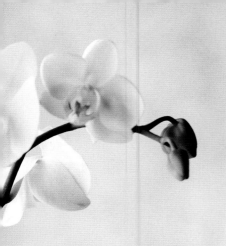

ENTERTAINING

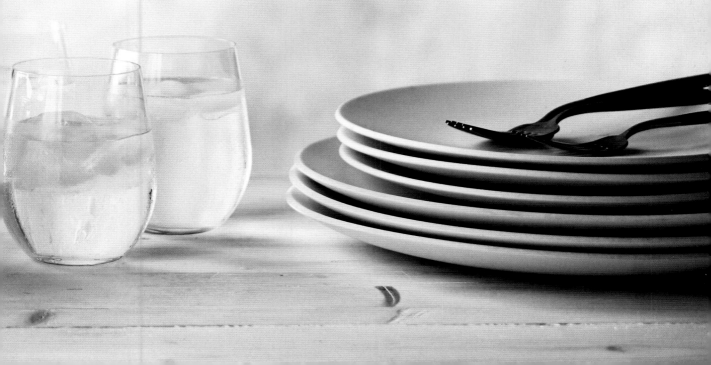

Baked rainbow trout with roasted vegetables and caper-parsley sauce

Serving up a whole fish to dinner guests looks impressive, and is easy to cook. You can buy the rainbow trout already cleaned and scaled, so all you need to do is stuff the cavity with flavour.

SERVES 4
PREP TIME 20 MINUTES
COOKING TIME 35 MINUTES

1 large orange-fleshed sweet potato, scrubbed and
    cut into 4 cm pieces
1 × 400 g tin low-salt chickpeas, drained and rinsed
1 parsnip, cut into thick strips lengthways
4 cloves garlic, lightly bruised
olive oil spray, for cooking
1 × 800 g or 2 × 400 g whole rainbow trout,
    cleaned and scaled
1 red onion, thinly sliced into rings
1 lemon, thinly sliced
large handful of dill
400 g Brussels sprouts, trimmed and halved
2 bunches broccolini
lemon wedges, to serve

CAPER-PARSLEY SAUCE
½ cup (140 g) reduced-fat natural Greek-style yoghurt
1 tablespoon baby capers in vinegar, rinsed, drained and
    chopped
1 handful flat-leaf parsley, finely chopped
1 tablespoon finely chopped dill

1. Preheat the oven to 220°C (200°C fan-forced). Line 2 large roasting tins with baking paper.

2. Place the sweet potato, chickpeas, parsnip and garlic in 1 lined pan. Lightly spray with oil and season with a little freshly ground black pepper. Roast for 20 minutes.

3. Meanwhile, place both fish side by side in the second lined pan. Stuff the fish cavities with the onion and lemon slices and dill sprigs.

4. After 20 minutes, remove the vegetables and chickpeas from the oven and turn the vegetables. Lightly spray the Brussels sprouts with a little oil and scatter over the vegetables and chickpeas. Return the pan to the oven, along with the pan of trout, and roast for a further 15 minutes or until the trout is just cooked through and the vegetables are tender and crisp around the edges.

5. Meanwhile, for the sauce, combine the yoghurt, capers, parsley and dill in a small bowl. Season with freshly ground black pepper to taste.

6. Steam the broccolini in a steamer basket over a saucepan of boiling water for 3–4 minutes or until tender and cooked to your liking.

7. Transfer the fish to a large serving platter and place the lemon wedges around it. Transfer the baked vegetables, chickpeas and broccolini to a large serving dish, and place on the table with the fish and sauce.

NUTRITIONAL ANALYSIS	ENERGY (KJ)	3010	CARBOHYDRATE (G)	52	SODIUM (MG)	446
TO SERVE 4 (PER SERVE)	PROTEIN (G)	63	SATURATED FAT (G)	7.7	FIBRE (G)	17

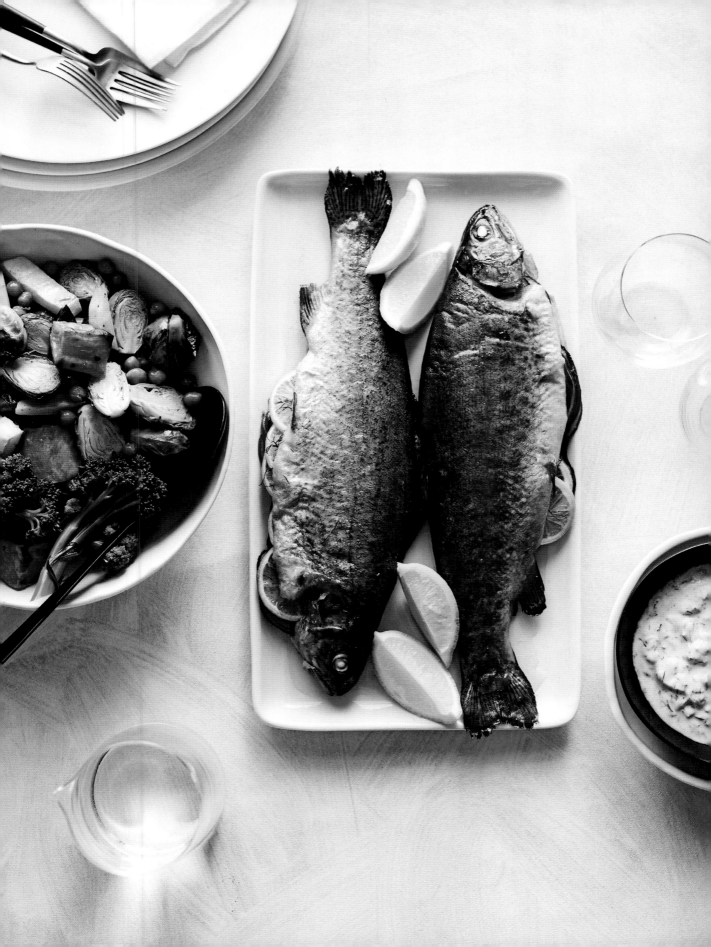

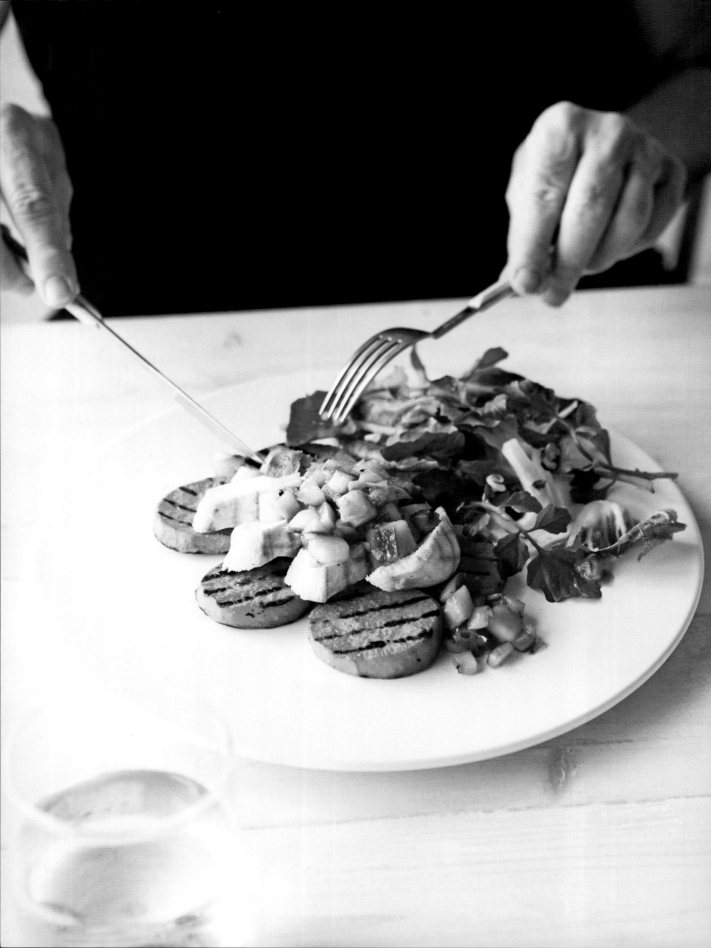

Chargrilled chicken with charred peach salsa

Cooked stone fruits go beautifully with chicken, and this charred peach salsa brings a delicious sweetness to the dish. If you have apricots that need eating, you could try substituting 8–10 apricots for the peaches in the salsa.

SERVES 4
PREP TIME 20 MINUTES
COOKING TIME 30 MINUTES, PLUS 5 MINUTES RESTING

1 large orange-fleshed sweet potato, cut into 5 mm-thick rounds
olive oil spray, for cooking
400 g skinless chicken breast fillets
1 tablespoon olive oil
½ teaspoon Dijon mustard
1 head radicchio, leaves torn into bite-sized pieces
1 small bulb fennel, trimmed and very thinly sliced (use a mandoline, if you have one)
100 g watercress, leaves picked
¼ cup (25 g) walnuts, lightly toasted

CHARRED PEACH SALSA
4 white peaches, halved and pitted
olive oil spray, for cooking
2 tablespoons red wine vinegar
½ small red onion, finely chopped
1 teaspoon lemon thyme leaves

1. Preheat the oven to 180°C (160°C fan-forced). Line a roasting tin with baking paper.

2. For the salsa, heat a chargrill pan or heavy-based non-stick frying pan over medium–high heat. Spray the cut sides of the peaches with olive oil and cook, cut-side down, for 3–4 minutes or until charred. Transfer to a plate to cool slightly, then roughly chop and place in a large bowl. Add the remaining salsa ingredients and set aside to macerate.

3. Meanwhile, lightly spray the sweet potato rounds with oil and cook in the same pan over medium heat, in batches if necessary, for 3–4 minutes on each side or until tender. Transfer to the lined tin.

4. Spray the chicken lightly with oil and cook in the pan for 2–3 minutes on each side or until seared. Place on top of the sweet potato in the lined pan. Roast for 8–10 minutes or until the sweet potato and chicken are cooked through. Cover loosely with foil and set aside to rest for 5 minutes.

5. Strain the salsa, reserving the liquid. Place the liquid in a small bowl and whisk in the olive oil and mustard until emulsified. (Alternatively, strain into a jar, seal and shake until combined.) Toss the radicchio, fennel and watercress together in a large bowl.

6. Thickly slice the chicken across the grain. Divide the sweet potato among 4 serving plates and top with one-quarter of the chicken and the peach salsa. Add the dressing to the salad and toss to combine. Share the dressed salad between the plates, scattered with the walnuts.

NUTRITIONAL ANALYSIS	ENERGY (KJ)	1731	CARBOHYDRATE (G)	41	SODIUM (MG)	104
TO SERVE 4 (PER SERVE)	PROTEIN (G)	30	SATURATED FAT (G)	1.8	FIBRE (G)	9

Italian-herb stuffed roast beef and cavolo nero with anchovy crumbs

The key to infusing the beef with the flavours from the stuffing is to ensure that you cut deep enough into the beef, but not so far that you cut it in half. Get it right, and you'll be rewarded with a mouthful of the herbs with every forkful of beef as you eat.

SERVES 4

PREP TIME 20 MINUTES

COOKING TIME 45 MINUTES, PLUS 15 MINUTES RESTING

1 × 400 g tin low-salt kidney beans, drained and rinsed

1 small handful flat-leaf parsley, chopped

1 tablespoon finely chopped fresh rosemary

1 teaspoon chopped thyme leaves

2 cloves garlic, crushed

1 teaspoon Dijon mustard

finely grated zest of 1 lemon

1 teaspoon olive oil

1 × 500 g lean beef fillet (the thickest section of the fillet), visible fat trimmed

olive oil spray, for cooking

1 bunch cavolo nero or curly kale, tough central stalks removed and leaves shredded

400 g baby carrots, scrubbed

340 g asparagus, trimmed

lemon wedges, to serve (optional)

½ quantity homemade red capsicum rouille (see page 242)

ANCHOVY CRUMBS

3 teaspoons olive oil

3 slices (200 g) stale sourdough bread, crusts removed, cut into 5 mm dice

2 anchovies, well drained and chopped

1 small handful flat-leaf parsley, finely chopped

1 small fresh red chilli, finely chopped

1. Preheat the oven to 180°C (160°C fan-forced).

2. Using a fork, roughly mash the kidney beans in a large bowl. Add half the parsley, the rosemary, thyme, garlic, mustard, lemon zest and olive oil, and mix until well combined.

3. Place the beef on a clean work surface and use a sharp knife to cut into the fillet along its length, cutting three-quarters of the way through; the aim is to open it out. Spread the bean mixture firmly over the cut surface. Fold the beef over to enclose the filling and secure with kitchen string tied at 2 cm intervals. Spray all over with olive oil.

4. Heat a flameproof roasting pan over high heat, lightly spray with oil and sear the beef, turning occasionally, for 5–6 minutes or until well browned all over. Transfer to the oven and roast for 35–40 minutes for medium–rare or until cooked to your liking. Cover loosely with foil and set aside for 15 minutes to rest.

5. Meanwhile, for the cavolo nero anchovy crumbs, heat a large heavy-based non-stick frying pan over medium–high heat. Add the oil, bread and anchovies and cook, stirring, for 4–5 minutes or until the bread is golden. Transfer to a bowl and set aside to cool.

6. Place the cavolo nero or kale in the same pan with ¼ cup (60 ml) water, then cook, covered, stirring occasionally, for 4–5 minutes or until softened, but still with a chewy bite. Remove the lid and cook for a further 1–2 minutes, until the water has evaporated.

7. Meanwhile, steam the carrots in a steamer basket over a large saucepan of boiling water for 3 minutes, then add the asparagus and steam for a further 2 minutes or until the vegetables are just tender.

8. Carve the beef, discarding the string, and divide among 4 plates, along with the carrots and asparagus. Add the parsley and chilli to the anchovy crumb, toss, then sprinkle over the cavolo nero or kale, and serve with a dollop of rouille and lemon wedges, if desired.

NUTRITIONAL ANALYSIS	ENERGY (KJ)	2488	CARBOHYDRATE (G)	31	SODIUM (MG)	564
TO SERVE 4 (PER SERVE)	PROTEIN (G)	58	SATURATED FAT (G)	6.7	FIBRE (G)	15

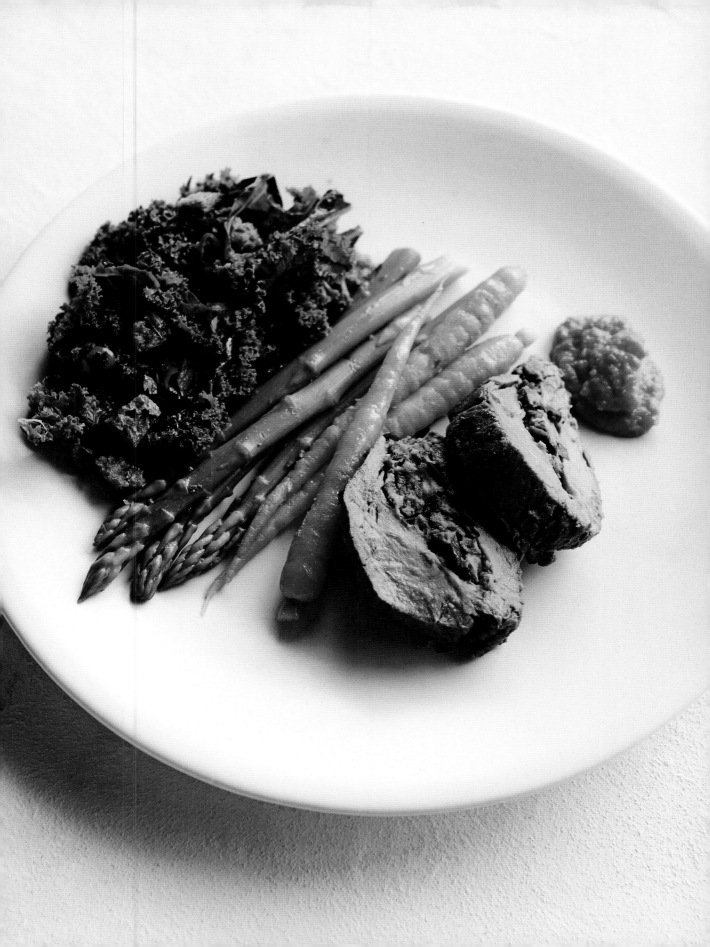

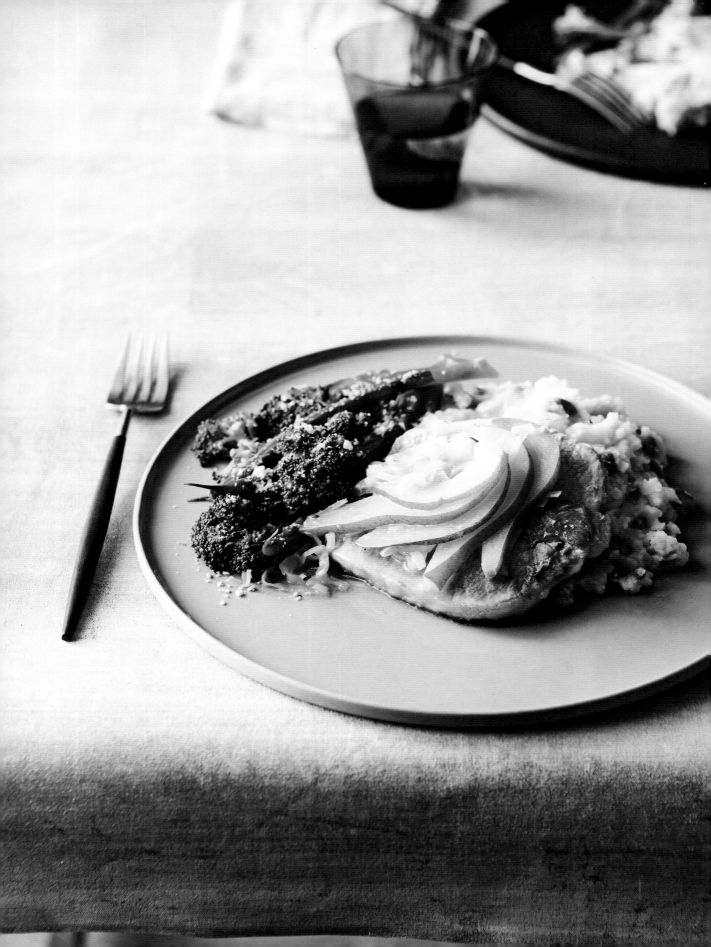

Pork steaks with pear and cider sauce and celeriac-borlotti bean mash

We all know and love that classic combination of pork and apple, and pear works just as well. The flavour is enhanced with the cider to give a wonderful stickiness to the juicy gravy, and is perfectly complemented by the nutty dukkah that coats the vegetables.

SERVES 4
PREP TIME 20 MINUTES
COOKING TIME 35 MINUTES

4 × 100 g butterflied pork loin steaks, trimmed of any visible fat
olive oil spray, for cooking
1 teaspoon olive oil
1 leek, white part only, well washed and thinly sliced
2 cloves garlic, crushed
2 pears, cored and thinly sliced
1 cup (250 ml) dry pear cider (or sparkling apple juice)
1 teaspoon Dijon mustard
½ cup (125 ml) homemade chicken stock (see page 288) or salt-reduced chicken stock
Steamed green beans and broccolini with homemade dukkah or nut-free dukkah (see page 291)

CELERIAC-BORLOTTI BEAN MASH
2 desiree potatoes (400 g), peeled and chopped
1 celeriac with leaves and stalk removed (550 g), peeled and chopped
½ cup (125 ml) buttermilk
2 teaspoons Dijon mustard
pinch of ground white pepper
1 × 400 g tin low-salt borlotti beans, drained and rinsed

1. For the mash, steam the potatoes and celeriac in a steamer basket over a saucepan of boiling water for 10–12 minutes or until very tender. Cool slightly, then transfer to a food processor, add the buttermilk and mustard, and process until smooth. Season lightly with freshly ground pepper, then return to the pan and stir in the borlotti beans. Cover to keep warm.

2. Meanwhile, heat a large heavy-based non-stick frying pan over medium–high heat. Lightly spray the pork steaks all over with oil and cook for 1–2 minutes on each side or until browned all over. Transfer to a warm plate, cover loosely with foil and set aside.

3. Heat the oil in the same pan over medium heat, add the leek and garlic and cook, covered, stirring occasionally, for 5 minutes or until softened. Add the pears and cook, stirring, for 2 minutes. Add the cider and cook for 2 minutes or until reduced slightly and the pear has started to soften. Stir in the mustard and stock and bring to the boil. Return the pork to the pan with any resting juices and simmer for 2–3 minutes or until just cooked through.

4. Divide the mash plus broccoli and beans with dukkah among 4 plates. Top with the pork steaks, and spoon the pear and cider sauce evenly over the pork.

NUTRITIONAL ANALYSIS	ENERGY (KJ)	2101	CARBOHYDRATE (G)	50	SODIUM (MG)	549
TO SERVE 4 (PER SERVE)	PROTEIN (G)	41	SATURATED FAT (G)	1.6	FIBRE (G)	17

Provençal fish stew with red capsicum rouille

Fish stock is easy to make and it's great to have a supply of it in the freezer. However, there are plenty of good shop-bought fish stocks out there that are tasty, low in salt and that will make this dish delicious.

SERVES 4
PREP TIME 20 MINUTES
COOKING TIME 40 MINUTES

8 baby potatoes (320 g), halved
1 tablespoon olive oil
200 g scallop meat (without roe)
200 g small cleaned squid tubes, sliced into rings
1 × 200 g mackerel fillet, cut into bite-sized pieces
1 bulb fennel, trimmed and thinly sliced
2 zucchinis (courgettes), cut into 5 mm dice
2 golden shallots, finely chopped
3 cloves garlic, crushed
2 tomatoes, chopped
½ cup (125 ml) dry white wine
2 cups (500 ml) salt-reduced fish stock
1 × 400 g tin low-salt butter beans, drained and rinsed
150 g baby spinach leaves
1 handful chopped flat-leaf parsley (optional)
4 slices wholegrain sourdough bread (optional), grilled

RED CAPSICUM ROUILLE
2 red capsicums (peppers), seeded, membranes removed, quartered
1 tablespoon olive oil
2 golden shallots, finely chopped

1. For the rouille, preheat the grill on high heat. Line a baking tray with foil. Place the capsicums, skin-side up, on the tray and grill for 8–10 minutes or until well charred and softened. Transfer to a bowl, cover with plastic film and set aside for 15 minutes to loosen the skin, then peel away and discard the skin. Chop the capsicum flesh and set aside. Meanwhile, heat the oil in a small heavy-based saucepan over medium heat and cook the shallots, stirring often, for 3–4 minutes or until softened. Add the capsicum and cook, stirring occasionally, for 3–4 minutes or until it starts to break down. Remove from the heat and set aside to cool slightly. Puree in a blender or with a stick blender until smooth, then transfer to a bowl and set aside.

2. Steam the baby potatoes in a steamer basket over a saucepan of boiling water for 10–12 minutes or until tender. Set aside.

3. Heat the olive oil in a large heavy-based saucepan over medium heat. Pat the scallop meat dry with paper towel and cook for 2–3 minutes on each side or until golden but not quite cooked through. Transfer to a plate and set aside. Repeat with the squid and the mackerel, pan-frying until just cooked through, then transferring to the same plate.

4. Add the fennel, zucchinis (courgettes), shallots and garlic to the pan, then cook, covered, over medium heat, stirring occasionally, for 10 minutes or until softened. Remove the lid, add the tomatoes and cook for 2 minutes or until it starts to collapse. Add the wine and cook for another 2–3 minutes or until reduced by half. Add the stock, steamed potatoes, butter beans and any juices from the plate holding the cooked seafood and bring to the boil. Remove from the heat and stir through the baby spinach until wilted. Return all the seafood to the pan, then cover and leave for 3 minutes to warm through.

5. Divide the seafood mixture among 4 shallow bowls, ensuring each bowl gets an even portion of seafood. Top with one-quarter of the rouille, scatter with parsley (if using), then serve with the grilled bread alongside, if desired.

NUTRITIONAL ANALYSIS	ENERGY (KJ)	2151	CARBOHYDRATE (G)	39	SODIUM (MG)	1146
TO SERVE 4 (PER SERVE)	PROTEIN (G)	42	SATURATED FAT (G)	3.5	FIBRE (G)	8

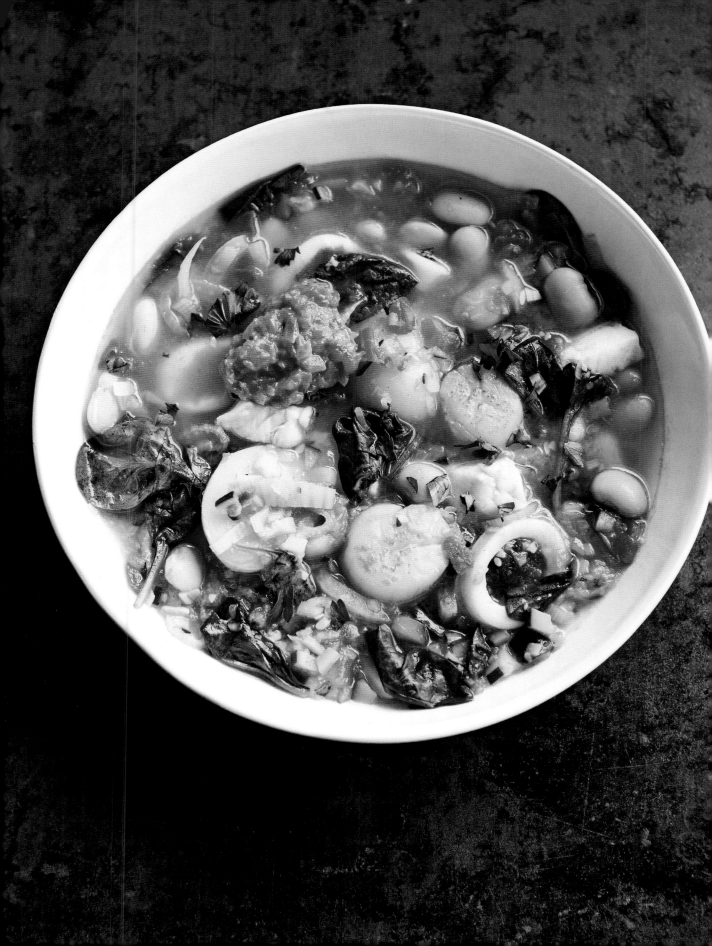

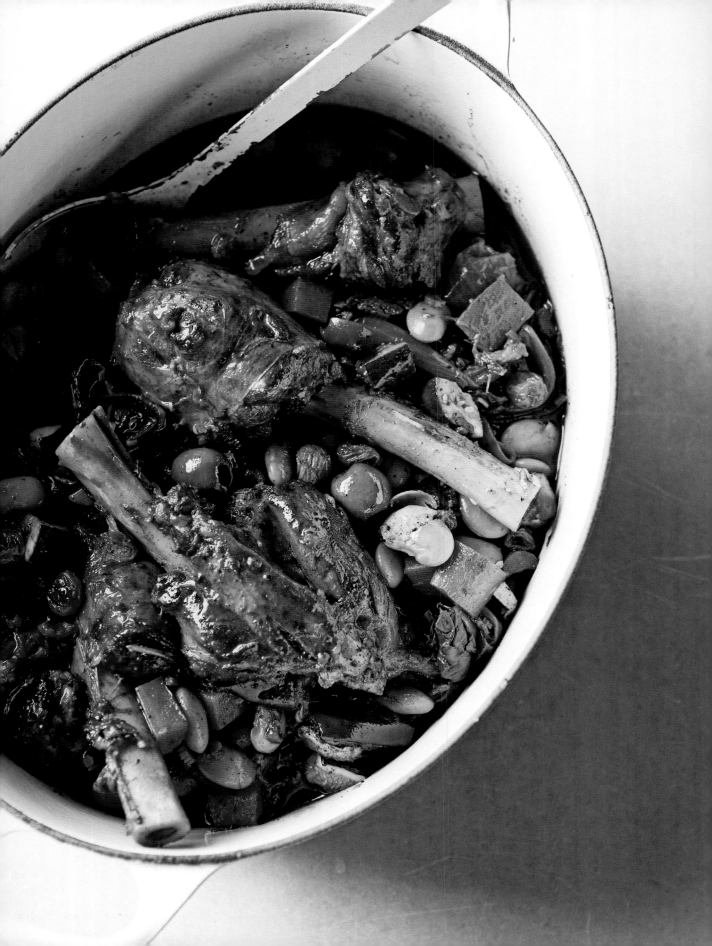

Braised lamb shanks with eggplant and zucchini

This casserole is rich in nutrients and juicy flavours – and who can resist lamb that falls off the bone? If you prefer, instead of saving half the spinach to serve as a salad, you can add all the leaves to the casserole dish to wilt and soak up those rich juices.

SERVES 4
PREP TIME 20 MINUTES
COOKING TIME 1 HOUR 45 MINUTES

4 × 180 g French-trimmed lamb shanks, visible fat removed
olive oil spray, for cooking
2 carrots, scrubbed and cut into 2 cm chunks
2 sticks celery, thinly sliced
1 onion, cut into thin wedges
1 large eggplant (aubergine), cut into 3 cm pieces
3 cloves garlic, bruised and peeled
3 teaspoons ras el hanout
1 cup (250 ml) dry red wine
1 cup (250 ml) homemade chicken stock (see page 288) or salt-reduced chicken stock
1 teaspoon sumac, plus extra to sprinkle
1 × 400 g tin low-salt butter beans, drained and rinsed
2 zucchinis (courgettes), cut into 2 cm chunks
¼ cup (35 g) raisins
⅓ cup (40 g) seeded green olives
200 g baby spinach leaves
4 thin slices wholegrain sourdough bread

1. Preheat the oven to 180°C (160°C fan-forced).

2. Heat a large heavy-based casserole dish over medium–high heat.

3. Lightly spray the lamb shanks with olive oil and cook, turning occasionally, for 5–6 minutes or until golden brown all over. Transfer to a plate. Add the carrots, celery sticks and onion to the pan and cook over medium heat, stirring occasionally, for 5 minutes or until the onion begins to soften. Add the eggplant, garlic and ras el hanout and cook, stirring, for 2–3 minutes or until fragrant.

Add the wine and cook for 30 seconds, stirring to dislodge any residue stuck to the base of the pan. Stir in the stock and sumac, and bring to the boil.

4. Return the lamb shanks to the dish and cover with a tight-fitting lid. Transfer to the oven to cook, stirring occasionally, for 1 hour. Add the butter beans and zucchinis, then cover and cook for a further 30 minutes or until the lamb is tender and begins to fall off the bone. Stir in the raisins, olives and half the spinach.

5. Place the casserole dish on a heatproof mat on the table and let your guests help themselves. Put the remaining spinach leaves in a salad bowl, and add to the table alongside a plate of the bread and a small bowl of sumac for sprinkling.

NUTRITIONAL ANALYSIS	ENERGY (KJ)	2082	CARBOHYDRATE (G)	28	SODIUM (MG)	732
TO SERVE 4 (PER SERVE)	PROTEIN (G)	46	SATURATED FAT (G)	5.6	FIBRE (G)	8

Slow-cooked lamb with green rice

Make sure you scrape all the juicy goodness from the casserole dish when you serve – you won't want to waste a drop of this delicious stew. The spicy green rice works well as an accompaniment for grilled meats, too; the coriander is what gives the green rice its colour and fragrance, while the jalapeño gives it a subtle kick.

SERVES 4

PREP TIME 20 MINUTES

COOKING TIME 2 HOURS 10 MINUTES, PLUS 15 MINUTES RESTING

1 teaspoon coriander seeds

1 teaspoon cumin seeds

1 × 500 g piece boned lamb leg, visible fat trimmed

olive oil spray, for cooking

1 lime, thinly sliced

1 × 400 g tin low-salt chopped tomatoes

2 bay leaves

3 carrots, peeled and sliced

250 g green beans, trimmed

GREEN RICE

2 cups (500 ml) homemade chicken stock (see page 288) or salt-reduced chicken stock

1 tablespoon sliced pickled jalapeño

1 handful roughly chopped coriander stems and leaves, plus extra leaves to serve

1 teaspoon olive oil

1 onion, finely chopped

2 cloves garlic, crushed

¾ cup (150 g) brown basmati rice

1 × 400 g tin low-salt black beans or red kidney beans, drained and rinsed

1. Preheat the oven to 180°C (160°C fan-forced).

2. Heat a small heavy-based frying pan over medium heat and toast the coriander seeds and cumin seeds in the dry pan for 1–2 minutes or until fragrant. Transfer to a mortar and use a pestle to coarsely crush them.

3. Heat a large flameproof casserole dish over medium–high heat. Lightly spray the lamb with oil and cook for 4–5 minutes or until well browned all over. Sprinkle the lamb with the crushed seeds, pressing them on to coat the meat, then lay the lime slices over the top. Add the tomatoes, bay leaves and a little water, if necessary, so there is about 1 cm of liquid in the base of the dish. Cover the dish with a layer of baking paper and the lid, and transfer to the oven to cook, stirring once or twice during cooking, for 2 hours or until the lamb is very tender.

4. When the lamb has been cooking for about 1½ hours, make the green rice: Warm the stock and jalapeño in a small heavy-based saucepan over low heat for 5 minutes. Stir in the coriander, remove from the heat and leave to cool slightly. Using a stick blender or blender, puree the mixture until smooth. Strain into a bowl, using a spatula to press some of the flavoursome green pulp through the sieve. You will need 1⅓ cups (330 ml) green stock. Discard the remaining pulp.

5. Heat the oil in a heavy-based saucepan over medium heat and cook the onion, partially covered, for 4–5 minutes or until tender. Add the garlic and rice and cook, stirring, for 1 minute or until fragrant. Add the green stock and bring to the boil, then reduce the heat to low and cook, covered, for 20–25 minutes or until the stock has evaporated and the rice is tender. Gently stir in the black beans or kidney beans. Set aside, covered, for 10 minutes.

6. Once the lamb is cooked and very tender, take the casserole dish out of the oven and leave to rest for 10–15 minutes. Discard the bay leaves. Then, using 2 forks, roughly shred (or 'pull') the lamb into bite-sized chunks. Stir to coat with the pan juices.

7. Meanwhile, steam the carrots and beans in a steamer basket over a saucepan of simmering water for 4–6 minutes or until just tender.

8. Divide the shredded lamb and sauce, green rice and vegetables among 4 shallow bowls. Scatter with the extra coriander.

NUTRITIONAL ANALYSIS					
TO SERVE 4 (PER SERVE)	ENERGY (KJ)	2142	CARBOHYDRATE (G)	32	SODIUM (MG)	766
	PROTEIN (G)	47	SATURATED FAT (G)	7.2	FIBRE (G)	10

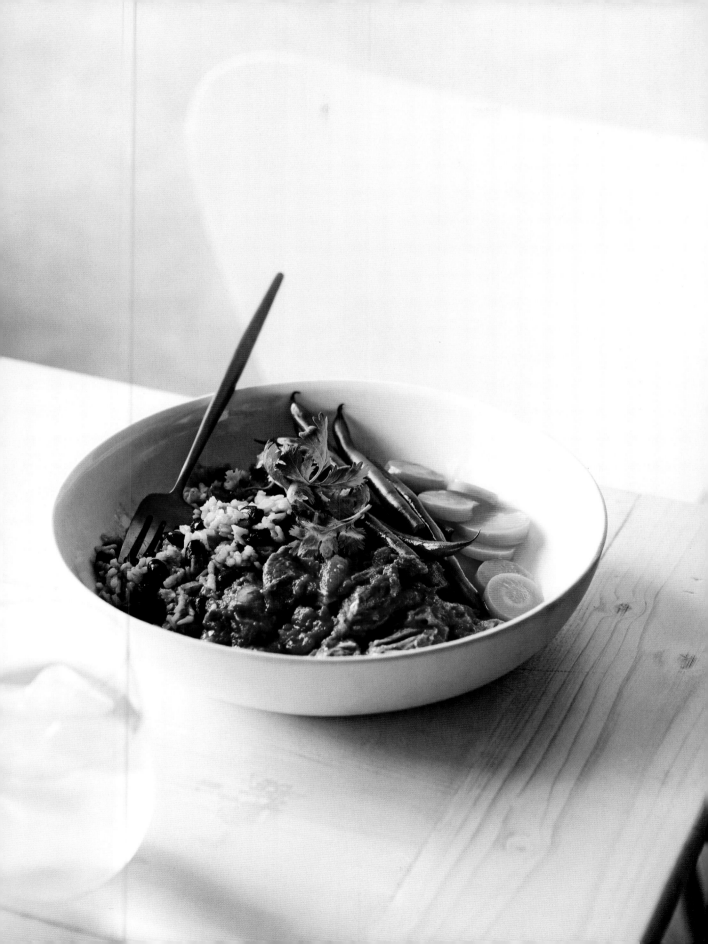

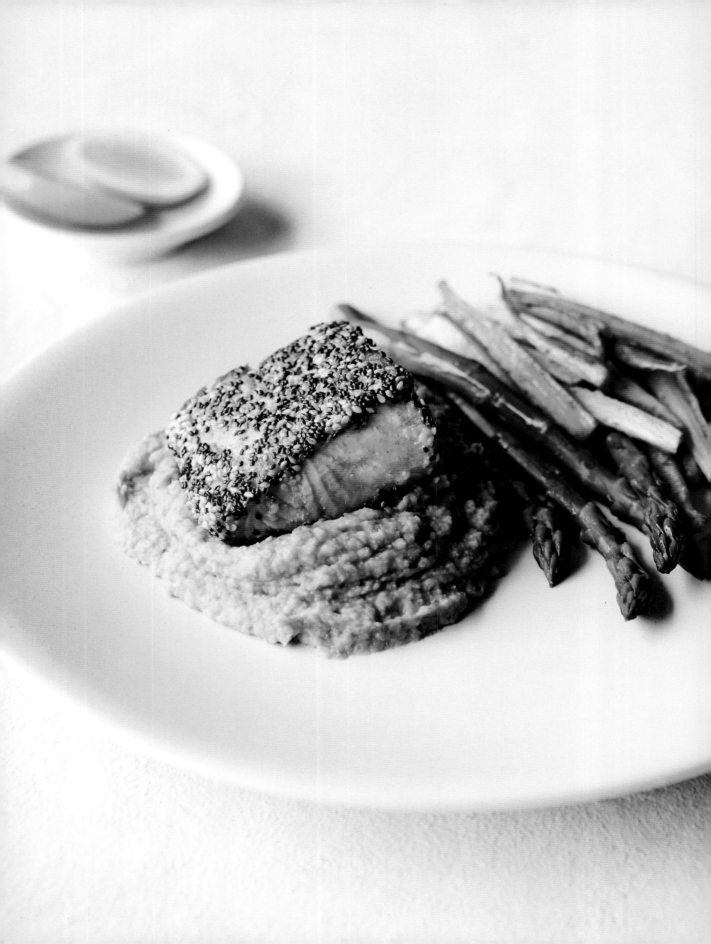

Salmon with parsnip fries and cannellini bean and pea puree

You can't help but smile when you eat this healthy take on fish, chips and mushy peas. The toasted seeds that coat the salmon give the fish a satisfying crunch and mouth-watering taste; the paprika-roasted parsnips are beautiful and golden to rival any chip, and the puree is packed with flavour from the beautiful stock.

SERVES 4
PREP TIME 20 MINUTES
COOKING TIME 30 MINUTES

2 parsnips, peeled and cut into batons
1 teaspoon sweet paprika
olive oil spray, for cooking
2 × 240 g pin-boned salmon fillets, skin on
1 tablespoon black chia seeds
1 tablespoon sesame seeds
1 teaspoon peanut oil
340 g asparagus, trimmed
lemon cheeks, to serve

CANNELLINI BEAN AND PEA PUREE
1 teaspoon olive oil
1 onion, finely chopped
2 cloves garlic, crushed
2 × 400 g tins low-salt cannellini beans, drained and rinsed
2 cups (240 g) frozen peas
½ cup (125 ml) homemade vegetable stock (see page 288) or salt-reduced vegetable stock

1. Preheat the oven to 210°C (190°C fan-forced). Line a baking tray with baking paper.

2. Scatter the parsnips over the lined tray in a single layer. Spray lightly with oil and sprinkle with the paprika. Roast, turning after 20 minutes, for 25–30 minutes or until tender and golden.

3. Meanwhile, for the cannellini bean and pea puree, heat the olive oil in a heavy-based saucepan over medium heat and cook the onion and garlic, stirring occasionally, for 3–5 minutes or until softened. Add the cannellini beans, peas and stock and bring to the boil. Set aside to cool slightly. Use a stick blender or food processor to puree until smooth. Set aside.

4. Cut each salmon fillet in half lengthways to give 4 long, thin pieces. Combine the chia and sesame seeds on a plate and carefully press each side of the fish in the seed mixture to coat evenly.

5. Heat the peanut oil in a heavy-based non-stick frying pan over medium–high heat. Cook the salmon, skin-side down for 2–3 minutes or until golden underneath, then turn and cook for a further 2 minutes for medium or until cooked to your liking.

6. Meanwhile, steam the asparagus in a steamer basket over a pan of simmering water for 3–4 minutes or until just tender.

7. Reheat the cannellini bean and pea puree gently over low heat, stirring occasionally, for 2–3 minutes to warm through.

8. Share the puree among 4 plates in generous dollops. Top with a portion of the salmon, and divide the asparagus and roasted parsnips between the plates. Serve with lemon cheeks on the side.

NUTRITIONAL ANALYSIS	ENERGY (KJ)	2263	CARBOHYDRATE (G)	47	SODIUM (MG)	992
TO SERVE 4 (PER SERVE)	PROTEIN (G)	44	SATURATED FAT (G)	2.9	FIBRE (G)	12

Spicy Italian mussels with tomato and pearl couscous

This is a terrific dish with generous portions of mussels. The bread is a brilliant
addition for mopping up the remnants of the scrumptious sauce.
Don't forget to add an empty bowl to the table for the discarded mussel shells.

SERVES 4

PREP TIME 20 MINUTES

COOKING TIME 25 MINUTES

1 tablespoon olive oil

1 bulb fennel, trimmed, quartered and thinly sliced

1 leek, white section only, well-washed and finely chopped

3 cloves garlic, crushed

½ cup (125 ml) red wine

1 × 800 g tin low-salt chopped tomatoes

1 × 400 g tin low-salt borlotti beans, drained and rinsed

1 large handful basil, including stalks

2 small fresh red chillies, thinly sliced

1 cup (250 ml) homemade chicken stock (see page 288)
or salt-reduced chicken stock

⅔ cup (100 g) pearl couscous

1.5 kg blue mussels, bearded and scrubbed

1 large handful flat-leaf parsley, chopped

150 g rocket

1 tablespoon homemade classic salad dressing
(see page 289)

1. Heat the olive oil in a very large, deep heavy-based
saucepan over medium heat. Cook the fennel, leek
and garlic, partially covered, stirring occasionally,
for 8–10 minutes or until softened.

2. Add the wine and simmer for 2 minutes or until
the liquid has nearly evaporated. Add the tomatoes,
borlotti beans, basil, chillies and stock and bring
to the boil. Add the couscous and mussels, then
cook, covered, giving the pan a shake occasionally,
for 5 minutes. Transfer the opened mussels to a
plate. Re-cover the saucepan and cook for a further
3–5 minutes or until the remaining mussels have
opened, then transfer the opened mussels to the
plate. Discard any mussels that haven't opened.
Continue to cook the tomato mixture until the
couscous is just tender. Return all the mussels in
their shells to the pan and stir to combine; add a
little hot water if the consistency
of the sauce needs adjusting.

3. Divide the mussel mixture evenly among 4 shallow
bowls and scatter with the parsley. Toss the rocket
with the dressing and serve alongside, with
sourdough, if you like.

NUTRITIONAL ANALYSIS	ENERGY (KJ)	1891	CARBOHYDRATE (G)	50	SODIUM (MG)	901
TO SERVE 4 (PER SERVE)	PROTEIN (G)	29	SATURATED FAT (G)	2.2	FIBRE (G)	5

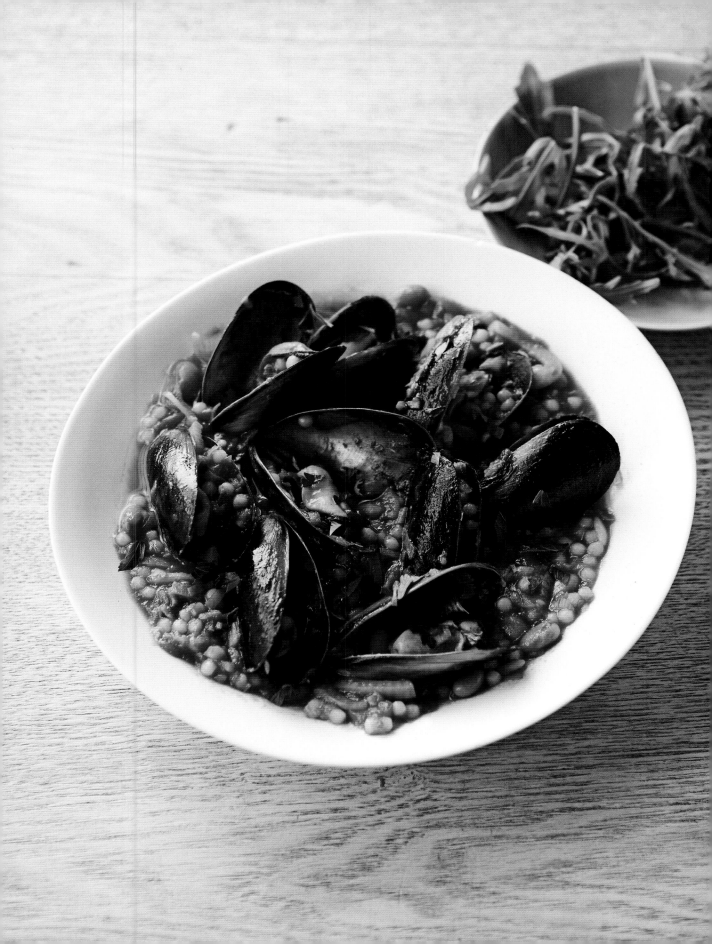

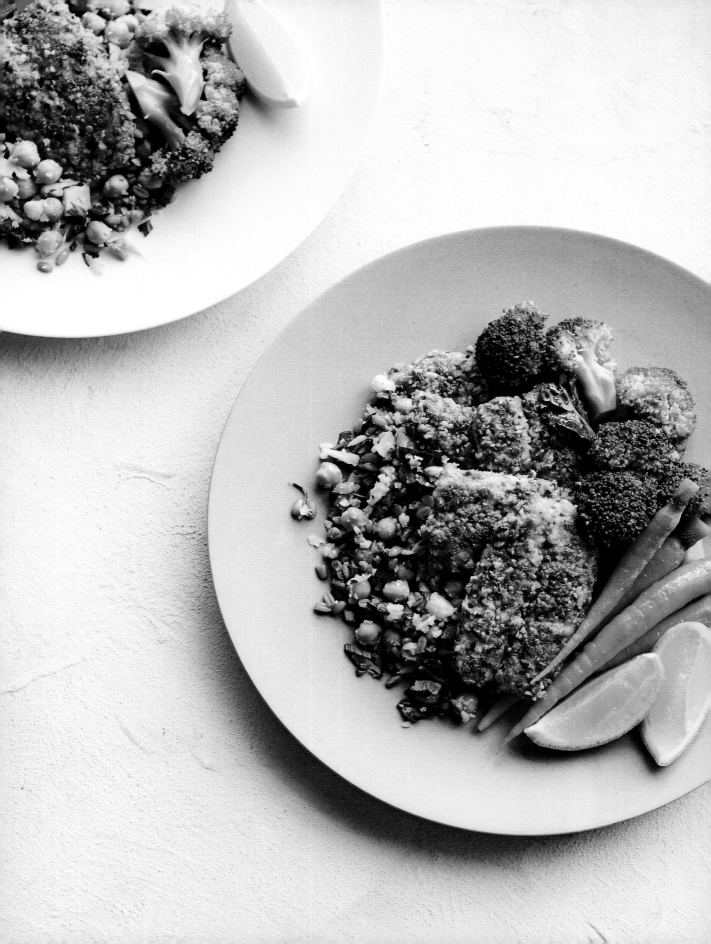

Dukkah-crusted butterflied sardines with freekeh and cauliflower pilaf

Sardines contain a wealth of goodness, including that all-important omega-3. And, because they're near the bottom of the deep-sea food chain, they contain very little mercury – so you can eat them to your heart's content.

SERVES 4
PREP TIME 20 MINUTES
COOKING TIME 25 MINUTES

3½ cups (350 g) roughly chopped cauliflower
¾ cup (150 g) cracked wholewheat freekeh
1 × 400 g tin low-salt chickpeas, drained and rinsed
1 handful flat-leaf parsley, roughly chopped
1 handful mint, shredded
1 tablespoon lemon juice
½ cup (60 g) dukkah or nut-free dukkah (see page 293)
2 eggs
500 g butterflied sardines, tails intact
olive oil spray, for cooking
600 g baby carrots, scrubbed
7 cups (600 g) broccoli florets
lemon wedges, to serve

1. Working in 2 batches, place the cauliflower in a food processor and pulse until it resembles grains of rice. Bring 8 cups (2 litres) water to the boil in a large heavy-based saucepan. Add the freekeh and return to the boil. Reduce the heat to medium, partially cover and simmer for 15–20 minutes or until the freekeh is tender but with some bite. Add the processed cauliflower and chickpeas and cook for a further 2 minutes or until the freekeh and cauliflower are tender. Drain well and return to the pan. Stir in the parsley, mint, lemon juice and freshly ground black pepper to taste. Cover to keep warm and set aside.

2. Meanwhile, place the dukkah in a small bowl. Crack the eggs into another small bowl, add 1 tablespoon water and whisk until combined. Working with one butterflied sardine at a time, dip first in the egg, shaking off the excess, and then in the dukkah mixture.

3. Heat a large heavy-based non-stick frying pan over medium heat. Lightly spray the coated sardines all over with olive oil and cook for 1–2 minutes on each side or until just cooked through.

4. Steam the carrots in a steamer basket over a large saucepan of boiling water for 2 minutes, then add the broccoli and steam for a further 3 minutes or until the vegetables are just tender.

5. Divide the pilaf among 4 serving plates. Top with one-quarter of the sardines, and share the vegetables between the plates. Serve with the lemon wedges alongside.

NUTRITIONAL ANALYSIS	ENERGY (KJ)	2358	CARBOHYDRATE (G)	35	SODIUM (MG)	324
TO SERVE 4 (PER SERVE)	PROTEIN (G)	47	SATURATED FAT (G)	4.9	FIBRE (G)	17

Caramelised leek, lentil, mushroom and thyme tarts

These little tarts are wonderfully easy to make and so tasty, packed as they are with sweetness from the caramelised leeks, richness from the mushrooms and creaminess from the feta. You can buy filo pastry fresh or frozen. If you don't cook with filo very often, buy the frozen pastry; you can then simply remove the number of sheets you need and keep the rest frozen until next time.

SERVES 4
PREP TIME 20 MINUTES
COOKING TIME 40 MINUTES

olive oil spray, for cooking
3 sheets filo pastry
1 teaspoon olive oil
1 leek, white section only, well washed and thinly sliced
2 portobello (flat field) mushrooms (100 g), stems trimmed, thinly sliced
2 cloves garlic, crushed
2 teaspoons chopped thyme leaves, plus extra to serve
1 × 400 g tin low-salt brown lentils, drained and rinsed
5 large eggs
½ cup (100 g) reduced-fat feta cheese, crumbled
100 g rocket or baby spinach leaves
homemade basic slaw (see page 291), to serve
1 avocado, stone removed, peeled and sliced

1. Preheat the oven to 180°C (160°C fan-forced). Grease four 10 cm fluted tart tins with a removable base with olive oil spray.

2. Layer the 3 sheets of pastry on a clean chopping board, lightly spraying oil between each layer. Cut the layered sheets into 8 even rectangles, then layer two rectangles into each tin, making sure the tins' bases and sides are completely covered, pressing the pastry gently into the side of each tin. Place the tins on a baking tray and bake for 5 minutes or until the pastry is just cooked through (it will not brown at this stage). Gently press the pastry down with paper towel if it puffs up during cooking.

3. Meanwhile, heat the oil in a large heavy-based non-stick frying pan over medium heat. Add the leek and cook, covered, stirring occasionally, for 5 minutes or until softened. Add the mushrooms and garlic and cook, covered, stirring occasionally, for 2–3 minutes or until the mushrooms begin to release their juices. Remove the lid and cook for a further minute or until most of the mushroom liquid has evaporated. Stir in the thyme and set aside to cool slightly.

4. Divide the mushroom mixture evenly among the tart cases, followed by the lentils, piling the lentils towards the centre of each tart. (It will seem like a lot of filling, but the egg will filter through to the base when you add it.) Whisk the eggs and a little freshly ground black pepper in a jug, then pour evenly and slowly over the filled tart cases. Sprinkle evenly with the crumbled feta.

5. Bake the tarts for 20–25 minutes or until the pastry and cheese are lightly browned and the filling is set. Set aside for 2–3 minutes to rest before removing the tarts from the tins and transferring the tarts to plates. Serve with rocket or baby spinach leaves, slaw and sliced avocado.

NUTRITIONAL ANALYSIS	ENERGY (KJ)	2054	CARBOHYDRATE (G)	22	SODIUM (MG)	581
TO SERVE 4 (PER SERVE)	PROTEIN (G)	28	SATURATED FAT (G)	8.4	FIBRE (G)	12

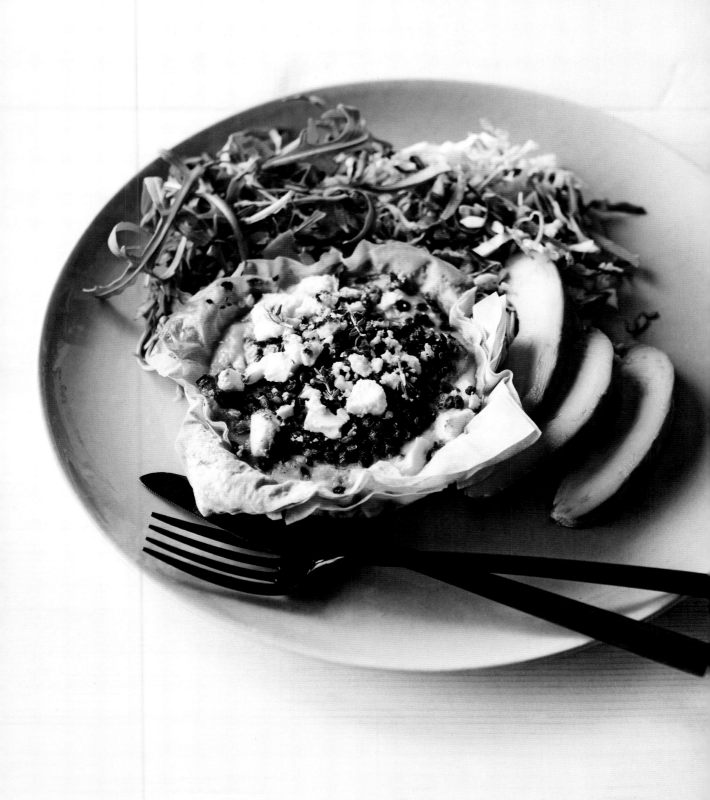

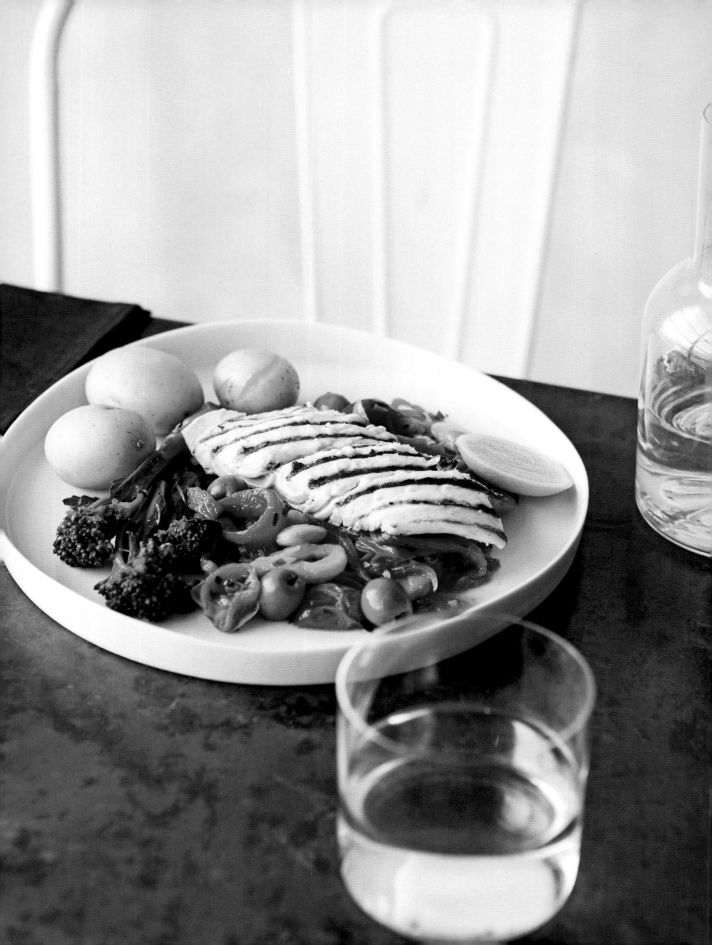

Grilled blue-eye trevalla with roasted capsicums, tomatoes and butter beans

Blue-eye trevalla is a versatile fish, similar to cod, that is suited to all methods of cooking. It can stand up to big flavours, being perfect for a fish stew or curry, but it is also delicious when cooked simply, as here, to let its mild and delicate flavour shine.

SERVES 4

PREP TIME 20 MINUTES, PLUS 15 MINUTES COOLING

COOKING TIME 40 MINUTES

2 red capsicums (peppers), seeded, membranes removed, quartered

2 yellow capsicums (peppers), seeded, membranes removed, quartered

1 tablespoon extra virgin olive oil

1 red onion, thinly sliced

3 cloves garlic, crushed

250 g cherry tomatoes, halved

¼ cup (40 g) seeded Sicilian green olives

1 tablespoon drained capers in vinegar, rinsed

2 anchovies, well drained and chopped

1 × 400 g tin low-salt butter beans, drained and rinsed

2 tablespoons finely chopped flat-leaf parsley

2 tablespoons red wine vinegar

10 baby new potatoes (400 g)

350 g broccolini, bases trimmed

4 × 150 g blue-eye trevalla fillets

olive oil spray, for cooking

lemon cheeks, to serve

1. Preheat the oven griller to high and line a baking tray with foil. Place the capsicums, skin-side up, on the lined tray and grill for 8–10 minutes or until well charred and softened. Transfer to a bowl, cover with plastic film and set aside for 15 minutes to steam. Peel away the skin and cut the capsicum into strips.

2. Meanwhile, heat the oil in a large heavy-based non-stick frying pan over low heat. Add the onion and garlic and cook, partially covered, for 8–10 minutes or until the onion is very tender.

Add the tomatoes, olives, capers and anchovies. Increase the heat to medium and cook, stirring occasionally, for 5 minutes or until the tomatoes start to collapse. Remove from the heat and stir in the capsicum strips, butter beans, parsley and vinegar. Season with pepper.

3. Steam the potatoes in a steamer basket over a pan of simmering water for 15 minutes or until tender. Steam the broccolini in a steamer basket over a saucepan of boiling water for 3–4 minutes or until just tender.

4. Meanwhile heat a chargrill pan or heavy-based non-stick frying pan over medium heat. Spray the fish fillets lightly with oil and cook for 3–4 minutes on each side or until golden and cooked through. (The cooking time will depend on the thickness of the fillets.)

5. Divide the capsicum mixture and broccolini among 4 serving plates. Top with the fish, and serve with the potatoes and lemon cheeks alongside.

NUTRITIONAL ANALYSIS	ENERGY (KJ)	1569	CARBOHYDRATE (G)	21	SODIUM (MG)	612
TO SERVE 4 (PER SERVE)	PROTEIN (G)	37	SATURATED FAT (G)	2	FIBRE (G)	9

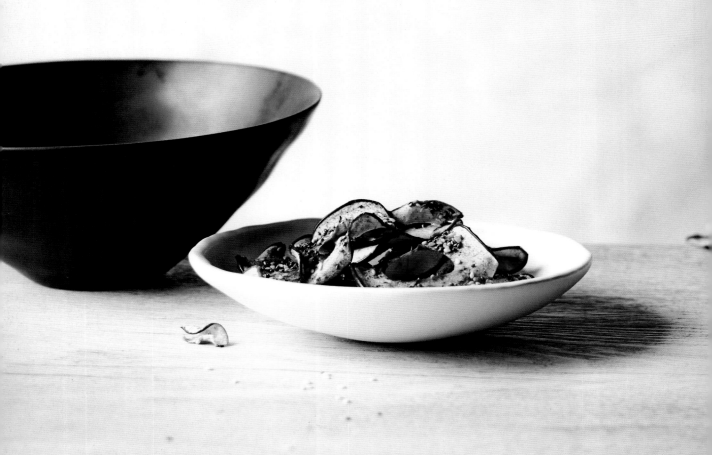

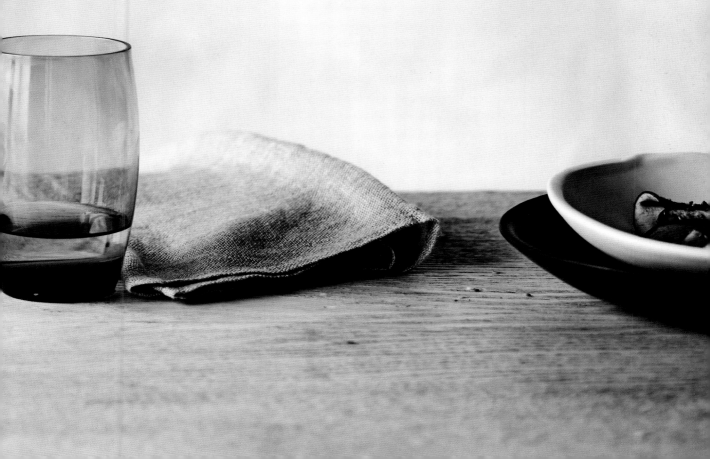

SNACKS

Cauliflower 'popcorn'

This healthy snack is quick, easy and extremely moreish either on its own or with the dipping sauce. Big and little hands alike will reach for the bite-size 'popcorn' – and keep coming back for more.

SERVES 4
PREP TIME 10 MINUTES
COOKING TIME 40 MINUTES

1 cauliflower, base trimmed, stalks and florets cut into
   2 cm chunks
olive oil spray, for cooking
2 tablespoons homemade dukkah or nut-free dukkah
   (see page 293)

PARSLEY, LEMON AND GARLIC SAUCE (OPTIONAL)
½ cup (140 g) reduced-fat natural Greek-style yoghurt
1 tablespoon finely chopped flat-leaf parsley
3 teaspoons hulled tahini
2 teaspoons lemon juice
½ small clove garlic, crushed

1. Preheat the oven to 200°C (180°C fan-forced). Line 2 large baking trays with baking paper.

2. Spread the cauliflower over the lined trays in a single layer, spray with oil and toss gently to coat in the oil. Sprinkle with the dukkah and roast, turning halfway through cooking, for 35–40 minutes or until tender and well browned around the edges.

3. Meanwhile, to make the sauce (if using), stir all the ingredients together in a small bowl. Cover with plastic film and refrigerate until ready to serve.

4. Serve the cauliflower 'popcorn' warm, with the sauce for dipping, if desired.

NUTRITIONAL ANALYSIS	ENERGY (KJ)	787	CARBOHYDRATE (G)	8	SODIUM (MG)	157
TO SERVE 4 (PER SERVE)	PROTEIN (G)	7	SATURATED FAT (G)	2.1	FIBRE (G)	5

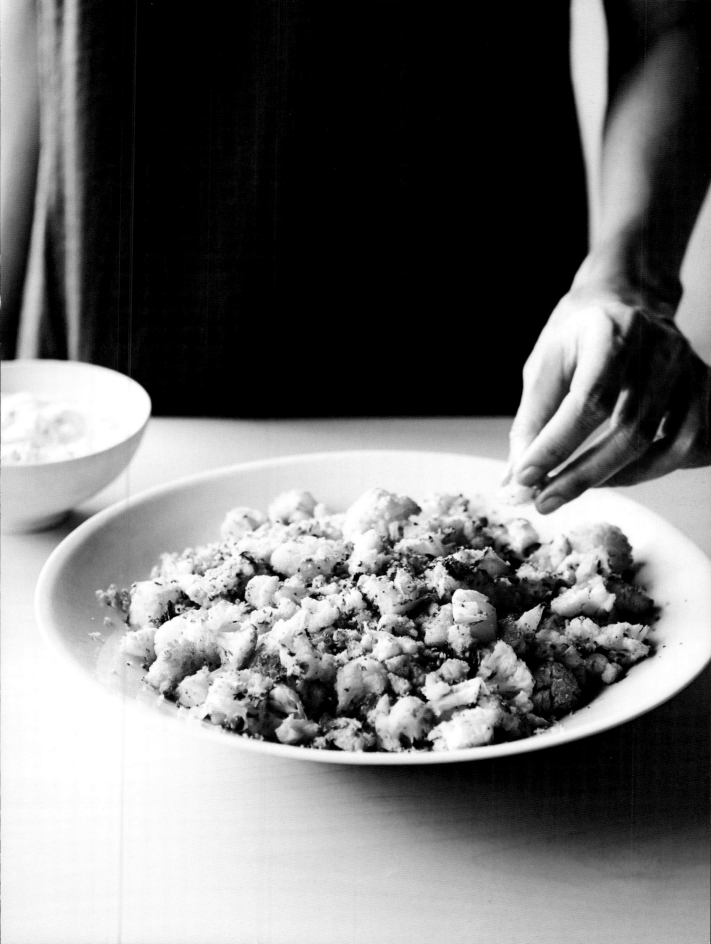

Delectable dips

These dips are all low enough in kilojoules to be served with a healthy selection of vegetables. Try them with baby carrots and radishes, celery sticks, cucumber sticks and any other vegetable options from your fridge.

Baba ganoush

MAKES ABOUT 1 CUP (ABOUT 240 G)
PREP TIME 5 MINUTES, PLUS 15 MINUTES COOLING
COOKING TIME 35–40 MINUTES

1 eggplant (aubergine)
1 tablespoon (or to taste) lemon juice
3 teaspoons hulled tahini
1 small clove garlic, crushed
1 handful mint leaves, shredded

1. Pierce the eggplant all over with a fork. Heat a heavy-based frying pan, chargrill pan or barbecue hotplate over medium–high heat. Cook the eggplant, turning occasionally, for 30–35 minutes or until charred in spots and tender. (Alternatively, cook for 15–20 minutes on the stovetop, then transfer to a lined tray in the oven at 180°C (160°C fan-forced) for a further 15–20 minutes or until tender.)

2. Set aside for 15 minutes or until cool enough to handle. Peel, discarding the skin, then roughly chop the flesh and place in a colander to drain.

3. Puree the cooled eggplant in a food processor with the lemon juice, tahini and garlic until smooth. Season with freshly ground black pepper and stir in the mint.

Black bean dip

MAKES ABOUT 1 CUP (ABOUT 300 G)
PREP TIME 5 MINUTES
COOKING TIME 10 MINUTES

2 teaspoons olive oil
1 red onion, chopped
1 clove garlic, roughly chopped
1 × 400 g tin low-salt black beans or kidney beans, drained and rinsed
2 teaspoons (or to taste) chopped pickled jalapeño chillies,
2 teaspoons lime juice
½ teaspoon ground cumin
1 handful coriander leaves, chopped
lime wedges, to serve (optional)

1. Heat the oil in a heavy-based non-stick frying pan over low–medium heat and cook the onion and garlic, stirring occasionally, for 8–10 minutes or until tender. Transfer to a bowl and set aside to cool.

2. Blend or process the onion mixture with most of the beans (reserve about 1 tablespoon), the jalapeños, lime juice and cumin until almost smooth, scraping down the side of the blender or processor bowl as necessary. Add a splash of water if needed to keep the mixture moving in the blender. Stir in the reserved beans and coriander. Serve with lime wedges to the side, if you like.

NUTRITIONAL ANALYSIS TO SERVE 4 (PER SERVE)

ENERGY (KJ)	213	SATURATED FAT (G)	0.3
PROTEIN (G)	2	SODIUM (MG)	9
CARBOHYDRATE (G)	3	FIBRE (G)	4

NUTRITIONAL ANALYSIS TO SERVE 4 (PER SERVE)

ENERGY (KJ)	435	SATURATED FAT (G)	0.4
PROTEIN (G)	6.1	SODIUM (MG)	42
CARBOHYDRATE (G)	11	FIBRE (G)	6

Cannellini bean, pea and parsley dip

MAKE ABOUT 1½ CUPS (ABOUT 450 G)
PREP TIME 5 MINUTES
COOKING TIME 10 MINUTES

---

1 teaspoon olive oil
1 small onion, finely chopped
1 clove garlic, crushed
1 × 400 g tin low-salt cannellini beans,
    drained and rinsed
½ cup (60 g) frozen peas, thawed
¼ cup (70 g) reduced-fat natural Greek-style yoghurt
3 teaspoons lemon juice
1 handful flat-leaf parsley, to serve

---

1. Heat the oil in a heavy-based non-stick frying pan over low–medium heat. Add the onion and garlic and cook, covered, stirring occasionally, for 5–6 minutes or until soft. Add the cannellini beans, peas and ¼ cup (60 ml) water and bring to the boil. Simmer, stirring, for 2–3 minutes or until the water has evaporated. Transfer to a bowl and set aside to cool.

2. Blend or process the bean mixture with the yoghurt and lemon juice until smooth, scraping down the side of the blender or processor bowl as necessary; add a little splash of water if needed to keep the mixture moving. Sprinkle with parsley, season with a little salt, if you like, then serve.

Pumpkin and red lentil dip

MAKES ABOUT 1 CUP (ABOUT 300 G)
PREP TIME 5 MINUTES
COOKING TIME 25 MINUTES

---

1 teaspoon olive oil
1 onion, roughly chopped
1 clove garlic, crushed
250 g kent or butternut pumpkin (squash),
    peeled and cut into 1.5 cm pieces
2 tablespoons red lentils, rinsed
½ teaspoon ground cumin
¼ teaspoon ground turmeric
2 tablespoons reduced-fat natural Greek-style yoghurt
1 handful coriander, roughly chopped
2 tablespoons pepitas (roasted pumpkin seed kernels),
    roughly chopped

---

1. Heat the oil in a small heavy-based saucepan over low–medium heat, add the onion and garlic and cook, covered, stirring occasionally, for 5–6 minutes or until soft. Add the pumpkin, lentils, spices and ¾ cup (180 ml) water and bring to the boil. Simmer, stirring occasionally, for 15–20 minutes or until the pumpkin and lentils are soft and collapse to form a puree; add a little more water if the mixture starts to stick to the pan. Transfer to a bowl and set aside to cool.

2. Swirl in the yoghurt and coriander to the pumpkin mixture, sprinkle with pepitas and serve.

NUTRITIONAL ANALYSIS TO SERVE 4 (PER SERVE)

ENERGY (KJ)	413	SATURATED FAT (G)	0.8
PROTEIN (G)	6	SODIUM (MG)	405
CARBOHYDRATE (G)	11	FIBRE (G)	5

NUTRITIONAL ANALYSIS TO SERVE 4 (PER SERVE)

ENERGY (KJ)	433	SATURATED FAT (G)	1.2
PROTEIN (G)	4	SODIUM (MG)	15
CARBOHYDRATE (G)	10	FIBRE (G)	3

Eggplant and zucchini 'fries'

These oven-baked bites are crispy on the outside and soft in the middle – just as the perfect fries should be. The spiced crumb crisps up beautifully and the paprika adds a little heat. Delicious.

SERVES 4
PREP TIME 20 MINUTES
COOKING TIME 15 MINUTES

2 zucchinis (courgettes), cut into 5 mm-thick batons
½ eggplant (aubergine), cut into 5 mm-thick batons
1 tablespoon plain flour
½ teaspoon ground coriander
½ teaspoon sweet paprika
¾ cup (50 g) fresh wholegrain breadcrumbs
1½ tablespoons polenta
2 tablespoons finely grated parmesan
1 extra-large egg
homemade parsley, lemon and garlic sauce
   (see page 212), to serve

1. Preheat the oven to 220°C (200°C fan-forced). Line 2 large baking trays with baking paper and place 2 wire racks on top of the trays.

2. Place the vegetable batons, flour and spices in a large zip-lock bag and shake to coat the vegetables in the flour mixture.

3. Combine the breadcrumbs, polenta and parmesan in a wide shallow bowl. Whisk the egg with 1 tablespoon water in another bowl.

4. Working with a few vegetable batons at a time, shake off the excess flour mixture and dip in the egg, then shake off the excess egg and toss in the breadcrumb mixture. Place in a single layer on the wire racks. Bake for 14–16 minutes or until tender and golden. Serve immediately with the sauce in a bowl to the side for dipping.

NUTRITIONAL ANALYSIS	ENERGY (KJ)	797	CARBOHYDRATE (G)	21	SODIUM (MG)	178
TO SERVE 4 (PER SERVE)	PROTEIN (G)	8	SATURATED FAT (G)	2.6	FIBRE (G)	3

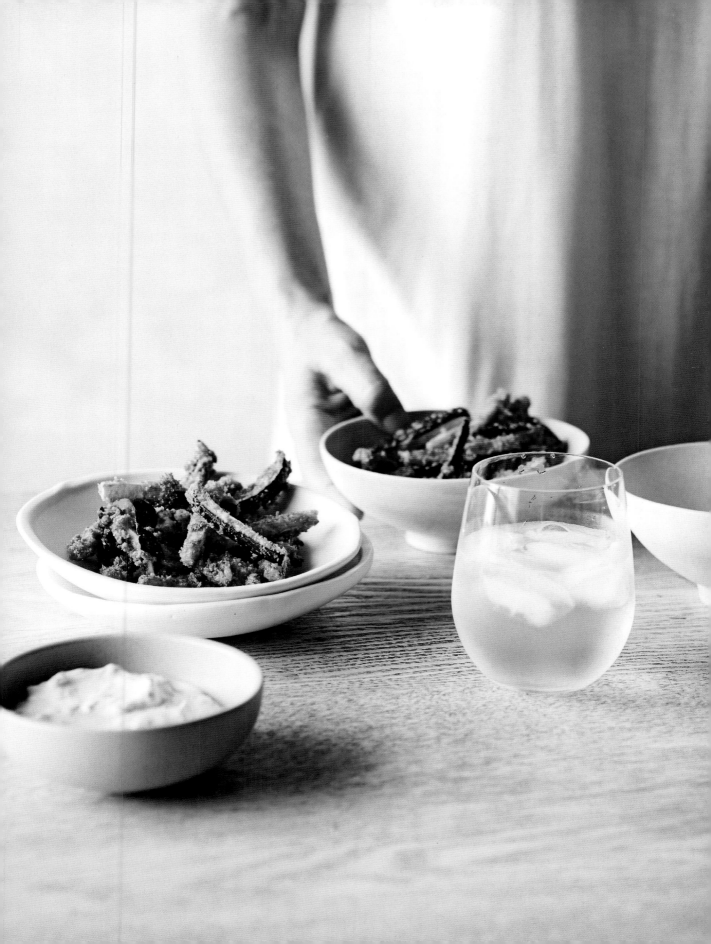

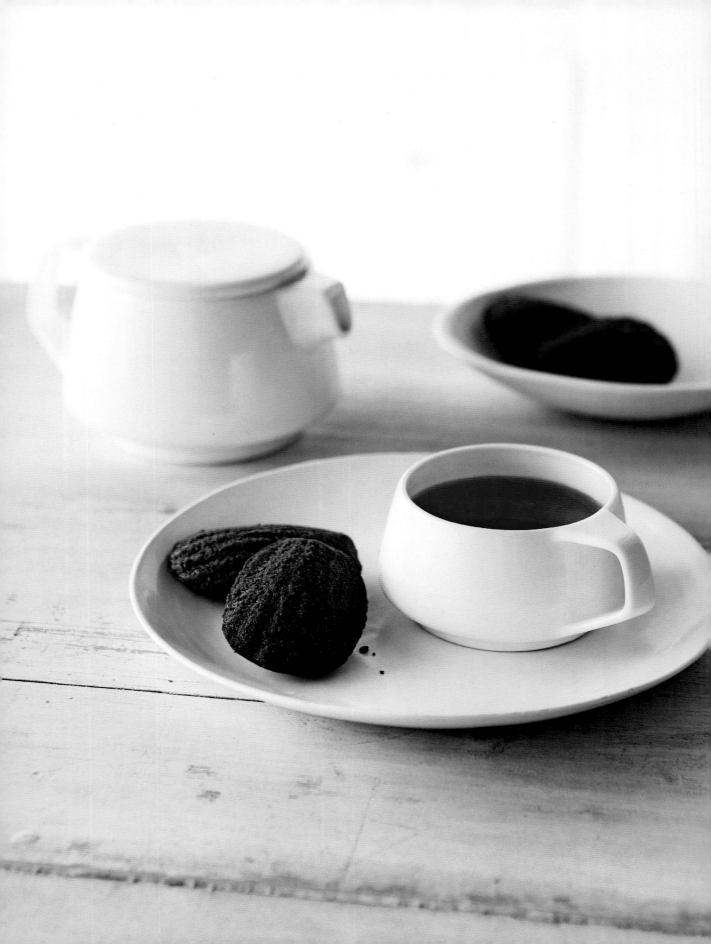

Chocolate and pistachio madeleines

These madeleines are gorgeously chocolately and a little bit earthy and not too sweet. They go perfectly with a cup of green tea, and will keep for a day or two, stored in an airtight container. Don't worry if you only have one madeleine tray – the mixture will hold between cooking the batches.

MAKES 20 (2 PER SERVE)
PREP TIME 10 MINUTES
COOKING TIME 10 MINUTES

olive oil spray, for greasing
½ cup (70 g) unsalted shelled pistachios
1 × 400 g tin low-salt red kidney beans, drained and rinsed
3 large eggs
¼ cup (55 g) soft brown sugar
1½ tablespoons macadamia oil
3 teaspoons vanilla extract
⅓ cup (35 g) Dutch-processed cocoa powder, sifted
2 teaspoons baking powder

1. Preheat the oven to 180°C (160°C fan-forced). Spray 2 non-stick madeleine trays with oil, or line 20 holes of a mini-muffin tray with paper cases.

2. Process the pistachios in a food processor until finely chopped. Transfer to a small bowl and set aside.

3. Process the kidney beans and 1 of the eggs in the food processor until smooth and creamy. Add the sugar, macadamia oil and vanilla, and process until smooth and creamy. Add the remaining eggs, ground pistachios, cocoa and baking powder, then process until combined.

4. Spoon about 1 tablespoon of the mixture into each oiled or lined hole, and bake for 8–10 minutes or until just firm to touch. Leave to cool for 3 minutes, then transfer to a wire rack to cool. Serve warm or at room temperature.

NUTRITIONAL ANALYSIS	ENERGY (KJ)	635	CARBOHYDRATE (G)	11	SODIUM (MG)	437
TO SERVE 4 (PER SERVE)	PROTEIN (G)	6	SATURATED FAT (G)	1.7	FIBRE (G)	3

Fruity yoghurt popsicles

Frozen banana makes these popsicles sublimely creamy. Keep a supply of frozen banana in zip-lock bags in the freezer for using in popsicles, smoothies and ice cream. You can use fresh bananas instead of frozen, but the mixture won't be as thick and will need to be par-frozen before the sticks are inserted, otherwise they will sink too low into the popsicles. The honey adds another layer of flavour into these fruity treats, but it can be omitted if desired.

MAKES 6
PREP TIME 20 MINUTES, PLUS 4 HOURS FREEZING
COOKING TIME NIL

125 g fresh or frozen raspberries
3 frozen bananas, chopped
½ cup (140 g) reduced-fat natural Greek-style yoghurt
2 teaspoons honey

1. Place a large bowl in the fridge to chill.

2. Drop 2–3 whole raspberries into each of six ⅓ cup (80 ml)-capacity popsicle moulds.

3. Process the banana and ¼ cup (70 g) of the yoghurt in a food processor, scraping down the side as necessary, until smooth and creamy. Drop about 1 tablespoon of the mixture into each popsicle mould and tap gently on the bench to settle it around the raspberries. Transfer about ¼ cup (3 tablespoons) of the banana mixture (this will be used for the final layer) to your chilled bowl, and place in the refrigerator or freezer to keep it cold, especially if the weather is hot.

4. Add the remaining raspberries, remaining yoghurt and the honey to the remaining banana mixture in the food processor, and process until smooth and creamy. Divide evenly among the moulds, then top with the reserved banana mixture. Insert the popsicle sticks and freeze for 3–4 hours or until frozen.

NUTRITIONAL ANALYSIS	ENERGY (KJ)	378	CARBOHYDRATE (G)	17	SODIUM (MG)	13
TO SERVE 4 (PER SERVE)	PROTEIN (G)	2	SATURATED FAT (G)	0.8	FIBRE (G)	2

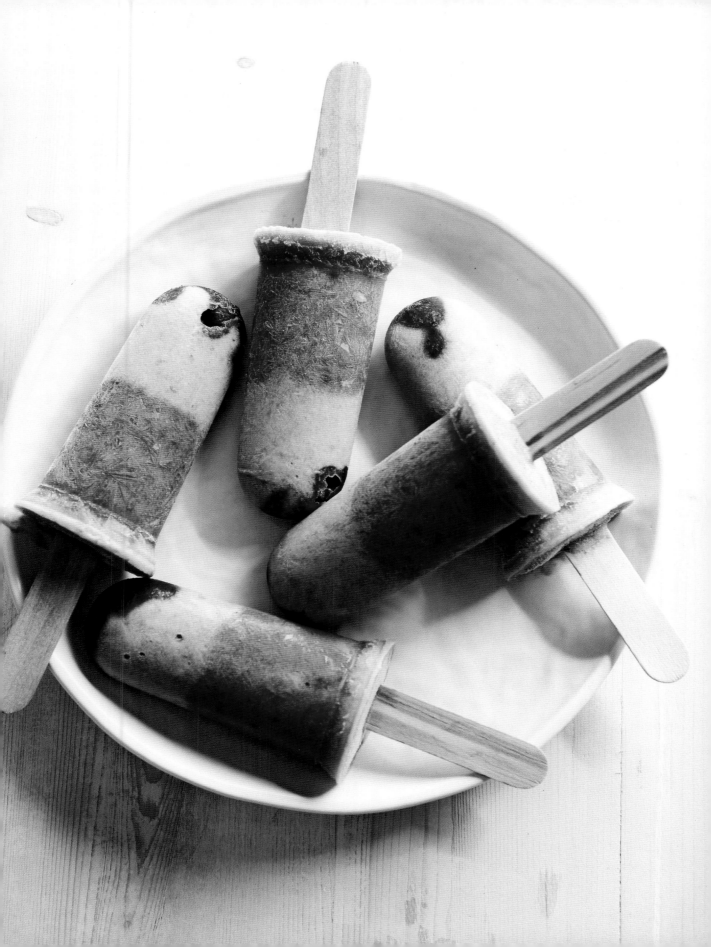

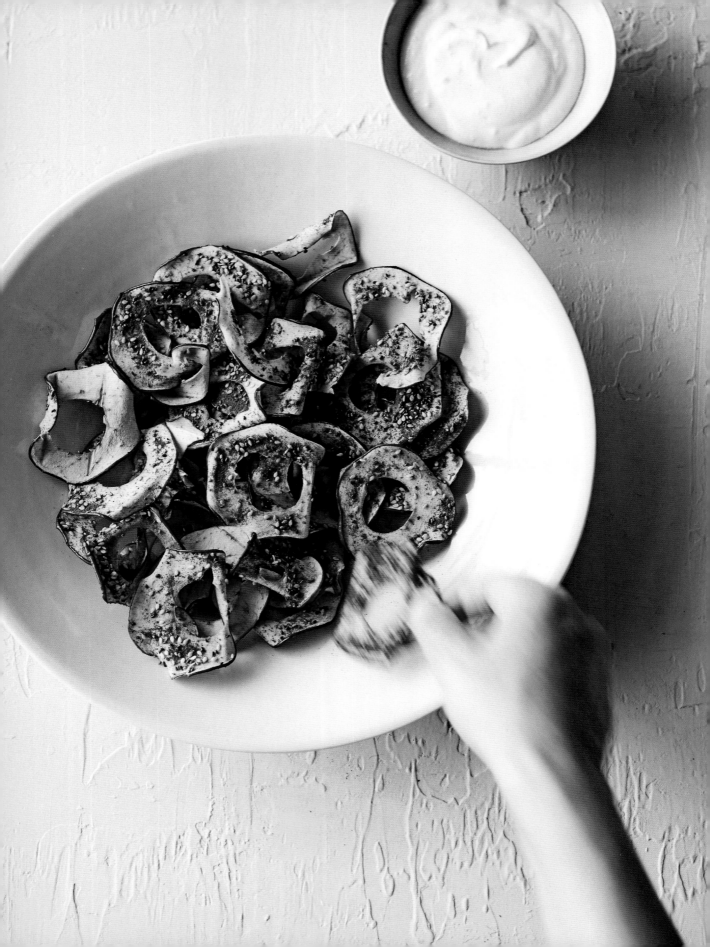

Spiced baked apple chips

These baked nibbles are at their best on the day they are made, when they are satisfyingly crisp. Store any leftovers in an airtight container and pack them in lunchboxes for devouring the next day. This recipe works well with pears, too.

SERVES 4

PREP TIME 10 MINUTES

COOKING TIME 2 HOURS

2 red apples

1 teaspoon mixed spice

2 teaspoons black chia seeds

2 teaspoons sesame seeds

2 cups (560 g) reduced-fat natural Greek-style yoghurt

1. Preheat the oven to 110°C (90°C fan-forced). Remove 1 or 2 oven racks from the oven and ensure they are clean.

2. Core the apples, then, with the apples on their sides, slice as thinly and evenly as you can with a very sharp knife. (If you have one, use a mandoline.) Arrange the slices in single layers on the clean oven racks. Sprinkle with the spice and seeds, then carefully return the racks to the oven.

3. Bake the apple for 1 hour, then carefully turn the slices over and swap the racks from top to bottom when you return them to the oven. Bake for a further hour or until the apple slices are quite dry. Transfer to a wire rack to cool completely.

4. Serve with yoghurt.

NUTRITIONAL ANALYSIS	ENERGY (KJ)	783	CARBOHYDRATE (G)	25	SODIUM (MG)	144
TO SERVE 4 (PER SERVE)	PROTEIN (G)	11	SATURATED FAT (G)	2.1	FIBRE (G)	2

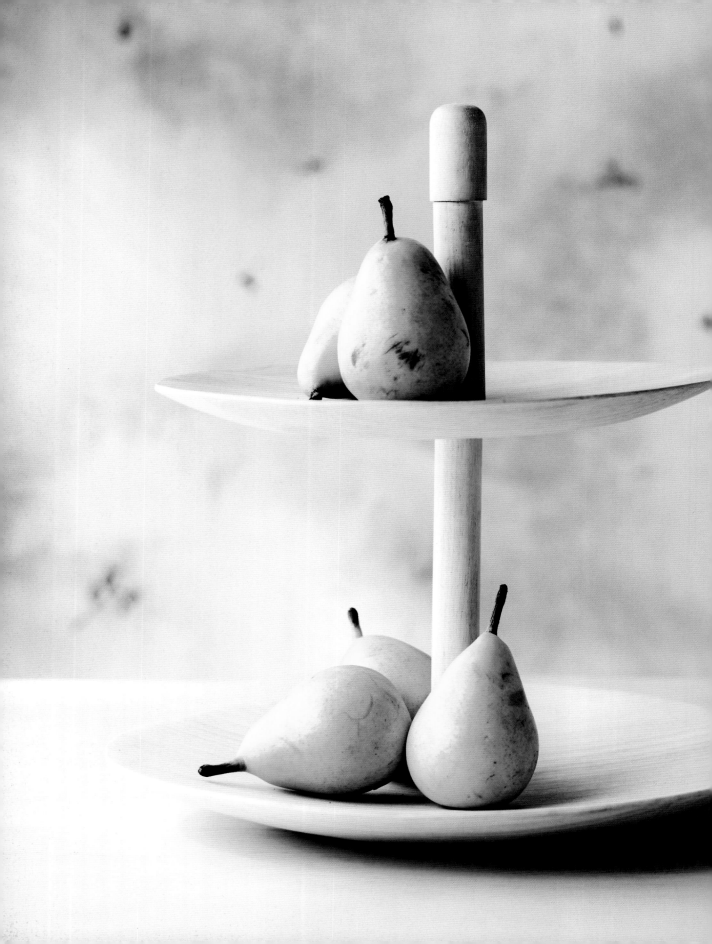

DESSERTS

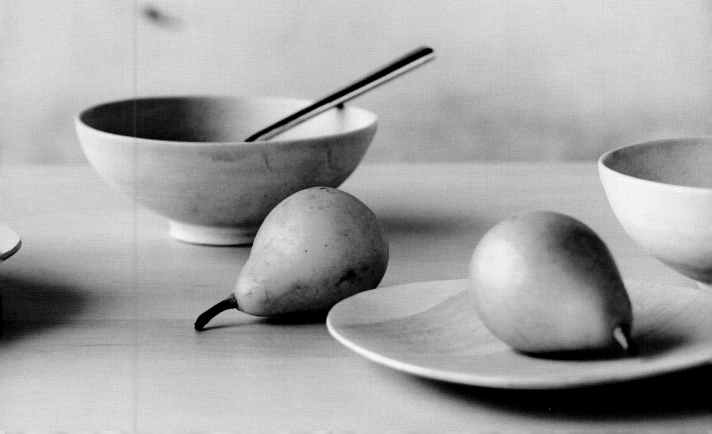

Berry tiramisu

This sweet treat is lighter than traditional tiramisu, but the sweetness of the berries and creaminess of the whipped ricotta make it feel just as indulgent, and taste delicious, too.

SERVES 4
PREP TIME 10 MINUTES, PLUS COOLING
COOKING TIME 10 MINUTES

1⅓ cup (200 g) frozen mixed berries
juice of 1 orange
2 cups (250 g) strawberries, hulled, and halved if large
⅔ cup (160 ml) strong black coffee, cooled
2 tablespoons Marsala
5 large (100 g) sponge finger biscuits (savoiardi),
     each broken into 4 pieces
Dutch-processed cocoa, to serve

WHIPPED RICOTTA
300 g firm, fresh low-fat ricotta
1 teaspoon vanilla bean paste

1. Place the frozen berries and orange juice in a small heavy-based saucepan over medium heat. Cook, stirring occasionally, for 2–3 minutes or until thawed. Strain the berries, reserving both the syrup and the berries.

2. Return the syrup to the pan and simmer over medium–high heat for 3–5 minutes or until thickened. Transfer the berries to a bowl, stir in the reduced syrup and fresh strawberries and set aside to cool.

3. For the whipped ricotta, place the ricotta and vanilla bean paste in a food processor or blender. Add about ¼ cup (60 ml) of the cooled syrup from the bowl containing the berries to the ricotta and process until smooth. Add a little more syrup to adjust the consistency, if required – it should be smooth and spoonable.

4. Combine the coffee and Marsala in a bowl. Dip half of the sponge finger pieces briefly in the coffee mixture, then divide among the bases of 4 glasses, bowls or jars. Share one-third of the whipped ricotta between the 4 glasses on top of the dipped sponge fingers, then do the same with about half of the berry mixture. Repeat with the remaining sponge fingers, half of the remaining whipped ricotta and all of the remaining berry mixture. Finish with a dollop of the remaining whipped ricotta and sprinkle with cocoa.

5. Serve immediately or cover and refrigerate for up to 4 hours before serving.

NUTRITIONAL ANALYSIS	ENERGY (KJ)	955	CARBOHYDRATE (G)	28	SODIUM (MG)	298
TO SERVE 4 (PER SERVE)	PROTEIN (G)	10	SATURATED FAT (G)	3.6	FIBRE (G)	3

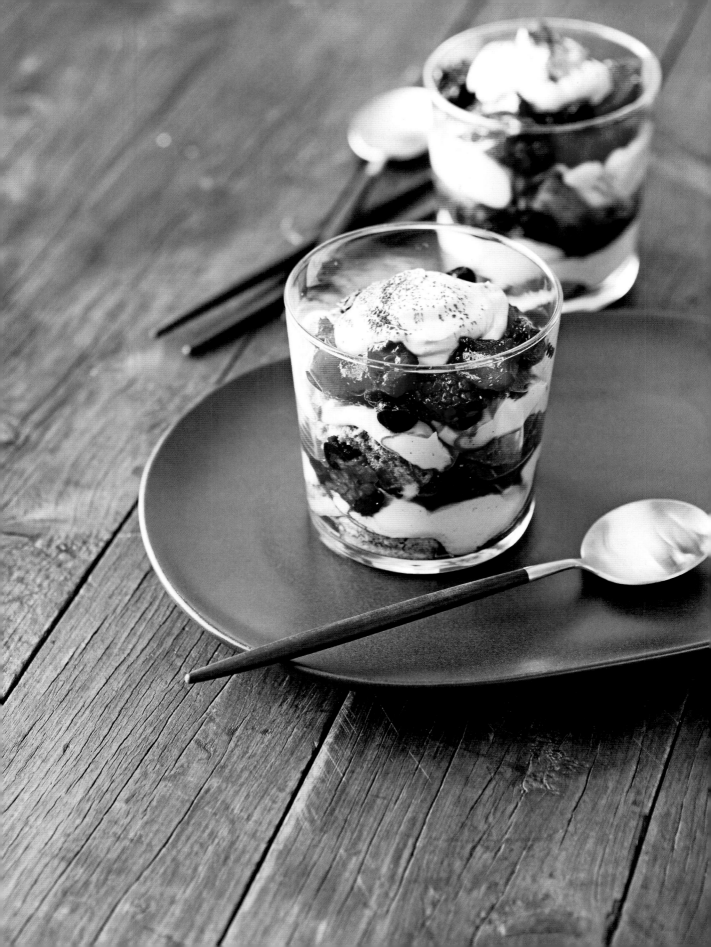

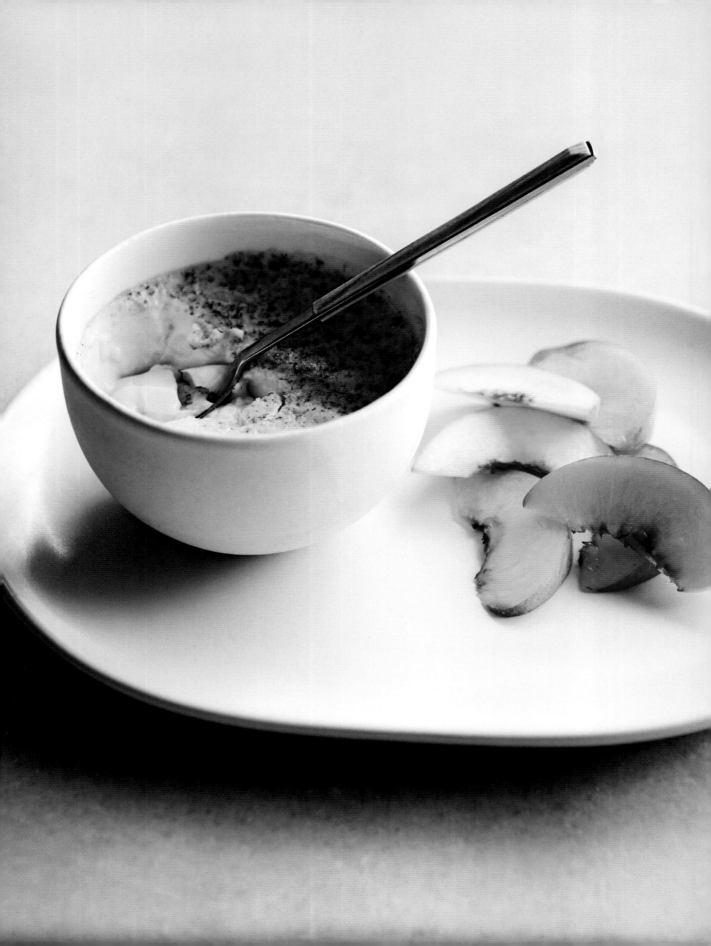

Baked custard with peaches

Poached fruit goes just as beautifully with these custards as fresh fruit.
Try with the poached strawberries and rhubarb from the breakfast pancake recipe (see page 125).

SERVES 4
PREP TIME 10 MINUTES
COOKING TIME 35 MINUTES, PLUS 30 MINUTES CHILLING

2 teaspoons cornflour
800 ml skim milk
1 teaspoon finely grated orange zest
2 large eggs
2 large egg whites
1 tablespoon honey
1 teaspoon vanilla bean paste
grated nutmeg, to sprinkle
2 white peaches
2 yellow peaches

1. Preheat the oven to 170°C (150°C fan-forced). Place four 1 cup (250 ml) ovenproof bowls or ramekins in a large roasting pan on top of a folded tea towel.

2. Place the cornflour and 1 tablespoon of the milk in a small heavy-based saucepan and whisk until combined. Whisk in the remaining milk and orange zest. Stir over medium heat and bring just to the boil. Whisk the eggs, egg whites, honey and vanilla bean paste together in a large heatproof bowl. Gently and constantly whisking, add the hot milk mixture in a slow, steady stream (so you don't introduce frothy bubbles), whisking until combined.

3. Fill the kettle with water and boil. Divide the custard mixture evenly among the bowls or ramekins in the roasting pan. Scoop off any froth with a spoon and sprinkle with the grated nutmeg. Place the pan on the oven rack and pour in enough boiling water from the kettle to come three-quarters of the way up the side of the ramekins.

4. Bake for 25–30 minutes or until the custards just wobble slightly in the centre. Remove and set aside in the pan for 10 minutes. Transfer the bowls or ramekins to a wire rack and leave to cool to room temperature, about 30 minutes, or refrigerate to chill before serving.

5. Cut the peaches into thin wedges and remove the pits. Share the white and yellow peach wedges between 4 plates, and place the ramekins of custard next to them for serving.

NUTRITIONAL ANALYSIS	ENERGY (KJ)	904	CARBOHYDRATE (G)	32	SODIUM (MG)	162
TO SERVE 4 (PER SERVE)	PROTEIN (G)	14	SATURATED FAT (G)	1.1	FIBRE (G)	4

Coconut and lime chia puddings

Generously layer the fruit between the creamy chia when dishing up to ensure you get mouthfuls of fruit with every spoonful, right to the last dram.

SERVES 4
PREP TIME 10 MINUTES, PLUS 1–2 HOURS CHILLING
COOKING TIME NIL

⅓ cup (60 g) white chia seeds
1 teaspoon finely grated lime zest
1 × 375 ml tin light and creamy evaporated milk
¼ teaspoon natural coconut essence
170 g honeydew melon, cut into 5 mm dice
170 g rockmelon (cantaloupe), cut into 5 mm dice
2 passionfruit, halved
2 tablespoons roughly chopped brazil nuts (optional)

1. Combine the chia seeds, lime zest, evaporated milk and coconut essence in a bowl and cover with plastic film. Refrigerate for 1–2 hours, stirring occasionally, until thickened.

2. Place the melon in a small bowl and add the passionfruit pulp.

3. Divide half of the chia mixture among 4 serving glasses or jars. Top with half of the fruit. Repeat with the remaining chia mixture and fruit. Sprinkle with the chopped brazil nuts, if using, and serve.

NUTRITIONAL ANALYSIS	ENERGY (KJ)	869	CARBOHYDRATE (G)	23	SODIUM (MG)	120
TO SERVE 4 (PER SERVE)	PROTEIN (G)	13	SATURATED FAT (G)	1.8	FIBRE (G)	8

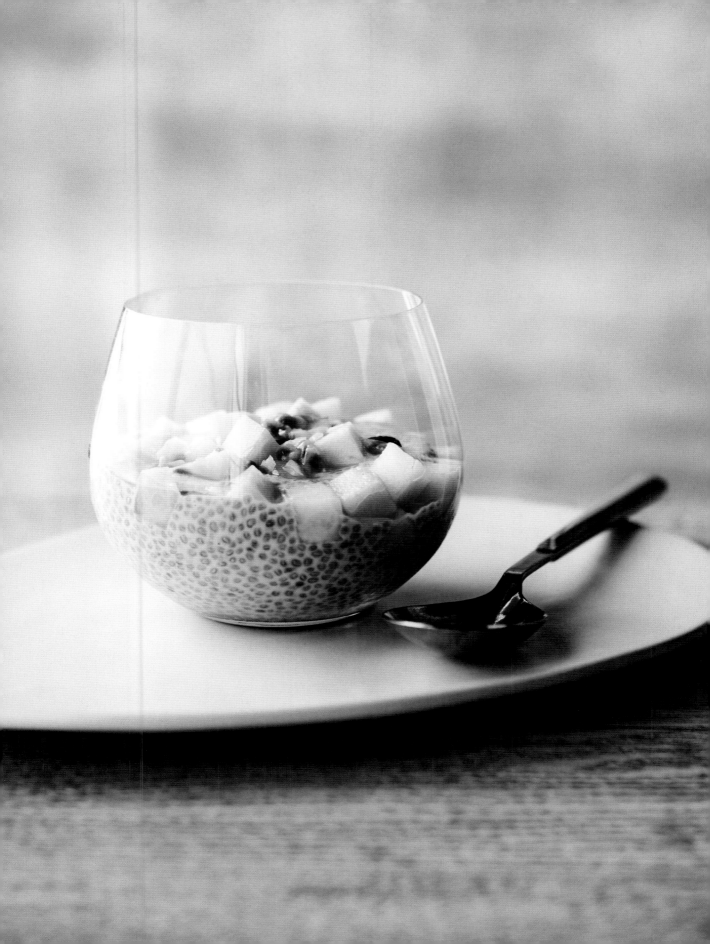

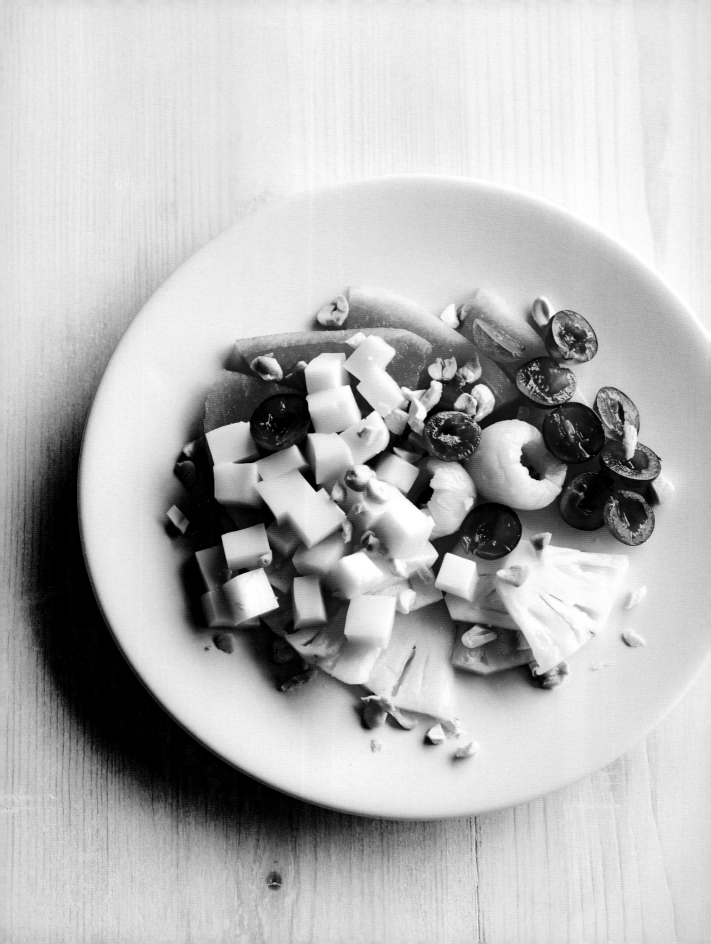

Milk and rosewater jelly with tropical fruit

A quirky and refreshing take on strawberries and cream, this creamy jelly melts in the mouth and goes wonderfully well with any fresh fruit.

SERVES 4

PREP TIME 20 MINUTES, PLUS 1–1½ HOURS CHILLING

COOKING TIME NIL

olive oil spray, for cooking

3 cups (750 ml) skim milk

7 teaspoons powdered gelatine

½ teaspoon (or to taste) rosewater

320 g peeled seedless watermelon, thinly sliced

200 g pineapple, thinly sliced

8 lychees, peeled and seeded

½ cup (90 g) red grapes, halved

2 tablespoons roughly chopped raw unsalted cashews

1. Lightly spray a 28 cm × 18 cm baking tin or shallow container with oil, then line with plastic film, smoothing out any wrinkles and allowing it to overhang the sides.

2. Pour ½ cup (125 ml) of the milk into a small microwave-proof bowl or jug and sprinkle the gelatine slowly and evenly over the surface. Whisk to combine. Set aside to absorb for 5 minutes. Microwave the mixture on high in 15-second bursts until the gelatine has dissolved and the mixture is smooth.

3. Pour the remaining skim milk into a heavy-based saucepan and stir, over medium heat for 1–2 minutes or until lukewarm. Whisk in the gelatine mixture and add the rosewater. Pour through a fine mesh sieve into the prepared tin or container and refrigerate for 1–1½ hours or until set. Use the overhanging plastic film to lift the jelly out of the tin, then cut it into cubes.

4. Divide the fruit among 4 plates, top with the jelly cubes and sprinkle with cashews to serve.

NUTRITIONAL ANALYSIS	ENERGY (KJ)	814	CARBOHYDRATE (G)	26	SODIUM (MG)	112
TO SERVE 4 (PER SERVE)	PROTEIN (G)	14	SATURATED FAT (G)	0.8	FIBRE (G)	3

Maple-baked pears
with whipped ricotta

When served warm, the maple-baked pears and syrupy juices make the whipped ricotta ooze on the plate. Eat immediately to savour the ooze. Alternatively, enjoy at breakfast with pancakes (see page 125) for an indulgent start to the weekend.

SERVES 4
PREP TIME 10 MINUTES
COOKING TIME 35 MINUTES

2 firm ripe pears, halved and cored
1 teaspoon macadamia oil
2 teaspoons pure maple syrup

WHIPPED RICOTTA
200 g firm, fresh low-fat ricotta
2 tablespoons skim milk, approximately
1 tablespoon pure maple syrup
1 teaspoon ground cinnamon

NUT AND SEED SPRINKLE
1 tablespoon flaked almonds
1 tablespoon roughly chopped unsalted macadamias
2 teaspoons sunflower seeds
1 teaspoon sesame seeds

1. Preheat the oven to 200°C (180°C fan-forced). Line a roasting pan or ovenproof dish with baking paper.

2. Place the pears, cut-side up, in the lined pan or dish. Drizzle with the macadamia oil and maple syrup, then cover with foil and bake for 15 minutes. Uncover, baste with the pan juices and bake for a further 15–20 minutes or until tender; the cooking time will depend on the ripeness of the pears. If extra browning is required, briefly place the pears under a hot grill until the desired colour.

3. Meanwhile, for the whipped ricotta, place the ricotta, milk, maple syrup and cinnamon in a food processor or blender and process until smooth. Add a little more milk to adjust the consistency, if required – it should be a smooth, spoonable consistency. Transfer to a small bowl, cover with plastic and refrigerate until ready to serve.

4. For the nut and seed sprinkle, heat a small heavy-based frying pan over medium heat. Add the nuts and seeds and toast, stirring, for 1–2 minutes or until fragrant, lightly coloured and the sesame seeds begin to pop. Transfer to a small bowl to cool.

5. Serve half a warm pear on each plate, topped with the whipped ricotta and any pan juices and finished with the nut and seed sprinkle.

NUTRITIONAL ANALYSIS	ENERGY (KJ)	847	CARBOHYDRATE (G)	21	SODIUM (MG)	132
TO SERVE 4 (PER SERVE)	PROTEIN (G)	8	SATURATED FAT (G)	2.5	FIBRE (G)	6

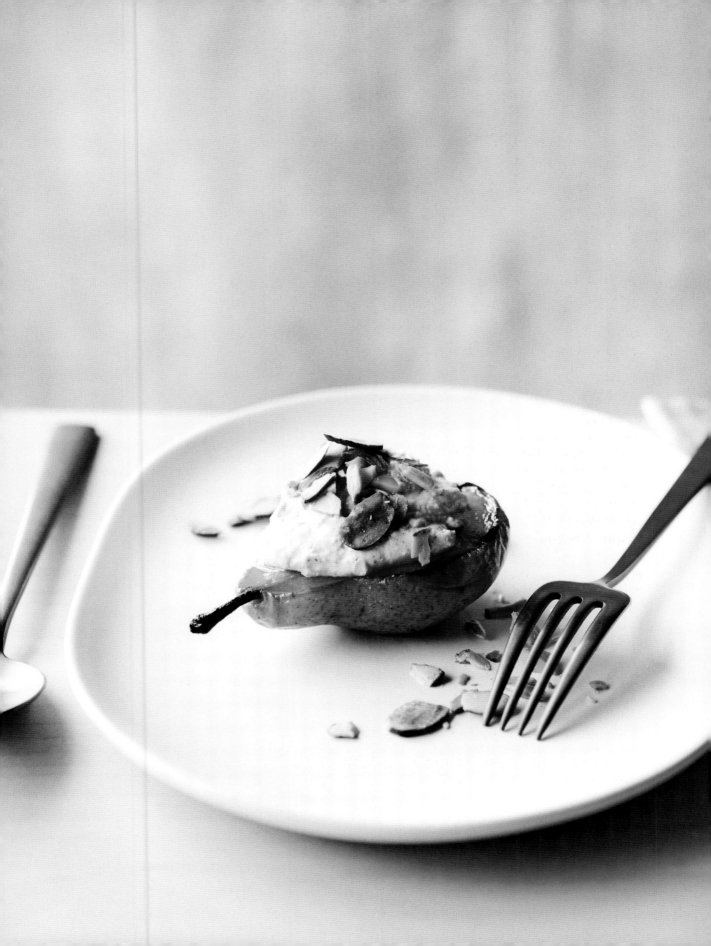

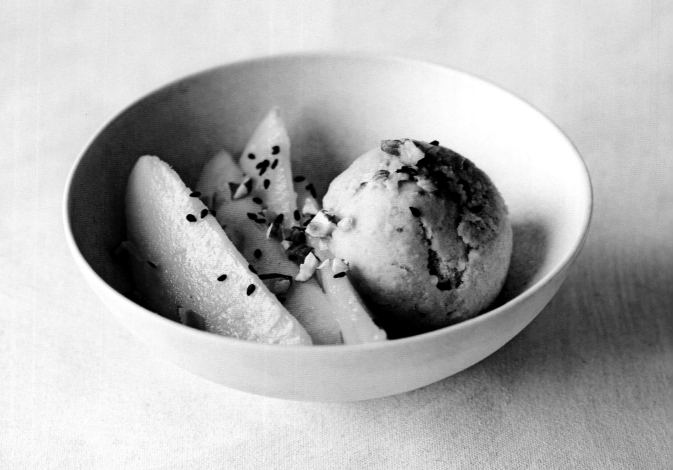

No-churn avocado, lime and cardamom ice cream

This ice cream is wonderfully creamy and not too sweet. If it is very firm from freezing overnight, remove it from the freezer 5–10 minutes – or transfer to the fridge for 15 minutes – before serving to allow it to soften.

MAKES ABOUT 1.25 LITRES/SERVES 12
PREP TIME 20 MINUTES, PLUS 2½–3 HOURS FREEZING
COOKING TIME NIL

5 frozen bananas, chopped
1½ teaspoons finely grated lime zest
1 avocado, peeled and stone removed
⅓ cup (80 ml) chilled light and creamy evaporated milk
2 tablespoons honey
1 teaspoon ground cardamom, plus extra to sprinkle
1 teaspoon roasted black sesame seeds, plus extra to sprinkle
½ mango per person, sliced
2 teaspoons per person roughly chopped unsalted roasted almonds, to serve

1. Place a 1.25 litre loaf tin or ice-cream dish in the freezer to chill.

2. Pulse the banana and lime zest in a food processor until grainy, then add the avocado, evaporated milk, honey and cardamom, and pulse until combined and smooth, scraping down the side of the bowl as necessary. Add a little more evaporated milk if needed to keep the mixture moving in the processor. Do not over-process; you don't want the mixture to melt.

3. Working quickly, transfer the ice cream to the chilled container. Scatter with the sesame seeds and extra cardamom. Cover and freeze for 2½–3 hours or until firm.

4. Serve 1 scoop of ice cream per person with half a sliced mango, sprinkled with the extra sesame seeds and roughly chopped almonds. Leftover ice cream will keep in an airtight container in the freezer for up to 2 weeks.

NUTRITIONAL ANALYSIS	ENERGY (KJ)	782	CARBOHYDRATE (G)	21	SODIUM (MG)	9
TO SERVE 4 (PER SERVE)	PROTEIN (G)	4	SATURATED FAT (G)	1.3	FIBRE (G)	5

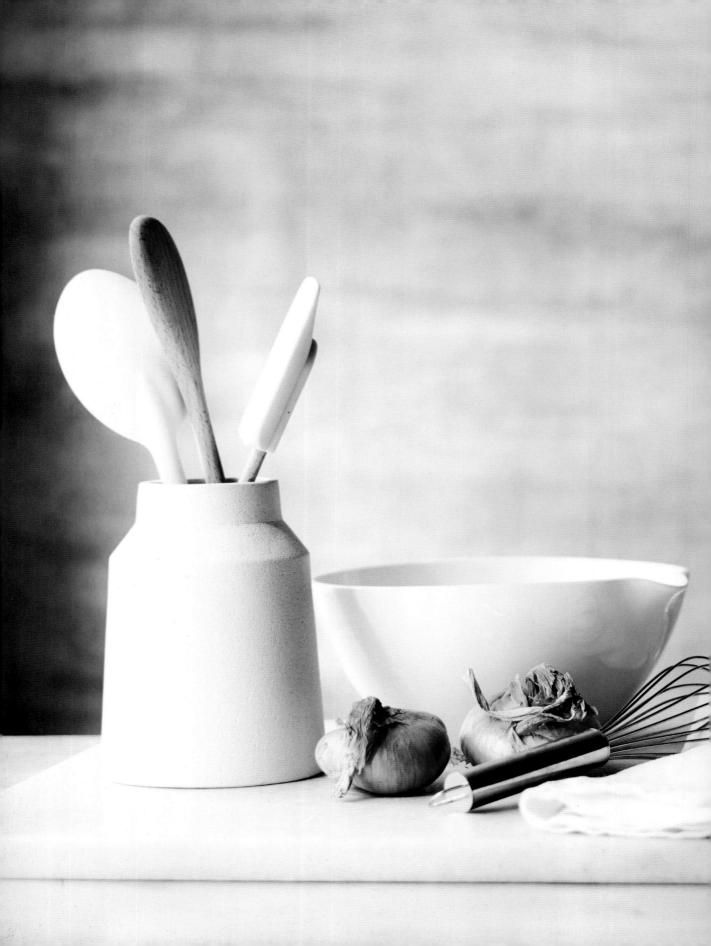

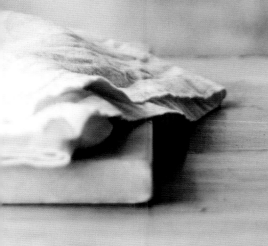

BASICS

Chicken stock

To save on freezer space you can boil the skimmed, strained stock until reduced down by half or even one-third and reconstitute it with water when you thaw it to use. You can also freeze it in ice-cube trays and use as a boost of flavour in sauces.

MAKES ABOUT 6 LITRES
PREP TIME 10 MINUTES
COOKING TIME 2 HOURS

2 kg chicken bones or carcasses
2 large carrots, roughly chopped
4 sticks celery, roughly chopped
2 large onions, roughly chopped
4 sprigs thyme
1 handful flat-leaf parsley sprigs
1 tablespoon black peppercorns
2 bay leaves

1. Wash the bones and drain well. Place them in a large heavy-based saucepan or stockpot with the carrots, celery sticks, onions, thyme, parsley, peppercorns and bay leaves, then add enough water to just cover the bones and vegetables – about 6 litres. (The amount of water needed is approximate – it will depend on the capacity of your saucepan.)

2. Bring the water slowly to a simmer, skimming off the impurities that rise to the surface. Reduce the heat to low–medium and simmer gently for 2 hours, occasionally skimming the surface to remove any fat; do not let the stock boil hard or it will be cloudy. Strain the stock, discarding the solids, then cool to room temperature.

3. Store the stock in an airtight container in the fridge for up to 3 days, or in portion-sized containers in the freezer for up to 2 months.

Vegetable stock

Mushroom and leek trimmings make good additions, if you have them on hand. Don't add strongly flavoured vegetables or herbs such as fennel, rosemary or dill to vegetable stock as the flavour will be overpowering.

MAKES ABOUT 4 LITRES
PREP TIME 10 MINUTES
COOKING TIME 1 HOUR

4 onions, roughly chopped
5 sticks celery, roughly chopped
4 carrots, roughly chopped
4 tomatoes, roughly chopped
6 sprigs thyme
1 large handful flat-leaf parsley sprigs
1 tablespoon black peppercorns
2 bay leaves

1. Place the onions, celery sticks, carrots, tomatoes, thyme, parsley, peppercorns and bay leaves in a large heavy-based saucepan or stockpot, then add enough water to just cover the vegetables – about 4 litres. (The amount of water needed is approximate – it will depend on the capacity of your saucepan.)

2. Slowly bring to a simmer, skimming off the impurities that rise to the surface, then reduce the heat to low and simmer gently for 1 hour; do not let the stock boil hard or it will be cloudy. Strain the stock, discarding the solids, then cool to room temperature.

3. Store the stock in an airtight container in the fridge for up to 3 days, or in portion-sized containers in the freezer for up to 2 months.

Beef stock

MAKES ABOUT 4 LITRES
PREP TIME 10 MINUTES
COOKING TIME 7–9 HOURS

2 kg beef bones, cut into large pieces
  (ask your butcher to do this)
2 onions, roughly chopped
2 carrots, roughly chopped
2 celery sticks, roughly chopped
2 tablespoons olive oil
1 tablespoon low-salt tomato paste (puree)
100 g button mushrooms or mushroom trimmings
3 sprigs thyme
2 teaspoons black peppercorns
1 bay leaf

1. Preheat the oven to 180°C (160°C fan-forced).

2. Place the bones, onions, carrots and celery sticks
   in a large roasting pan, drizzle with the oil, then
   roast for 1 hour or until well browned. Transfer to
   a large heavy-based saucepan or stockpot, then add
   the tomato paste, mushroom trimmings, thyme,
   peppercorns, bay leaf and enough water to just
   cover the bones and vegetables – about 5 litres.
   (The amount of water needed is approximate –
   it will depend on the capacity of your saucepan.)

3. Slowly bring to a simmer, skimming off any
   impurities that rise to the surface. Reduce the
   heat to low and simmer gently for 6–8 hours,
   occasionally skimming the surface to remove fat.
   Add water as needed if the level drops too much
   during cooking.

4. Strain the stock, discarding the solids. Cool to
   room temperature. Remove any fat that has
   solidified on the top.

5. Store the stock in an airtight container in the
   fridge for up to 3 days, or in portion-sized
   containers in the freezer for up to 2 months.

Classic salad dressing

MAKES ABOUT ¾ CUP (180 ML)
PREP TIME 10 MINUTES
COOKING TIME NIL

1 clove garlic, crushed
2 teaspoons Dijon mustard
¼ cup (60 ml) balsamic or red wine vinegar, or lemon juice
½ cup (125 ml) extra virgin olive oil

1. Place the garlic, mustard and vinegar or lemon
   juice in a bowl. Whisking constantly, slowly add
   the oil until well combined. Season to taste with
   freshly ground black pepper. Store in an airtight
   container in the fridge for up to 2 weeks.

**Use rice bran, macadamia or avocado oil instead of
olive oil, if you prefer. The dressing can be flavoured
in a variety of ways: Try adding a teaspoon or two of
honey and a little finely chopped rosemary for a salad to
accompany lamb. For an Asian-style dressing, use lime
juice, rice bran oil, finely chopped lemongrass and some
sesame oil. Or, for a Mediterranean twist, add some dried
currants, finely grated orange zest and chopped basil.
Toasted cumin seeds and chopped coriander also work
well with lemon juice and olive oil for a Middle Eastern-
inspired dressing.**

Wholemeal yoghurt seeded flatbread

These flatbreads are chewy and quite moreish. Have two pans cooking at once, or cook on a barbecue hot plate to speed the cooking process up. Once cooked, they can be frozen in a sealed container for up to 3 weeks. Thaw and reheat before serving.

MAKES 10

PREP TIME 5 MINUTES

COOKING TIME ABOUT 40 MINUTES (LESS IF USING 2 PANS OR BARBECUE FLATPLATE)

1 ²⁄₃ cups (250 g) wholemeal plain flour, plus extra for dusting
1 tablespoon linseeds
2 teaspoons chia seeds
2 teaspoons baking powder
pinch of salt (optional)
1 cup (280 g) reduced-fat natural Greek-style yoghurt

1. Place all the ingredients in a food processor and pulse until a dough forms. Transfer the dough to a lightly floured work surface.

2. Roll the dough into a long log shape and cut into 10 even pieces. Roll each piece into a ball and place on a baking tray, then cover with a clean tea towel. Roll out one dough ball at a time as thinly as you can, to form a 20 cm-diameter round, dusting with extra flour as needed to prevent sticking.

3. Heat a large heavy-based non-stick frying pan over low–medium heat and cook the flatbread for 2 minutes on each side, until charred in spots and slightly puffy; take care to not overcook. Transfer to a plate and cover with a clean dry tea towel while you repeat with the remaining dough balls.

4. Serve immediately. These are best served warm, so reheat in a warm pan or under a hot oven grill for a few seconds, if necessary.

Basic slaw

This slaw makes the perfect accompaniment to a whole host of meals. Use a food processor to shred and grate the vegetables for super-quick preparation.

SERVES 4
PREP TIME 20 MINUTES
COOKING TIME NIL

3 cups (240 g) finely shredded red cabbage
3 cups (240 g) finely shredded white cabbage
2 stalks celery, thinly sliced
2 carrots, peeled coarsely grated
½ cup (125 ml) buttermilk
2 tablespoons finely chopped chives
3 teaspoons Dijon mustard
2 tablespoons sunflower seeds
1 tablespoon pepitas (roasted pumpkin seed kernels)
1 tablespoon chopped walnuts

1. Combine the cabbage, celery and carrots in a large bowl. Whisk the buttermilk, chives and mustard together in a small bowl (or shake in a sealed screw-top jar). Add the dressing to the cabbage mixture and season with freshly ground black pepper. Toss until well combined.

2. Transfer the slaw to a serving platter or divide among 4 plates. Sprinkle with the seeds and walnuts, then serve.

Steamed green beans and broccolini with dukkah sprinkle

Sprinkling some spice mix over the vegetables brings another layer of flavour to this side dish. The simplicity of the lemon-juice 'sauce' enhances the flavours of the green veggies and dukkah. If preferred, you can leave off the lemon zest and just add the dukkah sprinkle.

SERVES 4
PREP TIME 5 MINUTES
COOKING TIME 5 MINUTES

400 g green beans, trimmed
350 g broccolini, stalks trimmed
1 lemon
⅓ cup (25 g) homemade dukkah or nut-free dukkah (see page 293)

1. Steam the beans and broccolini in a steamer basket over a saucepan of boiling water for 3–4 minutes or until tender.

2. Shred the zest from the lemon in long, thin strips, and cut the lemon into quarters.

3. Transfer the beans and broccolini to a serving platter or divide among 4 plates. Scatter evenly with the lemon zest, then sprinkle with the dukkah and serve with lemon wedges alongside.

Flour tortillas

These tortillas are easy to make and are best enjoyed while still warm.
You can make these in advance and freeze them in a sealed container for up to 3 weeks.

MAKES 12
PREP TIME 10 MINUTES, PLUS 25 MINUTES RESTING
COOKING TIME 20 MINUTES

1¾ cups (260 g) plain flour, plus 1 tablespoon extra for
   kneading
¼ cup (35 g) fine rice bran
1 teaspoon baking powder
½ teaspoon salt
1 tablespoon sunflower oil
⅔ cup (160 ml) lukewarm water, approximately

1. Sift the flour, rice bran, baking powder and salt
   into a large bowl. Make a well in the centre and
   add the oil and water. Mix until combined to form
   a soft dough; add a little more water if necessary.
   Cover with a clean tea towel and leave to rest for
   10 minutes.

2. Turn the dough out of the bowl onto a lightly
   floured work surface, then knead for 1–2 minutes
   or until quite smooth. Divide the dough into
   12 equal portions. Form each portion into a ball
   and flatten it with the palm of your hand. Place in
   a single layer on a baking tray lined with baking
   paper. Cover with plastic film and leave to rest
   for a further 15 minutes.

3. Heat a large heavy-based non-stick frying pan over
   medium–high heat. Roll out 1 dough portion on a
   lightly floured surface with a lightly floured rolling
   pin very thinly, to form a round (about 17 cm
   diameter). Repeat with the remaining dough.
   (Do not stack the uncooked dough on top of
   each other or the rounds will stick together.)

4. When the frying pan is very hot, place 1 dough
   round in the pan and cook for 1 minute or until
   the bottom is lightly browned in places and
   starting to bubble; reduce the heat if necessary.
   Flip to the other side and cook for 30 seconds or
   until the tortilla is soft and slightly puffy, with
   small golden-brown spots on the surface. Transfer
   to a plate, cover with a clean tea towel to stop from
   drying out and to keep warm, then repeat with the
   remaining dough rounds.

5. Serve immediately, or reheat briefly in a frying pan
   just before serving. Suitable for freezing.

Dukkah

This nutty, aromatic sprinkle is delicious as a dip just with bread and olive oil. But it also works well as a crumb for meats or a crumble for desserts. Make it once and you'll wonder how you ever cooked without it.

MAKES ABOUT ½ CUP (60 G)
PREP TIME 10 MINUTES
COOKING TIME 15 MINUTES

¼ cup (35 g) whole hazelnuts
2 tablespoons sesame seeds
2 teaspoons cumin seeds
2 teaspoons coriander seeds
pinch of sea salt (optional)

1. Preheat the oven to 180°C (160°C fan-forced) and line a baking tray with baking paper.

2. Place the hazelnuts in a single layer on the lined baking tray and roast in the oven for 10–15 minutes or until the skins have started to crack. Wrap them in a clean, dry tea towel and set aside.

3. Heat a small heavy-based frying pan over medium heat. Add the sesame seeds to the pan and toast, stirring often for 1–2 minutes or until the seeds are light golden. Transfer to a mortar and set aside.

4. Repeat the process with the cumin and coriander seeds, adding them to the mortar.

5. Rub the hazelnuts in the tea towel to remove the skins. Add the hazelnuts and salt, if using, to the mortar. Using the pestle, pound to a coarse, crumb-like consistency. (Alternatively, use a food processor to pulse the mixture.)

Nut-free dukkah

MAKES ABOUT ½ CUP (60 G)
PREP TIME 10 MINUTES
COOKING TIME 10 MINUTES

2 tablespoons sesame seeds
1½ tablespoons pepitas (roasted pumpkin seed kernels)
2 teaspoons cumin seeds
2 teaspoons coriander seeds
1½ tablespoons sunflower seeds
pinch of sea salt (optional)

1. Heat a small heavy-based frying pan over medium heat. Add the sesame seeds to the pan and toast, stirring often, for 1–2 minutes until the seeds are lightly golden. Transfer to a mortar.

2. Repeat the process, in batches, with the pepitas, cumin, coriander and sunflower seeds, adding them to the mortar. Add the salt, if using, and pound to a course, crumb-like texture. (Alternatively, the mixture can be pulsed in a food processor to the desired consistency.)

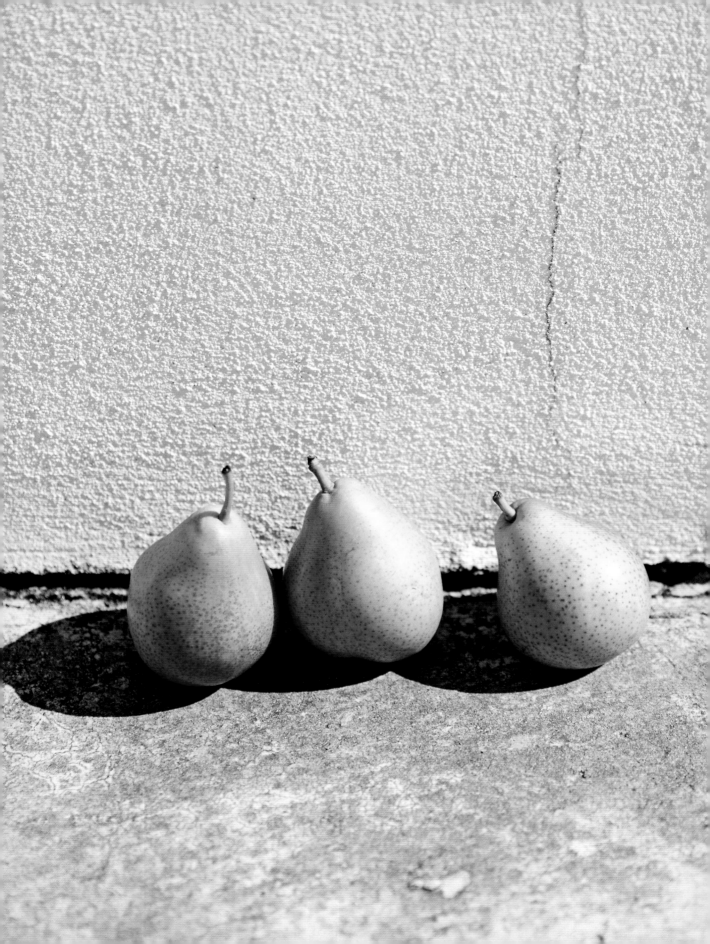

HEALTH TEST CHECKLIST

Various health tests become more important at different stages of our life. This checklist is a handy reference guide to the recommended health checks for every decade throughout your life.

People with a family history of a particular disease or certain risk factors may need to start some of these screenings at earlier times.

Whatever your situation, it is a good idea to discuss your own risk factors with your GP. Together, you can develop a personalised preventative health program that can be used in addition to the recommendations made below.

Tests and checks that become relevant upon the onset of adulthood (such as BMI, cholesterol, blood pressure, blood fats and sexually transmitted infections) should continue regularly throughout your adult life.

BIRTH TO 10 YEARS

- ☐ **Vaccinations** – The National Immunisation Program provides for vaccinations at birth, 2, 4, 6 and 12 months, then again at 18 months and 4 years. These vaccinations include hepatitis B, diphtheria, tetanus, acellular pertussis (whooping cough), haemophilus influenzae type b, inactivated poliomyelitis (polio), pneumococcal conjugate (13vPCV), rotavirus, meningococcal C, measles, mumps and rubella, and varicella (chickenpox).
- ☐ **Universal Child Health Check** – This is a government-funded GP assessment that happens at the age of 3. It is a check of the child's physical health, general wellbeing and development, allergies and toileting. This check aims to start medical interventions early if any issues are identified.

- ☐ **Weight, height, BMI and growth rate** – These factors should be measured regularly. In babies this is done under the guidance of the health centre nurse who will maintain a growth chart to track the development of your child. Typically this is done monthly for the first 6 months, every two months from 6 to 12 months and thereafter yearly.
- ☐ **Dental health** – Once a month, parents should lift their child's top lip to look for signs of tooth decay. Look for white lines on top of the teeth below the gums, or discolouration that can't be brushed away. Dentists recommend a first appointment within 6 months of the eruption of the first tooth, or by one year of age.

THE TEENAGE YEARS

- ☐ **Vaccinations** – School immunisation programs run for youth aged between 10–15 years. This includes the human papillomavirus (HPV), as well as booster shots for varicella (chickenpox), diphtheria, tetanus and acellular pertussis (whooping cough). In most local jurisdictions this is recommended in year 7 or 8 when the child is aged 12-13. Children not attending school should seek advice from a GP at this age.
- ☐ **Dental health** – A check-up and professional clean by a dentist should occur annually after the age of 12.
- ☐ **Sexual health** – Sexually active young people should be screened annually for chlamydia through a urine test. Young people who have unsafe sex with multiple new partners should also be tested for other sexually transmissible diseases.

- **Cervical screening** – The first human papillomavirus (HPV) test should start at age 18 years or two years after first becoming sexually active, whatever is later. This test replaces the two-yearly Pap test. The HPV test is done every five years.

IN YOUR 20s

- **Sexual health** – Sexually active young people should be screened annually for chlamydia through a urine test each year. Young people who have unsafe sex with multiple new partners should also be tested for other sexually transmissible diseases.
- **Blood pressure** – Blood pressure should be checked every two years throughout adulthood.
- **BMI and waist circumference measurement** – This check should occur every two years in overweight adults, and annually for those at increased risk (including Aboriginal or Torres Strait Islanders and people with diabetes, stroke, gout, liver, cardiovascular or gallbladder disease). To fall into the overweight category, waist circumference is above 94 cm for men and above 80 cm for women. Overweight is officially defined by a BMI above 25 kg/m². In Asian people the normal range is a little lower and 23 kg/m² is the cut off, whereas for Pacific Islanders the cut off is a little higher at 26 kg/m².
- **Breast self-check** – Women should perform a check on their breasts every month. Place a pillow under your right shoulder and your right arm behind your head. Using your left hand, move the pads of your fingers around your right breast gently in small circular motions covering the entire breast area and armpit. Use light, medium, and firm pressure. Squeeze the nipple; check for discharge and lumps. Repeat for the opposite side.
- **Testes self-check** – Men should perform a check on their testes every month – look and feel for unusual thickenings or lumps in the testicles.

IN YOUR 30s

- **Sexual health** – Sexually active adults should be screened annually for chlamydia through a urine test. People who have unsafe sex with multiple new partners should also be tested for other sexually transmissible diseases.
- **Cholesterol and glucose levels** – These tests can be ordered at the request of your doctor. It is recommended that all adults have these measurements by the age of 45 as part of an absolute risk assessment and by the age of 35 for Aboriginal and Torres Strait Islanders. However, we suggest testing for people in early adulthood if there is a family history of diabetes, or heart disease in close relatives aged under 60, or there are lifestyle associated clues such as being overweight.
- **BMI and waist circumference measurement** – This check should occur every two years in overweight adults, and annually for those at increased risk (including Aboriginal or Torres Strait Islanders and people with diabetes, stroke, gout, liver, cardiovascular or gallbladder disease). See 'In Your 20s' for a definition of 'overweight'. Overweight children are more likely to become overweight adults. There is considerable advantage in acting at an early stage, as efforts to prevent weight gain are generally more successful than attempts to lose weight later in life when habits and lifestyle are well established.
- **Vaccination** – The adult dTpa (diphtheria-tetanus-acellular pertussis) vaccine is recommended for pregnant women in their third trimester to protect them and their newborn against whooping cough. This is also advised for expectant fathers. It is also recommended that pregnant women have the influenza vaccination.

IN YOUR 40s

- **BMI and waist circumference measurement** – Check annually.
- **Eye health** – Check for glaucoma every two years from the age of 40, or from the age of 35 if you are at higher risk because of family history or other medical conditions.

- ☐ **Chronic disease** – A free, one-off health check is offered to people aged 45–49 years who are at risk of developing a chronic disease such as type 2 diabetes or heart disease. To be eligible, your doctor must identify at least one risk factor (such as lifestyle habits) or a family history.
- ☐ **Type 2 diabetes** – This check should occur every three years after the age of 40, or from age 18 for Indigenous Australians.
- ☐ **Fasting lipids/Hyperlipidaemia screening** – Checking cholesterol and blood fats in those without other cardiovascular risk factors is recommended every five years from the age of 45. If you're at high risk of cardiovascular disease, you should be tested every one to two years.
- ☐ **Stroke risk** – Everyone over the age of 45 should be screened for risk factors such as hypertension, dyslipidaemia and non-valvular atrial fibrillation.
- ☐ **Calculate absolute cardiovascular risk** – This check should be performed whenever your blood pressure, cholesterol and blood fats are measured.
- ☐ **Bone health** – Women should have their GP review fracture risk factors once they turn 45.

IN YOUR 50s

- ☐ **Bowel cancer** – A home faecal occult blood test (FOBT) should be done every two years from the age of 50 until 75.
- ☐ **Breast cancer** – Women should have a mammogram every two years from the age of 50.
- ☐ **Prostate cancer** – Men should have a PSA test if they have a family history of prostate cancer.
- ☐ **Hearing test** – A hearing test only needs to happen if you are having symptoms such as reduced hearing.
- ☐ **Vaccinations** – Consider having an annual influenza and/or pneumococcal vaccination if you are at high risk. Consider having the whooping cough vaccination if you are a new or expectant grandparent who will have close contact with the newborn until the age of two months.
- ☐ **Bone health** – Review fracture risk factors for

both women and men. These include frailty, osteoporosis, difficulty with balance.
- ☐ **Eye health** – Have an eye examination every two years between the ages 50 and 65 years.

IN YOUR 60s

- ☐ **Bone health** – Have the bone density scan (known as a bone mineral densitometry [DEXA]) if you are over the age of 65 years or if you have risk factors.
- ☐ **Eye health** – Have an annual eye check from the age of 65.
- ☐ **Vaccinations** – An annual influenza injection, pneumococcal polysaccharide vaccination and single dose of Herpes-zoster is recommended for people in their 60s and older. The whooping cough vaccination is also advised for new or expectant grandparents who will have close contact with the newborn until the age of two months.
- ☐ **Falls** – Have yourself screened for risk factors for falls every 12 months by your GP.
- ☐ **Dementia screening** – Dementia screening is only recommended at this age if you have symptoms or risk factors.

IN YOUR 70s

- ☐ **Vaccination** – Consider having an annual influenza vaccination.
- ☐ **Cervical screening** – A woman who has had two normal Pap tests within the last 5 years may stop having this test at the age of 70 years.

RESOURCES

NATIONAL HEART ORGANISATIONS

Baker IDI Heart and Diabetes Institute
bakeridi.edu.au
(03) 8532 1111

We are a medical research institute with a mission to reduce death and disability from cardiovascular disease, diabetes and related conditions through research, education and health care delivery. Health information on topics such as blood pressure, cholesterol, diabetes, with a link to the Australian Type 2 Diabetes Risk Assessment tool, and details about our clinical services can be accessed via our website. Information about current clinical trials are also available on our website.

Heart Foundation
heartfoundation.org.au
1300 362 787

The website gives advice on heart conditions and risk factors, heart procedures and medical tests, warning signs for heart attacks and guidance on living with heart disease. There is information on the importance of getting active, deciphering food labels and healthy recipes. You can also find links to local activities in your area, such as the Heartmoves program and walking groups. The 1300 number provides free personalised information and support on heart health, nutrition and a healthy lifestyle from their experts.

OTHER NATIONAL ORGANISATIONS

National Stroke Foundation
strokefoundation.com.au
1800 787 653

The website provides risk factors for stroke, emergency information and rehabilitation. You can find your nearest pharmacy offering free blood pressure checks by clicking on 'Health Check Finder' under the 'About Stroke' tab. The StrokeLine 1800 number also provides information on stroke prevention, treatment and recovery.

Diabetes Australia (Vic)
diabetesvic.org.au
1300 136 588

The website provides advice on living with diabetes, complications, nutrition and prevention, including a link to the Australian Type 2 Diabetes Risk Assessment tool to measure your risk. You can also find details on the free lifestyle modification program, called The Life! Program, as well how to get involved in clinical research trials.

Cancer Council
cancer.org.au
13 11 20

The Cancer Council offers information on treatments, ways to reduce your risk and early detection for most cancers. There is a link to help you find a specialist, a glossary on the different medical specialists a cancer patient will meet, and information on how to find emotional support. The website's homepage also has a UV measure, which tells you the time of day you need sun protection in your specific city. Other features include oncologists who regularly post blogs, a range of patient stories and the sister website – cancer-connections.com.au – is a peer-based support and information service for people living with or affected by cancer. The support line (number listed above) provides information, emotional and practical help from trained staff.

Nutrition Australia
nutritionaustralia.org

Nutrition Australia is an independent, member organisation that aims to promote the health and wellbeing of all Australians. The website has a range of resources and fact sheets on nutrition.

GENERAL HEALTH

Better Health Channel
betterhealth.vic.gov.au
The Better Health Channel is a modern day encyclopedia of health, providing information on a huge variety of illnesses, injuries, conditions, tests and treatments. It can be searched by body part or alphabetically. It also features videos by experts on commonly searched topics, recipes, tips on getting active, links to events and online health calculators.

Federal Department of Health and Ageing
healthyactive.gov.au
eatforhealth.gov.au
1800 020 103 (Department of Health)
The Healthy Active website provides tools and strategies for healthy eating and exercise, as well as links to national health campaigns and projects such as the 'Stephanie Alexander Kitchen Garden' program and 'Get Set 4 Life – Habits for Healthy Kids'. It also contains physical activity and nutrition guidelines for different age groups.
The Eat for Health site provides the Australian dietary guidelines, tips for making healthy food choices, games and calculators to help you estimate your kilojoule and nutrient needs.

Your Brain Matters
yourbrainmatters.org.au
1800 100 500 (National Dementia Helpline)
This is the website of Alzheimer's Australia, and it offers evidence-based strategies for lifestyle changes to help you stay brain healthy at any age, with the aim of reducing your chance of developing dementia. It features the latest medical research news, videos and risk reduction information in 29 languages.

Jean Hailes for Women's Health
jeanhailes.org.au
1800 532 642
The Jean Hailes website is a comprehensive offering of advice, information, research and support covering hundreds of topics concerning women's health and wellbeing. It features fact sheets, links to clinical research trials, online education, podcasts, recipes and tools to plan for better health, such as the Weekly Activity Diary to plan your week in a more healthy and balanced way. The regular updates in the 'News' tab analyses international research findings to explain what they mean for real women.

LiveLighter
livelighter.com.au
LiveLighter is a program developed in Western Australia which aims to encourage Australian adults to lead healthier lifestyles. It encourages people to make changes to what they eat and drink, and to be more active.
LiveLighter aims to help people understand why they need to take action and what simple changes they can make in order to 'LiveLighter'.

MENTAL HEALTH, ADDICTIONS AND DRUGS

Beyond Blue
beyondblue.org.au
1300 224 636
The website gives information about treatments, recovery, staying well and where to find support for people experiencing anxiety, depression, suicide, grief or self-harm. Friends, family and work colleagues of someone with a mental illness can also get advice on how to offer support, as well as looking after their own wellbeing.
People in some states have access to a free coaching program called NewAccess. There are links to national helplines and mental health professionals, and the 24/7 hotline (number listed above) connects you with a trained mental health professional. It also has an online forum, found under the 'Connect with Others' tab, to seek advice or support from others around the country.

Black Dog Institute
blackdoginstitute.org.au
Expert information on depression and bipolar disorder for the public and professionals,

including information on getting help for mood disorders and suggestions on ways of staying well.

e-couch
Ecouch.anu.edu.au
A self-help interactive program with modules for depression, generalised anxiety and worry, social anxiety, relationship breakdown, and loss and grief. It provides self-help interventions drawn from cognitive, behavioural and interpersonal therapies as well as relaxation and physical activity.

headspace
Headspace.org.au
Information, support and advice for young people 12–25, and their families, on general health; mental health and wellbeing; alcohol and other drugs; education, employment and other services. Headspace has centres around Australia that provide access to youth-friendly health professionals.

mentalhealthonline
mentalhealthonline.org.au
Information about anxiety disorders, a free automated psychological assessment and self-help treatment programs, plus access to low-cost, therapist-assisted programs that run for over 12 weeks.

MoodGYM
moodgym.anu.edu.au
A popular interactive program, which incorporates cognitive behaviour therapy for depression. MoodGYM has been extensively researched and its effectiveness has been demonstrated in randomised controlled trials.

Partners in Depression
partnersindepression.com.au
An innovative information and support group program for people who love, live with or support someone experiencing depression.

Parenting Strategies
parentingstrategies.net
Developed by researchers from Victorian universities, this website gives parents information to help manage issues including alcohol and drug misuse, depression, anxiety and other mental health problems in both primary school-aged children and teenagers. The site also has a survey parents can complete to get personalised feedback about their parenting practices in relation to alcohol, with the experts linking them to specific topics of an online parenting program.

Drinkwise Australia
drinkwise.org.au
9682 8641
Despite being developed by the alcohol industry, this website gives information about safe drinking levels, the effects of alcohol and links to support services. There is a calculator to measure standard drinks, as well as advice aimed at parents and teenagers.

Quit
quit.org.au
13 78 48
Support for people preparing to give up smoking, those wanting to stay cigarette-free and advice on managing relapses. By calling the Quit Line (on the number listed above) you can request a quit support pack, get free support from a trained coach, and access a link to the Quit Txt program that sends you an instant text message reply with strategies when you are close to relapse.

GLOSSARY

ACE inhibitors – a class of blood-pressure-lowering medications, also used to treat heart failure.

aerobic exercise – physical exercise of any intensity which increases oxygen consumption during exercise and improves cardiovascular fitness.

aneurysm – a swelling in an artery roughened by plaques, usually in the upper abdomen.

angina – a pressing or squeezing pain in the front of the chest, back, neck or arms, caused by a partial blockage of the blood vessels supplying the heart.

arteries – blood vessels with muscular walls that take blood away from the heart to the rest of the body.

atherosclerosis – hardening of the arteries due to a build-up of plaques.

atrial fibrillation – a particular form of irregular heart rhythm, which may require anti-clotting medications to reduce the chance of stroke.

absolute risk – the number of heart attacks/strokes per 100 people per 5 or 10 years. High-risk people may have a 20% chance of having a heart attack or stroke over 10 years. Risk factors, such as cholesterol, blood pressure, diabetes, smoking and HDL cholesterol are taken into account in the equation.

Alzheimer's disease – a form of dementia characterised by tangles of a protein called amyloid in the brain tissue.

blood pressure – the force of blood pressing against the walls of the arteries as they deliver blood from the heart to all parts of the body, expressed as the systolic pressure over the diastolic pressure and measured in mmHg.

blood glucose – the level of sugar in the blood stream. Fasting levels are measured as a test for detecting diabetes.

blood cholesterol – the total amount of cholesterol in the blood, including those carried in LDL, HDL and other particles.

Body mass index (BMI) – a measure of normal or excess body weight. It is calculated as weight in kilograms/ height (in meters) squared.

calcium blockers – drugs used to reduce high blood pressure by reducing the resistance of the blood vessels and reducing the force of the heart's contraction.

carotid arteries – arteries that supply the head and brain with blood.

congenital – something you're born with.

coronary heart disease – narrowing or blockage of the arteries that supply the heart with blood and oxygen.

cholesterol – an essential part of the functioning and structure of all our cells, which is naturally tightly regulated by the body. There are two sources of cholesterol in the blood – that which is found in foods and that which is made in the body. There are several types of proteins that carry cholesterol in the body – LDL (low-density lipoproteins, known as 'bad') and HDL (high-density lipoproteins, known as 'good') cholesterol.

coronary arteries – the main arteries supplying blood to the heart. Narrowings in these arteries are bypassed or stented (a metal cage that keeps the artery open) as a treatment for coronary disease.

cortisol – a hormone we can't live without. It keeps our blood pressure up and protects us against stress. It is made from cholesterol.

cardio-metabolic diseases – the combination of lifestyle-related health problems that often occur together, including heart and vascular disease, diabetes, obesity, high blood pressure.

cardiovascular disease – heart, stroke and vascular disease.

chronic kidney disease – any problem affecting the kidney that diminishes their function over the long term.

diastolic blood pressure – the second number in a blood-pressure reading, which represents the pressure against the walls of the arteries when the heart is relaxing and filling with blood.

diuretic – a medication that increases the amount of urine passed and lowers blood pressure.

dementia – the general term to describe diminished cognitive function of the brain.

endorphins – natural hormones produced in the body. Some endorphins affect mood and brain function.

epigenetics – a chemical change affecting DNA that may turn the function of a particular gene on or off. Epigenetics provides a way in which environment and genes interact.

fatty acids – chains of carbon and hydrogen that are a major source of energy. Three fatty acids make up triglyceride, the fat on meat and under our skin.

gestational diabetes – diabetes occurring during pregnancy.

HDL cholesterol – high-density lipoproteins or 'good' cholesterol, high levels of which reduce the risk of heart disease.

heart attack – a colloquial term for blockage of an artery leading to the heart that destroys part of the heart muscle.

hypertension – high blood pressure.

hyperglycaemia – a condition where blood glucose levels are too high.

heart failure – a term used to describe inability of the heart to pump sufficient blood to supply the needs of the body. It can be the result of any condition that damages the heart and reduces its capacity to pump blood.

insulin – a hormone that controls glucose levels in the blood.

LDL cholesterol – low-density lipoproteins or 'bad' cholesterol, high levels of which increase the risk of heart disease.

lipoproteins – small globules that contain proteins, cholesterol and other fats.

mmHg – the unit for blood-pressure measurements; all blood-pressure readings your doctor gives you will be in mmHg, so you can always compare the numbers directly without worrying about the units.

musculoskeletal conditions – muscle, joint and bone conditions.

metabolic – the chemical processes in our body.

metabolic syndrome – a common combination of factors that affect risk of cardiovascular disease including some or all of obesity (especially in the abdomen), diabetes, high blood pressure and resistance of the tissues to the actions of insulin.

plaque – a fatty and cellular deposit that builds up on the inner wall of the arteries, eventually leading to atherosclerosis.

pancreas – the gland behind the stomach that produces insulin.

peripheral arterial disease – a disease of the arteries that supply blood to the limbs that causes pain in the buttocks or legs. It can lead to gangrene and amputation.

resistance exercise – exercise using weights or other resistance often used to improve skeletal muscle size and function, which also improves lipids, blood pressure and insulin sensitivity.

systolic blood pressure – the first number in a blood-pressure reading, which represents the pressure when the heart is contracting and pushing blood away from the heart to the rest of the body.

statins – medications used to reduce blood LDL-cholesterol levels.

triglycerides – fats circulating in the blood and used for energy. Leftovers are stored as body fat. High levels of triglycerides are a risk factor for heart disease.

trans fat – a dietary fat that occurs naturally in small amounts in some foods, such as dairy products and red meat, but is also produced when vegetable oils are hardened, or hydrogenated.

type 1 diabetes – diabetes due to failure of the pancreas to produce insulin and requiring insulin replacement therapy.

type 2 diabetes – diabetes associated with normal or high production of insulin by the pancreas but which is insufficient to maintain normal glucose levels. Often associated with obesity.

wellbeing – an overall picture of a person's happiness. To achieve an overall wellbeing, we collectively need to invest in all aspects of life; the physical, the psychological and the emotional.

ABOUT THE AUTHORS

PROFESSOR GARRY JENNINGS AO

Professor Garry Jennings AO is Senior Director at Baker IDI and Chief Medical Advisor at the National Heart Foundation.

Garry is the past Director and Chief Executive Officer of Baker IDI. He is also past President of the Association of Australian Medical Research Institutes, the High Blood Pressure Research Council of Australia, the Asia Pacific Society of Hypertension and Head of a WHO Collaborating Centre for Research and Training in Cardiovascular Health.

A cardiologist, Garry has a distinguished career in clinical practice and was previously Director of Cardiology at The Alfred Hospital, Melbourne and Chair of the Division of Medicine.

His research interests cover the causes, prevention and treatment of cardiovascular disease and he has received national and international awards. In 2014 he received the Bjorn Folkow award from the European and International Societies of Hypertension for 'outstanding research on the pathogenesis of hypertension'.

DR MARLIES E ALVARENGA

Dr Marlies E Alvarenga is an Adjunct Senior Lecturer in the School of Public Health, Monash University and a Consultant Clinical Psychologist at Monash Cardiovascular Research Centre and MonashHEART, Monash Health & Department of Medicine (SCS at Monash) as well as The Australian Centre for Heart Health in Melbourne.

She is past director of the Monash Psychology Centre. She is the founder of the first Psychocardiology Clinic in South East Asia and Oceania within the Department of Cardiology at Monash Medical Centre. Her main area of research interest is in cardiac neurosciences, where she studies the link between stress, mental illness and increased risk of heart disease. Dr Alvarenga's other area of interest is in applied treatments for improving mental health in cardiac patients. In addition, she also lectures and supervises in cardiac psychology at various universities. Dr Alvarenga is also an active practising clinician.

PROFESSOR MURRAY ESLER AM

Professor Murray Esler AM FAA FRACP is a cardiologist and medical scientist based at Baker IDI, where he is the NHMRC Senior Principal Research Fellow. He is also a Consultant Cardiologist at the Alfred Hospital and an Adjunct Professor of Medicine at Monash University. He is a Fellow of the Australian Academy of Science.

Murray's research interests include the human sympathetic nervous system; stress, and its effects on the heart and blood pressure; the causes and treatment of high blood pressure and heart failure; and neurotransmitters of the human brain. He is the author of more than 400 papers on these topics.

PROFESSOR PAUL NESTEL AO

Professor Paul Nestel AO MD FRACP FTSE FCSANZ is on the Senior Faculty of Baker IDI. He has been involved in nutrition-related research and nutrition-relevant health policies for several decades.

He was Chief of CSIRO's Division of Human Nutrition for 10 years, and chaired the Oversighting Committee, National Food & Nutrition Policy of the Commonwealth Government in 1992. He was a member of a Working Group on Food Processing for the Prime Minister's Science Council, a member of NHMRC National Nutrition & Food and Health Committee, Chairman of National Heart Foundation's Diet & Heart Disease Committee, President of the International Union of Nutrition Congress 1992, and Chair of the National Nutrition Committee for the Australian Academy of Science.

Paul has been an academic holding two professorships of Medicine and serving as Deputy Director of the Baker Heart Institute, Melbourne.

He has published 460 peer-reviewed research and health policy papers, many in the area of nutrition.

Paul is also a recipient of the Order of Australia and the Centennial Medal.

BRIGID O'CONNELL

Brigid O'Connell has been a journalist for more than 13 years at various print media outlets in Australia. Most recently, she has been the health reporter for the Herald Sun since 2008. She has won a Melbourne Press Club Quill Award for best Suburban Reporting, and Special Commendation in the United Nations Media Peace Awards.

Brigid also teaches journalism at Deakin University, and is a qualified personal trainer. She was involved in the writing of the manuscript.

PROFESSOR ANNA PEETERS

Anna Peeters is Professor of Epidemiology and Equity in Public Health & Head of Obesity and Population Health in the School of Health and Social Development at Deakin University.
Anna is a NHMRC Career Development Fellow and the immediate past president of the Australia New Zealand Obesity Society (2011–14). She has been awarded the prestigious World Obesity Federation Andre Mayer Award for 2014 and a Churchill Award in 2014.
Anna is a public health researcher, and is particularly interested in the provision of information to facilitate objective and equitable choices in public health by policy makers, practitioners and the public. She sits on a number of national and international advisory boards and steering committees, including the Parent's Voice, the Victorian government's Equity Focussed Health Impact

Assessment advisory group and WorkHealth advisory group, and on the World Cancer Research Fund's Policy Advisory Group.
Anna's research program aims to build the evidence base for public health policy regarding the prevention of obesity and its consequent diseases.

REBECCA STIEGLER

Rebecca completed a Master of Science in Nutrition & Dietetics and is an Accredited Practising Dietitian. She has specialised in diabetes for over 8 years and has co-convened the Dietitians Association of Australia (DAA) Diabetes Interest Group. Rebecca also has a strong interest in research and has presented at the DAA and Australian Diabetes Society / Australian Diabetes Educator Association national conferences as well as providing training programs on chronic disease management to health professionals. She has also published articles on dietary and lifestyle management for the prevention of cardiovascular disease and type 2 diabetes. She also co-authored *The Baker IDI Healthy Cholesterol Diet and Lifestyle Plan*. Rebecca grows most of her own fruit and vegetables in her backyard garden and loves using them when cooking, especially trialling the cookbook recipes.

INDEX

PENGUIN BOOKS

UK | USA | Canada | Ireland | Australia
India | New Zealand | South Africa | China

Penguin Books is part of the Penguin Random House group of companies
whose addresses can be found at global.penguinrandomhouse.com.

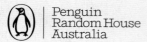

Penguin
Random House
Australia

First published by Penguin Random House Australia Pty Ltd, 2017

10 9 8 7 6 5 4 3 2 1

Design by Daniel New and Adam Laszczuk © Penguin Random House
Australia Pty Ltd
Food photography by Chris Chen
Food styling by Cass Stokes
Recipe development by Caroline Griffiths
Food preparation by Leanne Kitchen
Project management by Katrina O'Brien and Natalie Mendan
Edited by Carolyn Leslie and Niki Foreman
Colour separation by Splitting Image Colour Studio, Clayton, Victoria
Printed and bound in China by RR Donnelley Asia Printing Solutions Limited

National Library of Australia Cataloguing-in-Publication entry

   Title: The Baker IDI Wellness Plan :
    scientific secrets for a long and healthy life / Baker IDI Heart and
    Diabetes Institute.

   ISBN: 9780143573210 (paperback)

   Notes: Includes index.
   Subjects: Lifestyles--Health aspects--Handbooks, manuals, etc.
   Nutrition--Handbooks, manuals, etc.
   Health attitudes--Handbooks, manuals, etc.
   Longevity--Health aspects--Handbooks, manuals, etc.
   Self-care, Health--Handbooks, manuals, etc.
   Well-being--Health aspects--Handbooks, manuals, etc.

   Other Creators/Contributors:
   Baker IDI Heart and Diabetes Institute, author.

   612.68

penguin.com.au

ACKNOWLEDGEMENTS

The Baker IDI Wellness Plan is the result of work by:
Professor Garry Jennings AO, Senior Director,
Baker IDI Heart and Diabetes Institute
Dr Marlies E. Alvarenga, MonashHeart and
Baker IDI Heart and Diabetes Institute
Professor Murray Esler AM, NHMRC Senior Principal
Research Fellow, Baker IDI Heart and Diabetes Institute
Professor Paul Nestel AO, Senior Scientist,
Baker IDI Heart and Diabetes Institute
Brigid O'Connell, journalist
Professor Anna Peeters, Professor of Epidemiology
and Equity in Public Health & Head of Obesity
and Population Health, Deakin University and
Baker IDI Heart and Diabetes Institute
Rebecca Stiegler, Accredited Practising Dietitian,
Baker IDI Heart and Diabetes Institute.

Personal acknowledgements
Professor Garry Jennings, Professor Murray Esler and
Professor Anna Peeters each have a contractual agreement
and receive research support from the National Health
and Medical Research Council of Australia.
Dr Marlies E. Alvarenga: For Noah, Eliza, Luca, Reno & Penny.
Penguin would like to thank Natalie Mendan from Baker IDI for
her diligence and commitment.

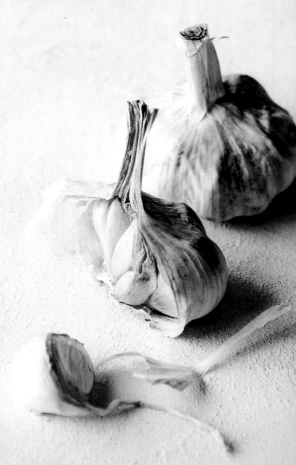